THE COMPLETE
FAMILY GUIDE TO
ALTERNATIVE
MEDICINE

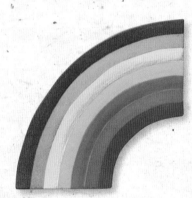

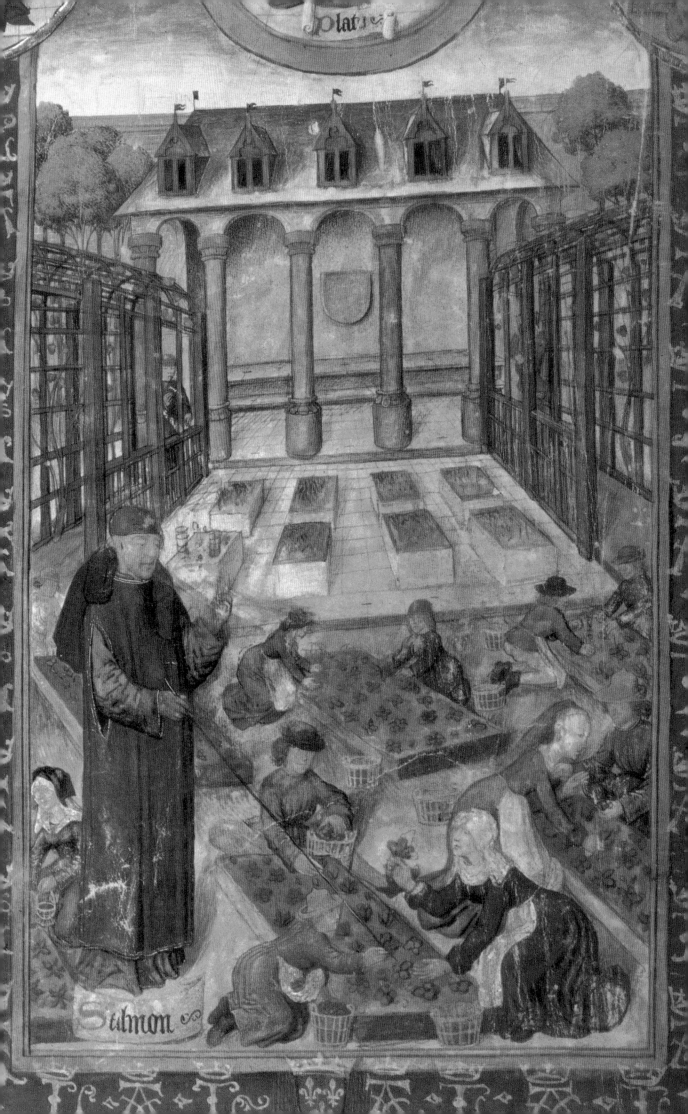

THE COMPLETE
FAMILY GUIDE TO
ALTERNATIVE
MEDICINE

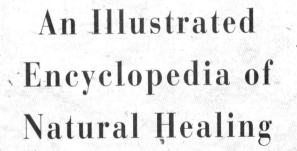

An Illustrated
Encyclopedia of
Natural Healing

Consultant Editor C. Norman Shealy M.D. Ph.D.

General Editor Richard Thomas

ELEMENT

Shaftesbury, Dorset • Rockport, Massachusetts • Brisbane, Queensland

© Element Books Limited 1996
First published in Great Britain 1996 by
ELEMENT BOOKS LIMITED
Shaftesbury, Dorset SP7 8BP

Published in USA in 1996 by
ELEMENT BOOKS INC.
PO Box 830, Rockport, MA 01966

Published in Australia in 1996 by
ELEMENT BOOKS LIMITED
for JACARANDA WILEY LIMITED
33 Park Road, Milton, Brisbane 4064

First Published October 1996
Reprinted November 1996

NOTE FROM THE PUBLISHER
*Any information given in this book is not intended to
be taken as a replacement for medical advice. Any
person with a condition requiring medical attention
should consult a qualified practitioner or therapist.*

Consultant Editor: **C. Norman Shealy M.D. Ph.D.**
General Editor: **Richard Thomas**

Designed and created with The Bridgewater Book Company

ELEMENT BOOKS LIMITED
Editorial Director: **Julia McCutchen**
Managing Editor: **Caro Ness**
Production Director: **Roger Lane**
Production Control: **Sarah Golden**

THE BRIDGEWATER BOOK COMPANY
Art Director: **Peter Bridgewater**
Designer: **Jane Lanaway**
Page Makeup: **Chris Lanaway**
Mac Artworker: **Amanda Payne**
Editorial Consultants: **Book Creation Services, London**
Managing Editor: **Anne Townley**
Editor: **Viv Croot**
Picture Research: **Lynda Marshall**
Three-dimensional Models: **Mark Jamieson**
Studio Photography: **Guy Ryecart**
Medical Illustrations: **Michael Courtney**
Illustrators: **Paul Allen, Lorraine Harrison,
Ivan Hissey, Andrew Kulman,
Mainline Design, Andrew Milne**

Printed and bound in the USA by Rand McNally, Versailles, Kentucky.

British Library Cataloging in Publication data available
Library of Congress Cataloging in Publication
data available

ISBN 1 85230 873 7 U.K. HARDBACK
ISBN 1 85230 901 6 U.S. PAPERBACK

Contents

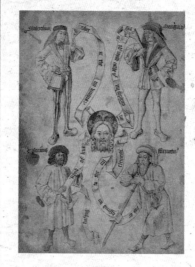

Contributors and Acknowledgments   6
Foreword   7
How to Use This Book   8
Introduction   10

PART ONE
THE THERAPIES

Diagnosis and Therapy Systems   *16–37*

NATURAL DIAGNOSTIC TECHNIQUES   *16–22*
Oriental Diagnosis   *18*
Western Diagnosis   *20*

COMPLETE THERAPEUTIC SYSTEMS   *23–37*
Naturopathy   *24*
Oriental Systems   *30*
Shamanism   *37*

Individual Therapies   *38-127*

Physical Therapies   *38–101*

BODYWORK   *38–55*
Chiropractic   *39*
Osteopathy   *42*
Cranial Osteopathy   *44*
Rolfing   *46*
Myotherapy   *46*
Rosen Technique   *47*
Bowen Technique   *47*
Massage   *48*
Aromatherapy   *50*
Reflexology   *52*
Polarity Therapy   *55*

BALANCE AND MOVEMENT   56–65
Western Forms   56
Eastern Traditions   59

PLANT, FOOD, AND MINERAL THERAPIES   66–89
Herbal Medicine   67
Dietary and Nutritional Therapies   74
Homeopathy   82
Flower and Tree Remedies   86

ORIENTAL THERAPIES   90–97
Acupuncture   90
Acupressure   94
Shiatsu   96

ENVIRONMENTAL THERAPIES   98–101
Clinical Ecology   98
Geopathic Therapy   100

Psychological Therapies   102–20

PSYCHOTHERAPY AND COUNSELING   103–9

HYPNOSIS AND HYPNOTHERAPY   112

RELAXATION THERAPIES   116

Energy Therapies   121–27

HEALING   121–24
Reiki   123
Radionics   124

CRYSTAL AND GEM THERAPIES   125

LIGHT AND SOUND THERAPIES   126

PART TWO
THE AILMENTS

The Ailments   130–261

Infections and Immunity   130–41

Body Systems   142–219

PROBLEMS OF THE HEAD   142–53

PROBLEMS OF THE RESPIRATORY SYSTEM   154–63

PROBLEMS OF THE HEART AND BLOOD   164–71

PROBLEMS OF THE MUSCLES, BONES, AND JOINTS   172–87

PROBLEMS OF THE NERVOUS SYSTEM   188–95

PROBLEMS OF THE SKIN   196–203

PROBLEMS OF THE DIGESTIVE AND URINARY SYSTEMS   204–19

Problems of the Mind   220–31

Sexual and Reproductive Problems   232–47

Children's Ailments   248–53

First Aid   254–61

PART THREE
QUICK REFERENCE AND INFORMATION

A–Z of Ailments   264
A–Z of Therapies   270
Glossary   276
Useful Addresses   278
Further Reading   284
Index   285

Contributors

Consultant Editor
C. Norman Shealy M.D. Ph.D.

General Editor
Richard Thomas

Carol Bosiger

Jane Butterworth

Amanda Cochrane

Maggie Comport

Gerry Cooney

Anthea Courtenay

Moira Crawford

Taj Deoora

Pippa Duncan

Nigel Howard

Eve Hunter

Anne Kubota

Sheila Lavery

Alison MacKonochie

Janette Marshall

Simon Martin

Christine McFadden

Sheena Meredith

Anna Rushton

Enid Segall

Cathy Steven

Alex Thomas

Denise Winn

Jacky Young

Acknowledgments

Picture Credits:

Bridgeman Art Library: pp.2, 23B, 66BL (Bibliothèque Nationale, Paris), pp.4, 11, 36TR (British Library, London), p.243 (Hermitage, St. Petersburg), p.214T (Lincolnshire County Council), p.71C (Private Collection), p.102 (Rijksmuseum, Kroller-Muller, Otterlo), p.112TL (Norrkoping Museum, Sweden); British Chiropractic Association: p.39TL; British School of Osteopathy: p.42T; Center for Reiki Training: p.123T;Silvio Dokov: p.60TL, 60CL; Inge Dougans: p.54; E.T.Archive: p.37T (Bibliothèque Nationale), p.67BR (British Library), p.60TR (British Museum), p.13TR (National Palace Museum, Taiwan), pp.66C, 121B (V&A, London); Faculty of Homeopathy: Homeopathic Trust, London: p82TL, 82C; Fortean Picture Library: p.106L; Hulton-Deutsch Collection: pp.10B, 104T, 105BC, 112T, 112CR; Hutchison Library: pp.137B, 214B; Images Colour Library: pp100B, 220B; Mansell Collection: pp.36BL, 113T, 201C; Michael Holford: p.37L; Caroline Myss: p.20T; National Portrait Gallery, London: p.192TR; Philips Medical Systems: p.192BL; Anthea Sieveking: p.211; Rudolf Steiner House: p.23T; Science Photo Library: pp.7BR, 36T, 39CL, 80B, 93, 99B, 113BR, 131, 136TL, 140TL, 140R, 152T, 152C, 158R, 166, 177, 180, 200BL, 202, 217, 234, 237, 247, 249, 251TR, 253; Society of Teachers of Alexander Technique: p.57T; Jeremy Thomas: p.29CL; Richard Thomas: p.21; United Kingdom Polarity Therapy Association/Tony Hutchings: p.55; Werner Forman Archive: pp.32, 33, 34T, 235T; Trevor Wood: p.207BR; Zefa Pictures: pp.5, 25, 26T, 34B, 35, 51, 61T, 72T, 92BL, 98T, 100T, 107T, 108T, 116, 117B, 119, 120T, 127TL, 154, 170, 186B, 196L, 209BR, 233T, 241, 244B, 246, 250T

Special thanks go to:

Caroline Dorling and **Flint House**, Lewes, East Sussex
for help and advice in the preparation of this book

Jan O'Boyle – Yoga
Sarah Bristow – Shiatsu
Margaret Burrowes – Feldenkrais
Amanda Clarke – Osteopathy
Agni Ecroyd and Jill Dunley – The Trager Approach
Susan Geall – Herbalism
Marsha Goodwin – Healing
Wendy Hart – Crystal Therapy
Emma Ridley – Massage
Paul Smith – Alexander Technique
William Wheen – Chiropractic and Craniosacral Therapy
Keith Wright – Acupuncture and Acupressure

for help and advice with photography of the therapies

Tom Aitken, Glyn Bridgewater, Rebecca Carver, Judith Cox, Nina Downey, Carly Evans, Marianne Hillier-Brook, Nicola Hobbs, Julia Holden, Simon Holden, Susan and Gina Jamieson, Janice Jones, Arthur Larkin, Pippa Losh, Sarah Martin, Chloe McCausland, Clare Packman, Sally-Ann Russell, Stephen Sparshatt, Sarah Stanley, Sue Wheatley, Oliver Wheen, Robin Yarnton

for help with photography

Dr. Hugh Anderson
Brighton University
Daniel Froggat
James and Jenny Herold
The Plinth Company Limited, Stowmarket, Suffolk
Winfalcon's Healing Centre and Holistic Shop,
Brighton, East Sussex

for help with properties

Foreword

"Alternative medicine" is something of a misnomer when describing many of the therapies contained in this book because people have been relying on acupuncture, Chinese medicine, herbal medicine, and massage for centuries whilst so-called "conventional" medicine, allopathic medicine, has only been in existence for a relatively short time. Furthermore, these therapies do not necessarily replace conventional medicine but complement or support it. Allopathic medicine has always tended to isolate a problem and treat it, often without any reference to the root cause. Alternative medicine treats nothing in isolation, stressing instead the importance of the holistic approach; seeing the mind and body as inseparable and capable of self-repair if the individual is ready to take an active part in his or her own healing and general welfare.

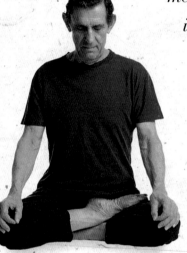

The half lotus position, a classic pose for meditation, can also help to concentrate on breathing and lengthening the spine. The mind is better able to focus when breathing is controlled.

In the last few years "alternative medicine" has become increasingly popular as more and more of us decide to take control of our own health. This is merely a long overdue acknowledgment that allopathic medicine has ignored the most important aspect of healing: the untapped power of positive thinking and the body's innate ability to heal itself.

Look at yourself! The way your body works defies belief. You are a miracle beyond imagination, far greater than that of drugs or surgery. If you realize this and that the responsibility of maintaining your own health lies with you, you will be capable of anything. You must learn to be guardian of your own health and welfare. How you choose to do so is up to you but the fact that you have decided to read this book may prompt the realization that each of you is extraordinary and therefore capable of creating miracles to match the miracle of life within you.

C. NORMAN SHEALY

The lethal bushmaster snake *Lachesis muta*, whose venom is the source for the homeopathic remedy Lachesis.

How to Use This Book

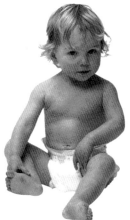

The Complete Family Guide to Alternative Medicine has been designed thematically to let you approach the subject matter via therapies or ailments. It is divided into three parts.

Part one, **The Therapies**, offers a review of the alternative therapies that are current and available today. The section opens with an introduction covering the diagnostic techniques used in alternative therapies and how they differ from orthodox medicine. There follows a résumé of complete therapeutic systems from both east and west. Finally, the therapies themselves are addressed, grouped into categories depending on their characteristics: bodywork, plant, mineral, and food therapies, psychotherapies, environmental therapies, and energy therapies.

Part two, **The Ailments**, discusses the common illnesses and conditions and lists which alternative therapies are useful and how they can help. The section opens with a general introduction to infection and immunity and is then subdivided into body systems to make it easy to locate specific ailments. Children's illnesses are covered in a separate category and there is a special section on first aid. Throughout this part of the book are scattered "special" spreads which deal with a wide-ranging subject which cannot be confined to a body system category: pain and cancer, are examples.

Part three, **The Quick Reference Library**, offers two A–Z listings for at-a-glance information. The A–Z of Ailments covers common complaints and conditions and indicates the therapies that can help them. The A–Z of Therapies covers major therapies and lists the conditions they can help. An extensive list of internationally sourced useful addresses directs you to associations or institutes that can help you find a qualified therapist. A reading list and an index complete this section.

Fumitory
Fumaria officinalis

Special Note on Homeopathic and Herbal Remedies
Throughout the book, the names of homeopathic remedies are given in the abbreviated form you will find on the commercially available remedies over the counter. Recommended potencies (6c or x, 12c or x, and 30c or x) are given where relevant. Herbs are given their common names in the main text, but are specified in addition by their scientific latin names when illustrated.

This spread is an example from the first section of the book, in which complete therapeutic systems as well as individual therapies are discussed.

main text describing the history, approach, principles, and elements of the therapy or system

box copy emphasizing a specific point of interest about the therapy or system

caution and contraindication box warning when the therapy or system is inadvisable

left hand sidebar to locate the overall category

specially commissioned plaster figures

This is a a sample of a spread from part two which concentrates on one major ailment and uses a more discursive approach.

right hand sidebar to pinpoint exactly where you are within the overall category

cross reference bar leads to further information about the therapies specified and helps you to navigate easily between the first and second parts of the book

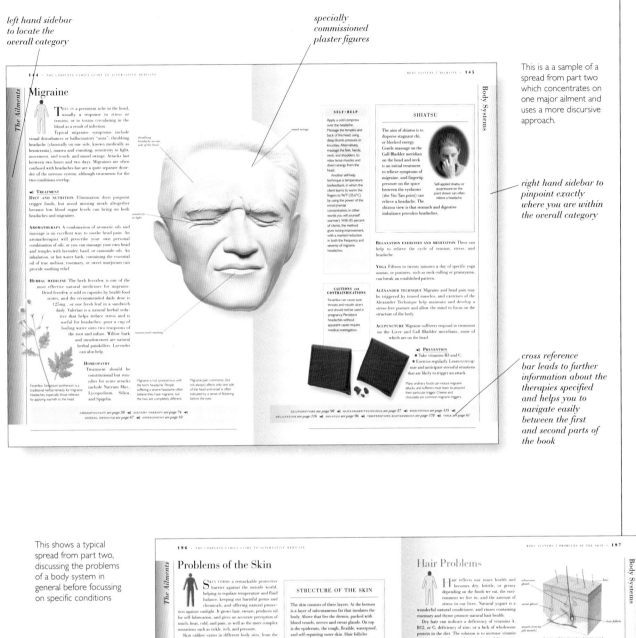

This shows a typical spread from part two, discussing the problems of a body system in general before focussing on specific conditions

specially commissioned medical artwork

main text describes the causes, symptoms, and onset of the ailment or condition and any special characteristics

therapies listed in order of usefulness in the case

self-help box offering tips to help you help yourself

Introduction

Few of the so-called "natural" therapies you will read about in this book are new developments. The majority of the treatments involved, from massage to the use of herbs and water, are probably as old as the human race itself. Others, such as traditional Chinese medicine and Ayurveda (traditional Indian medicine) go back thousands of years into the mists of time.

INTRODUCING THE "GENTLE" ALTERNATIVES

The rise of modern "scientific" medicine in the last 200 years resulted in many of these ancient practices being pushed aside, sometimes even suppressed. But in recent years that trend has been dramatically reversed, and natural therapies are becoming as popular and widespread as they ever were. Today's natural therapists usually see themselves as the latest in a long tradition – including the modern-day shamans ("witch doctors") of Africa, the United States, and Australia.

This trend seems as much to do with many people's growing disillusionment and even distrust of conventional medicine, with its reliance on powerful drugs and impersonal "high-tech" equipment, as a general movement toward more natural and less harmful ways of living.

The return of traditional medicine (conventional medicine is new medicine, not traditional) has brought with it a host of new ideas to add to those from ancient times. From homeopathy, founded at the start of the 19th century, osteopathy, and chiropractic, developed at the end of the same century, to those created in the 20th century – including radionics, radiesthesia, aromatherapy, reflexology, a mass of psychological and manipulative therapies, nutritional medicine and the more recently popular "energy" therapies such as crystal, electrocrystal, and color therapy – the list increases almost daily as new approaches are developed.

Choosing the right therapy can be a daunting task. This book sets out to make that choice a lot clearer and easier, whether it is finding out more about a therapy, or what treatment is likely to work best for what condition.

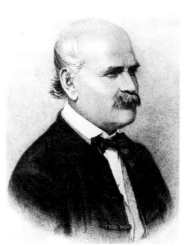

Ignaz Semmelweiss (1818-65), the Hungarian physician whose life-saving hygiene methods were denigrated by orthodoxy.

WHY GO TO A NATURAL THERAPIST?

A natural health practitioner is, or should be, someone who understands not only you and your problem but is also familiar with the host of safe and gentle treatments available. They should be prepared to give you plenty of time to explore these options.

This person may be a medical doctor but is just as likely to be a nonmedical practitioner of natural, holistic, alternative, or complementary therapies – that is unconventional medical techniques to treat disease.

People often turn to a natural therapist as a last resort. They have tried the conventional route and it hasn't worked. For various reasons – and it is usually because their problem was not helped or, sadly, perhaps even made worse – their needs have not been met. But whatever the reasons, people seem to get a high level of satisfaction when they do go to practitioners of natural therapy. In Britain, for example, where no therapist is legally required to train to practice nonmedical therapy or "heal", surveys in recent years have consistently shown satisfaction levels of 60-80 percent.

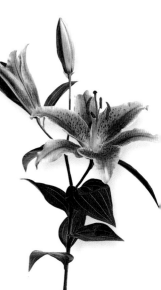

The passion flower *Passiflora Incarnata,* the herbal remedy for insomnia.

WHAT IS ALTERNATIVE MEDICINE?

There is quite a discussion (not to say argument, even among alternative therapists themselves) about whether or not all alternative therapies operate under one common idea or principle. In separate reports published in the early 1990s both American and British medical authorities have stated that alternative therapies are a mixture of different beliefs and techniques with nothing in common at all. But this is untrue. The natural approaches more or less all understand, accept, and operate under the principles outlined below.

• The body has a natural ability to heal itself and remain stable (this is known also in medicine as homeostasis).

• The human being is not simply a physical machine, like a car, but a subtle and complex blend of body, mind, and emotions (or spirit or soul as some prefer to call it) and all or any of these factors may cause or contribute to problems of health. In other words, every individual is not a random collection of moving parts but a fully integrated "whole." The term "holistic medicine" has been coined to describe treating the individual as a "whole being" composed of body, mind, and emotions, as opposed to the allopathic principle where physical symptoms are treated in isolation, using the same textbook solutions for everyone.

• Environmental and social conditions are just as important as an individual's physical and psychological makeup and may have just as big an impact on his or her health.

• Treating the root cause or causes of a problem is more important than treating the obvious immediate symptoms. Treating symptoms only may simply cover up the real underlying problem.

• Each person is an entirely original individual and cannot be treated in exactly the same way as every other person.

• Healing is quicker and more effective if the person takes central responsibility for his or her own health and has an active involvement in the healing process. (However, a good therapist should also recognize when someone needs to "let go" and place themselves in the hands of another.)

• Good health is a state of emotional, mental, spiritual, and physical "balance." (Balance is

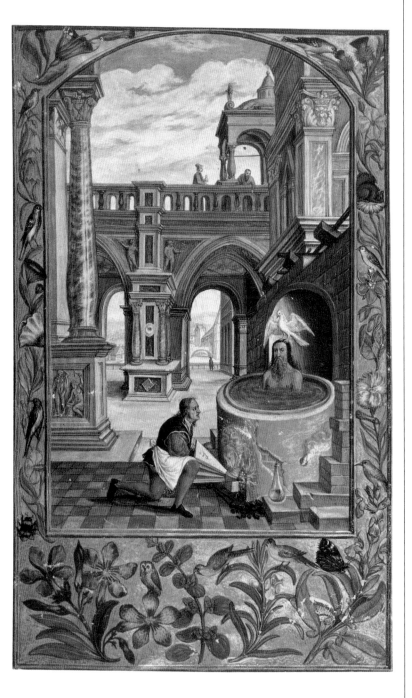

Healing baths and water treatments have long enjoyed a place in the repertoire of traditional medicine. The water may be hot or cold, and herbs or minerals may be added for their specific effect.

fundamental to the basic notion of health in natural therapy. Ill-health, say its exponents, is the result of being in a state of imbalance, or "disease." (The Chinese express this as the principle of yin and yang.)

• There is a natural healing "force" in the universe (the Chinese call this chi or qi – pronounced "chee" – the Japanese ki, and in India it is prana. In the West it used to be called by its Latin description *vis medicatrix naturae*, meaning "natural healing force," shortened today to "life force"). Anyone can "tap into" or make use of this force, and it is a natural health practitioner's job to activate it in the client or help the client activate it in him or herself.

It is natural therapists' belief in the Oriental ideas expressed particularly in the last two principles – and also often their use of those terms – that has caused so much controversy among so many doctors trained in the Western scientific method. But many doctors now feel that the essence of the natural therapies is, or should be, at the core of what makes good medicine in a return to the earliest principles followed, practiced, and preached by the ancient healers of Greece, Asia Minor, and China.

To summarize: the best approach is the one that is the softest and gentlest, that avoids dangerous and traumatic procedures, that treats the client as a "whole" individual, that encourages the body's natural healing processes to do their job, and in which the client takes a positive and active part in his or her own recovery and health maintenance.

Alternative medical therapies can be used to treat young and old alike.

HOW ALTERNATIVE THERAPIES DIFFER

Alternative therapies are considered to fall very roughly into two main categories: physical therapies and psychological therapies. Some people consider there is also a third category that can be termed "energy" therapies.

• Physical therapies are those that work obviously and directly on the body in a very physical way, both outside and in. Examples are chiropractic,

osteopathy, herbalism, nutritional therapy, massage, and aromatherapy.

• Psychological therapies aim to help the body through the mind and emotions. Examples are counseling, psychotherapy, hypnotherapy, relaxation therapy, meditation, visualization, and biofeedback.

• "Energy" therapies are often based on Eastern ideas of health and disease (or dis-ease) and work on the idea that illness is the result of an imbalance or interruption in the body's natural energy or "life force" at a very fine or subtle level. Examples are homeopathy, acupuncture, shiatsu, and reflexology.

There are, however, many therapies that fall into more than one of the above headings. That is, they have a "multilevel" effect, treating both body and mind as well as, in some people's view, the soul or spirit of a person. The best examples of this are therapies such as yoga and t'ai chi, but others would be massage and meditation.

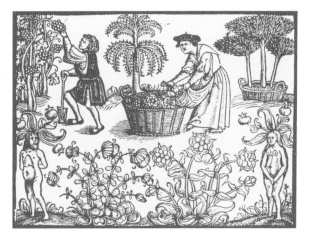

The ancient lore of traditional medical practices have been passed down from generation to generation by word of mouth and written treatises.

WHAT TO EXPECT FROM A NATURAL THERAPIST

Most natural health practitioners will treat you for the precise way you are feeling at the time you see them. If, for example, you are suffering from a cold or influenza at the time of your appointment, your practitioner will want to treat that as well as the back pain or the depression you made the appointment for in the first place. The principle here is that there is a reason for the infection and it should be cleared first since it may be linked to the basic problem. You are likely to find this common approach whether you are seeing an osteopath for a back problem, a reflexologist for your energy levels, or an aromatherapist for relaxation. They will all adjust your treatment for that visit, to encourage your body to heal itself in the best way possible. Most therapists will encourage you to "take control" of the problem, using terms such as "taking responsibility for yourself."

Moxibustion, a traditional Chinese therapy, aims to correct imbalances in the body's natural energy system.

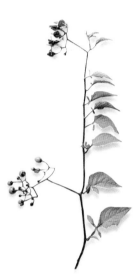

Bittersweet *Solanum dulcamara*, a herbal remedy for skin disease and rheumatic disorders. The stems are made into ointment.

Treating the body as well as the mind, yoga is an increasingly popular practice in the West.

THE SIGNIFICANCE OF "TAKING CONTROL"

Research shows conclusively that actively participating in your own healing is an important factor in the success of most alternative therapies – whether the problem is one as commonplace as influenza or as serious as heart disease. A good practitioner will always encourage you to take on a positive role, even if it is a matter of just recommending a simple change in lifestyle.

The realization that even small changes in lifestyle can contribute to an individual's health can come as a total revelation to many people who have struggled for years with a persistent problem. This book will open the way to making sure that little problems never become large ones – and encourage the first steps toward learning to live healthily, energetically, and, as far as possible, with neither doctors nor drugs.

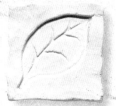

NATURAL DIAGNOSTIC TECHNIQUES

COMPLETE THERAPEUTIC SYSTEMS

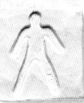

PHYSICAL THERAPIES

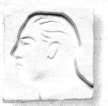

PSYCHOLOGICAL THERAPIES

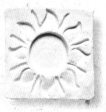

ENERGY THERAPIES

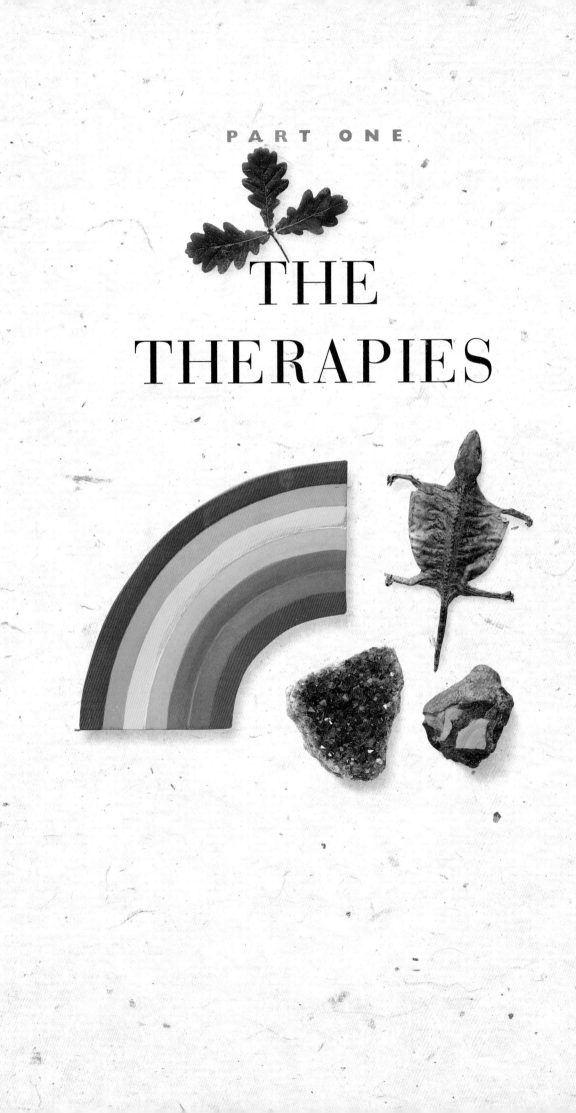

PART ONE

THE
THERAPIES

NATURAL DIAGNOSTIC TECHNIQUES

DIAGNOSTIC methods used in natural therapeutics differ from therapy to therapy, but one thing alternative practitioners generally have in common is that they spend a great deal of time in consultations, especially at the initial examination. In many cases the first consultation may last an hour, or even longer. Holistic systems of medicine usually depend for diagnosis on assimilating a whole range of signs, symptoms, and general information which may seem totally unrelated to the complaint but builds up to form a picture of the client, predisposing conditions in the client, and external factors that may have contributed to the present complaint.

The practitioner will talk through a person's case in detail and make notes on a wide range of influences. He or she will probably ask about diet and food preferences, temperament, and liking for warmth or cold, sleep patterns, digestion, lifestyle, environment, social life, mental and emotional state. By contrast, conventional doctors in the West will make a diagnosis on the basis of physical tests and questions about symptoms, rarely being concerned to explore other influences.

The approach of alternative medicine generally involves a greater reliance on intuition and also the use of testing methods that are unproven in conventional scientific terms. Often these methods are tests of a physical kind, such as muscle-testing, but they can also involve such techniques as dowsing and "aura reading," based on psychic powers. In many cases, however, "conventional" modern equipment is also used. Blood pressure may be taken and X-rays or ultrasound scans used.

The differences in approach can be summed up as subjective versus objective methods. Conventional doctors rely mainly on diagnostic techniques that are considered to be objective in which their personal opinions play no part. Alternative therapists trust more in their own subjective judgment and responses. However, in all the major forms of therapy (such as homeopathy, acupuncture, or herbalism), this subjective evaluation is set against a background of rigorous training and experience and systematic theory.

Although all alternative therapists will ask questions about symptoms and take a detailed case history, the real aim is to find out what has caused the problem in the first place and to treat that. The belief is that if the root cause of the problem is removed, the symptoms themselves will disappear.

Particular aspects of diagnosis include those listed below and right.

ORIENTAL SYSTEMS Acupuncturists, Chinese herbalists, Ayurvedic practitioners, and practitioners of other forms of Oriental medicine strive to discover what disharmonies, deficiencies, and excesses are involved in a person's "energy" systems.

Herbal remedies have the authority of tradition behind them. Tansy *Tanacetum vulgare* is a versatile herb that can be taken internally or externally.

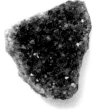

amethyst

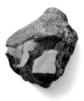

malachite

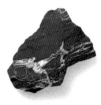

red jasper

The energy of crystals may be used as a diagnostic tool or a therapeutic treatment.

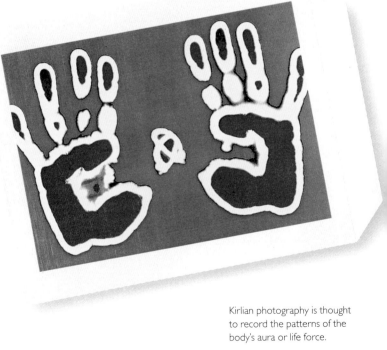

Kirlian photography is thought to record the patterns of the body's aura or life force.

SUMMARY OF ALTERNATIVE DIAGNOSTIC TECHNIQUES

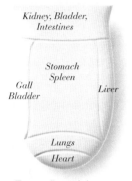

Kidney, Bladder, Intestines

Stomach
Spleen

Gall Bladder　　　*Liver*

Lungs
Heart

Tongue diagnosis is important in Chinese medicine.

Testing techniques in alternative medicine differ widely, not only between those who favor either physical or psychic means but also between East and West. Among a wide range of diagnostic techniques used by alternative therapists worldwide the following are the most common:

ORIENTAL DIAGNOSIS (PAGES 18–19)

Oriental methods of diagnosis concentrate mainly on personal touch and observation and very little on machinery or "outside" tests. They include

- *pulse-taking*
- *abdominal touch*
- *observational diagnosis*
- *tongue diagnosis*
- *"listening" diagnosis*
- *urine analysis*
- *questioning.*

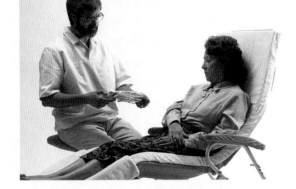

WESTERN DIAGNOSIS (PAGES 20–22)

Western diagnosis uses a combination of both ancient skills and modern "high-tech" machinery and tests. Among those most used are

- *dowsing (or radiesthesia)*
- *radionics*
- *aura reading*
- *Kirlian photography*
- *muscle-testing (or applied kinesiology)*
- *iridology*
- *reflexology*
- *hair analysis*
- *VEGA and MORA devices.*

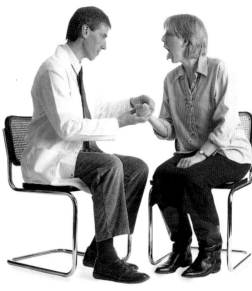

Before any needles are applied, an acupuncturist diagnoses the problem using questions, observation, tongue examination, and other techniques.

HOMEOPATHY The practitioner needs to analyze the patient into one of the major types recognized by the system. The patient will be asked many questions about his/her tastes, preferences, and responses.

CHIROPRACTIC The chiropractor uses X-rays to check for fracture or other underlying skeletal conditions.

OSTEOPATHY An osteopath checks the whole musculo-skeletal framework of the body, paying particular attention to the spine.

Reflexology uses the responses that occur when the feet are touched to discover the site of the problem in the patient's body.

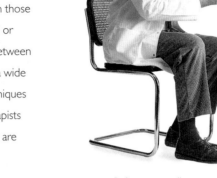

Oriental Diagnosis

IN TRADITIONAL Oriental diagnosis, the practitioner uses all the senses of touching, looking, listening, smelling, as well as questioning. The aim is to determine the relative balance of energy in the body as a whole rather than concentrating on isolated symptoms.

❧ **PULSE-TAKING** This is the most common form of touch diagnosis in Chinese medicine. The procedure takes much longer than that used in Western medicine. Three fingers are used on each wrist to measure a total of 12 different pulses. The speed, depth, and overall quality of the pulses are all considered important. Each pulse is correlated with a particular acupuncture meridian (energetic pathway) and internal organ. There are 14 different pulse characteristics that may be found at each location, signifying different types of disharmony. These are described in terms such as "empty," "full," "floating," and "slippery," as well as "rapid" and "slow."

❧ **ABDOMINAL TOUCH DIAGNOSIS** This is used in Japanese traditional medicine, with some practitioners believing that all the organs can be both diagnosed and treated by applying pressure to different parts of the abdomen. It is thought that each part of the abdomen relates to a particular internal organ. If one part of the abdomen is soft and weak to the touch, it is likely that the corresponding internal organ is not working properly.

❧ **OBSERVATIONAL DIAGNOSIS** This begins the moment a client walks into the surgery as the practitioner looks for signs of imbalance in the posture and movement of the person as well as on the face. The color and texture of the skin, and even the presence of lines and blemishes, can give important clues about the person's health. For example, a gray tint to the skin could indicate weak kidney function, while a very red end of the nose may be a sign of heart problems.

❧ **TONGUE DIAGNOSIS** This is also widely used, with the practitioner examining the shape of the tongue, its color and coating as part of the diagnosis. As with the abdomen, each part of the tongue corresponds to different internal organs, and its appearance, the color, thickness, and quality of the coating, all give information about the state of health of each organ.

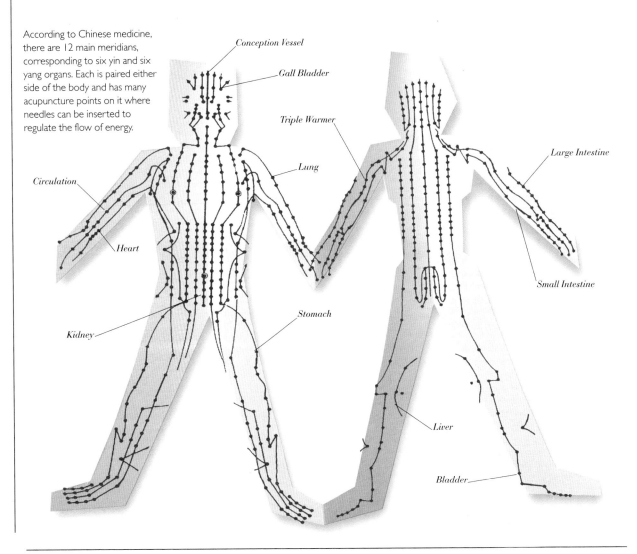

According to Chinese medicine, there are 12 main meridians, corresponding to six yin and six yang organs. Each is paired either side of the body and has many acupuncture points on it where needles can be inserted to regulate the flow of energy.

Conception Vessel

Gall Bladder

Triple Warmer

Lung

Large Intestine

Circulation

Heart

Small Intestine

Kidney

Stomach

Liver

Bladder

NATURAL DIAGNOSTIC TECHNIQUES / ORIENTAL DIAGNOSIS • **19**

Natural Diagnostic Techniques

❧ LISTENING

This involves listening to the sounds of the voice and of the body. A loud voice can be a sign of an excess condition, and a weak voice can suggest a deficiency condition. In a similar way, the person's breathing can give an indication of his or her condition. Obviously, a gurgling abdomen is a clear sign that all is not well with the person's digestion. Smells are sometimes regarded as embarrassing in the West, but the Oriental practitioner will pay attention to body odors and the smell of the breath.

❧ URINE ANALYSIS

In Chinese medicine it is important to note whether the urine is scant and dark or plentiful and pale. It may be clouded and may have a peculiar smell. In Tibetan medicine urine analysis incorporates both listening and smelling diagnosis and has been refined to a highly accurate diagnostic tool. The appearance and odor, and even the sound of the urine when it is vigorously stirred, are all noted and interpreted. A strong odor can indicate too much heat in the body, and if a lot of noisy bubbles are produced when the urine is stirred, this is taken as a sign of mental confusion and restlessness in the client.

❧ QUESTIONING

This may cover medical history, symptoms, psychological state, and even external influences such as diet and the weather. All of these provide

TONGUE DIAGNOSIS

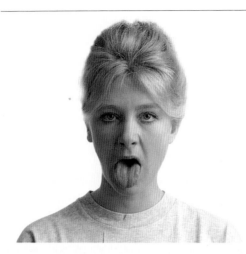

In Chinese medicine, each organ in the body and its accompanying meridian and set of functions is represented by an area on the tongue or an aspect of the tongue. Color, size, moisture, and ability to move, all indicate the balance of health in the body. For example, a pale red tongue is normal, a red tongue indicates internal heat, a pale tongue shows deficiency, a blue-black tongue signifies internal cold. The color and thickness of the tongue's coating is also important.

important information, but for a skilled Oriental medical practitioner, it is the senses that are crucial in diagnosing the client's condition.

❧ PERSPIRATION

Daytime sweat indicates a yang deficiency, and sweating at night suggests a yin deficiency. The area of the body affected, and the quantity and quality of the sweat, give further indications for the diagnostic process.

❧ SLEEP PATTERNS

Such problems as inability to sleep, continually waking and sleeping, waking because of unpleasant dreams, waking too early, and sleeping too much, all form part of the overall picture.

❧ TASTE

A preference for hot drinks indicates a "cold" problem and vice versa, and food preferences also indicate the nature of the disease. The patient may have a characteristic taste in the mouth, such as bitter or sweet.

three fingers to take pulse

pulses represent meridians and organs of the body

Pulse-taking is a long process in acupuncture as each wrist is thought to contain six pulses, one for each meridian, and each has to be checked in turn.

Diagnosis and Therapy Systems

Western Diagnosis

Most Western alternative therapists will start an initial consultation by taking a detailed case history. Homeopaths and many naturopaths, for example, will rely on little else, believing that the answers to the problem will be revealed by close questioning regarding a client's entire lifestyle, past and present.

Some therapists practice a therapy they say will diagnose as well as treat a problem – both radionics and reflexology are said to do this – but others use a range of further tests if questioning alone is not considered enough.

Diagnostic tests in Western alternative medicine fall roughly into one of two broad categories: the physical and the psychic.

❧ PHYSICAL DIAGNOSTIC METHODS Common diagnostic methods that concentrate on testing a person's physical state include
* muscle-testing or "applied kinesiology" – this is a way of testing for food allergies and intolerances *(see also pages 28, 74–5, 99, 202)*
* hair mineral analysis – chemical analysis of hair is often used to reveal nutritional deficiencies in the body, particularly of minerals
* iris diagnosis – here a diagnosis is formed by careful observation of the iris of the eye, also known as "iridology" *(see page 22)*.

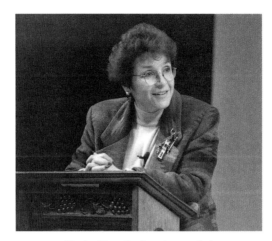

Carolyn Myss, the American medical dowser who has enjoyed an impressive record of success in diagnosing the site and nature of people's illnesses.

❧ PSYCHIC METHODS AND "ENERGY" DEVICES IN DIAGNOSIS Popular psychic methods of diagnosing include dowsing, radionics, and "aura" reading, while among those claiming to measure levels of "subtle energy" in the body are Kirlian photography, MORA and VEGA devices, and polycontrast interface photography (PIP).

PSYCHIC METHODS
Certain people have the gift of dowsing, which is comparable to water dowsing. Dowsing for water, oil, and minerals using rods or twigs has long been accepted as a valid way of finding something normally hidden from view.

Dowsing for medical purposes began in the West in the 1920s when the French Abbé Mermet began using a pendulum hung on a thread to locate and diagnose illness. His theory was that all substances, including the human body, emit radiations that can be identified. He called this form of medical dowsing radiesthesia (meaning "sensitivity to radiations").

Today many natural therapists use dowsing to aid assessment. Held over the body's "energy centers" or chakras *(see page 121)*, the pendulum's swing is said to indicate strengths and weaknesses in the energy system. It may also be used to give yes/no answers (by swinging clockwise or anticlockwise) to specific questions about the person's health status and requirements.

Accurate dowsing requires good training and extreme honesty. A dowser with strong opinions about diet, for instance, can unconsciously influence the pendulum in their hand to respond to their own beliefs rather than the patient's condition and thus invalidate the assessment.

The pattern of a heart, shown on a conventional ECG (electrocardiogram). This records the electrical changes in the heart muscle. Psychic dowsers believe that they can read the body's energy picture directly and "see" such patterns .

this pattern represents one heartbeat

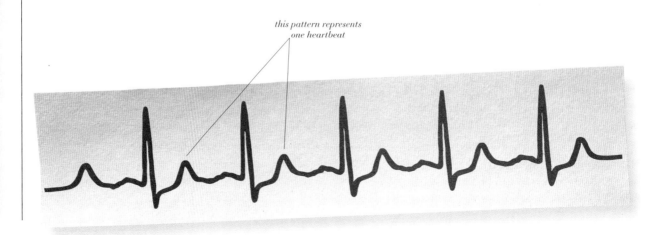

RADIONICS

Radionics uses instruments to measure different aspects of a person's energy state from a "witness" – a hair clipping or drop of blood – often at a distance, accompanied by a questionnaire completed by the client. This covers the energy system, nutrition, mental/emotional problems, chemical and environmental poisoning, lifestyle, and so on as a basis for radionic treatment. Practitioners do not claim to produce a medical diagnosis, preferring the word "analysis" instead. *(See also page 124.)*

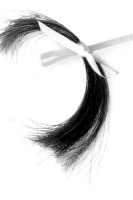

A lock of hair can be used by a radionics practitioner to make an analysis of a person's energy state.

AURA DIAGNOSIS

The aura is said to be an energy field or magnetic field surrounding a person's body, which certain sensitive people can discern by clairvoyance, touch, or an inner "knowing." Most healers "scan" the energy field with their hands, sensing areas of heat, cold, pain, tingling, and so on that indicate problems. A few claim they can actually see and interpret the colors of the aura and can pick up the effects of past traumas and potential future problems. Some diagnose at a distance, using a photograph or simply the person's name as a link. Accuracy varies, but healers have been known to find problems missed by conventional medical diagnosis. *(See also pages 121–2.)*

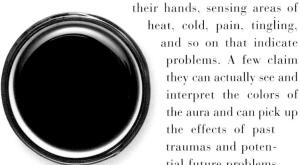

Testing the blood is a standard diagnostic technique in orthodox medicine; it can also be used in radionics.

KIRLIAN PHOTOGRAPHY

Developed by a Russian engineer, Kirlian photographs are said to show the energy radiations emitted by living things, including plants and animals. A healthy person emits strong radiations, while weak radiations are said to show imbalances requiring treatment. Usually the subject's hands are photographed. The resulting print shows flares of energy, areas of blockage, and so on that the trained practitioner interprets.

VEGA AND MORA DEVICES

VEGA and MORA are two of the best-known examples of a large number of "high-tech" devices, many originating in Germany, that claim to be able to make a diagnosis based on various "energy" principles, particularly those of acupuncture.

POLYCONTRAST INTERFACE PHOTOGRAPHY (PIP)

A diagnostic aid developed over seven years by Harry Oldfield, a pioneer of the clinical use of Kirlian photography and electrocrystal therapy *(see page 125)*, PIP consists of a video camera attached to a specially programmed computer. The way in which the computer then interprets this light in the colors that appear on the screen is all down to computer mathematics. According to Oldfield, it shows a person's subtle energy field in full, moving color. Particular colors and patterns indicate states of health or illness. Oldfield believes these can also reveal latent weaknesses before physical symptoms manifest, so that appropriate preventive action can be recommended, or a medical checkup sought.

✥ **SPECIAL NOTE** There is little independent scientific evidence to support many of the methods described in this section. They should be used in conjunction with a full conventional medical diagnosis.

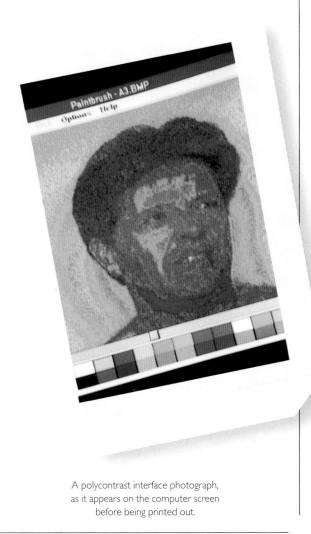

A polycontrast interface photograph, as it appears on the computer screen before being printed out.

Diagnosis and Therapy Systems

Iridology

According to iridologists, the iris of the eye represents a kind of map of the human glands, organs, and systems of the whole human body. Problems show up on the iris as spots, flecks, white or dark streaks, and so on. Texture and color indicate the person's general state of health.

Some iridologists claim they can find tendencies toward inherited disease and possible future problems, and some even address emotional and spiritual health problems this way. Common conditions that iridologists claim to be able to diagnose include arthritis, heart disease, skin problems, and allergies.

Iridology was developed in the 19th century by the Hungarian Dr. Ignatiz von Peckzely, who as a boy noticed changes in the eye of an owl with a broken leg as the owl made its recovery. He published his theories in 1881, and soon after a Swedish doctor, Nils Lilinquist, added his own observations.

But iridology did not become widely popular until Dr. Bernard Jensen pioneered its use in the United States. In 1950 he published a chart that showed the location of every gland and organ reflected in each eye. The left eye, he said, corresponds with the left-hand side of the body, the right with the right-hand side. Generally speaking the upper organs (for example, the brain) are at the top of the iris, and the lower ones (for example, the kidneys) at the bottom. The bodily systems – digestion, blood and lymph, glands and organs, muscles, skeleton, and skin – appear in six rings around the pupil.

Some practitioners examine the iris with a flashlight and magnifying glass. Others take color photographs or transparencies (slides) that are magnified and read.

Because iridology is a purely diagnostic tool, it is best to see a practitioner who is also qualified in some form of treatment to benefit properly. Iridology, or "iris diagnosis," is widely used by many natural therapists to aid diagnosis and assessment, particularly in the United States, Germany, and Australia.

Many iridologists also practice nutritional therapy *(see page 76)* and will prescribe herbal remedies or nutritional supplements to help the condition that they detect. The aim is to pinpoint the underlying causes of generalized symptoms such as joint pain or bowel problems, both of which may be the result of an allergy, and to support and rebalance the whole body system.

According to the iridology theory, specific parts of the body are reflected in the iris, the colored part of the eye, with the right and left eye almost mirroring each other.

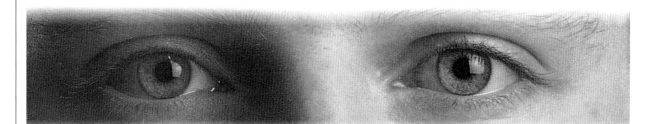

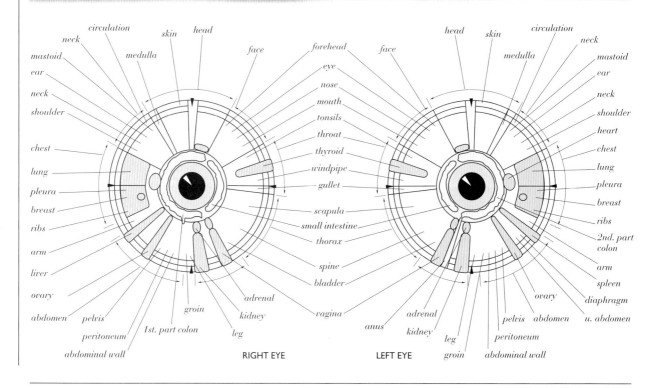

RIGHT EYE

LEFT EYE

COMPLETE THERAPEUTIC SYSTEMS

WHAT IS a useful definition of a complete therapeutic system? It may be described as a system based on an all-encompassing philosophy or set of beliefs and a comprehensive range of treatments, therapies, and remedies. Until very recently most people in industrialized Western countries would have considered conventional Western medicine just such a self-contained system, and in a way it is. But developments that have taken place over the last 20 years, particularly the growing interest in the traditional Oriental systems of healing, have changed that.

Western medicine of the future may well incorporate some of the traditions of the rich and varied systems that have survived for centuries in India, China, Japan, and Arabia.

INTRODUCTION TO WESTERN SYSTEMS
Though few people in the West know it, a complete system of healing did manage to survive the onslaught of Western science that came with the Industrial Revolution in the 18th and 19th centuries. It was called "Nature Cure" at first and, later, "naturopathy," and today it is thriving.

But what still fewer people realize is that modern naturopathy descends directly from

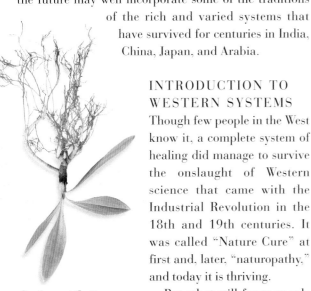
Gentian root *Gentiana lutea* provides a fortifying herbal remedy.

that tradition of complete systems of medicine learned by the Greeks from the Orient, and passed to the West by the Arabs during the European "Dark Ages." Although that tradition seems never to have included some of the methods and much of the philosophy and terminology we think of as peculiarly Oriental, it included almost everything else.

STEINER

Rudolf Steiner (1861–1925) was an Austrian social philosopher who established the doctrine of anthroposophy, a word he coined from the Greek words for man and divine wisdom. Steiner could be described as a pioneer of the alternative medicine movement. Trained as a scientist and a mathematician, he was influenced by ideas from ancient Greece and traditional Hindu beliefs, and his doctrine was an attempt to bring together the spiritual and the material sides of life and revive the human ability to use their spiritual perceptions to heal themselves. Steiner founded a school in which his theories became practice.

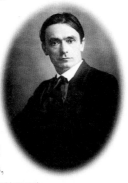

Most important, it included all the elements of body, mind, and emotions that are now seen as vital to any system of medicine that claims to be complete, and a common thread seems to run through many of the systems described in the following section. They all incorporate principles from the same ancient source.

For example, both homeopathy, which was founded by the 18th-century German doctor Samuel Hahnemann, and anthroposophical medicine, started by the 19th-century Austrian philosopher Rudolf Steiner, owe most of their basic ideas to the practices and principles of ancient Greece and the Orient.

Homeopathy is now a major part of naturopathic medicine in most countries where naturopathy is established (although there is a case for it being seen as a complete system in its own right) while anthroposophical medicine, hugely influential in the 1920s and 1930s (and still popular in parts of Europe and the United States), has largely been absorbed by newer and more accessible systems.

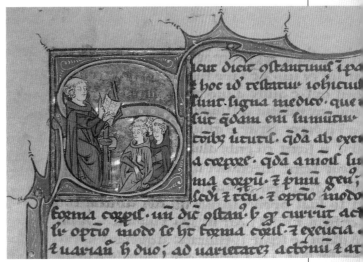

The Hippocratic oath, established by Hippocrates of Cos (c.460–360 B.C.). Hippocrates' ideas on the significance of diagnosis, the importance of diet, and the sparing use of drugs all have a resonance today.

Diagnosis and Therapy Systems

Naturopathy

NATUROPATHY is an umbrella term used in most Western countries to cover a range of therapies coming under the heading of "natural medicine." Originally coined by the German pioneer Benedict Lust, naturopathy means, literally, "natural treatment," and today its practitioners are generally those trained at specialist colleges in a range of skills that include acupuncture, herbalism, homeopathy, osteopathy, hydrotherapy, massage, nutrition, and diet.

Lust came up with the term "naturopathy" after he, and his fellow-countryman Henry Lindlahr, emigrated to the United States early in the 20th century. But he based his ideas almost entirely on those of a 19th-century German predecessor Vincent Preissnitz, who founded "Nature Cure," and the Austrian Dominican friar Father Kneipp. Nature Cure, and "natural hygiene," are still terms used by practitioners who claim to follow this form of natural medicine first recommended by Hippocrates.

Germany, where *heilpraktikeren* ("health practitioners") enjoy a status similar to that of doctors, remains the true home of naturopathy, but the United States is where it is most firmly established. Pioneers there and in Britain include Herbert Shelton, John Bastyr, Stanley Lief, and James C. Thomson. They have built naturopathy up over the course of more than half a century so that it is now the closest thing in the West to an alternative system to conventional medicine, on a par with the various complete systems of medicine in the Orient.

Training in naturopathy is becoming standard for those interested in practicing natural medicine in its widest sense (except, ironically, in Britain where the trend is proving slow to be accepted by those who run the natural therapies). Countries such as the United States, Australia, Canada, Germany, Israel, New Zealand, and South Africa now run full three- to four-year courses leading to a recognized degree or diploma.

✒ THE BASIS OF NATUROPATHIC MEDICINE

Naturopaths believe that four basic components make for good health:
* clean air
* clean water
* clean food from good earth
* exercise and "right living."

All naturopathic treatments concentrate on various of these elements, and often all of them combined, to restore health and vitality.

THE NATUROPATHIC PHILOSOPHY

Naturopaths usually follow three main principles when prescribing any treatment.

✒ *The body has the power to heal itself, so treatment should not be given to alleviate symptoms but to support the self-healing mechanism or vis medicatrix naturae (Latin for "natural healing force" or "vital force").*

✒ *The symptoms of disease are not part of the disease itself but a sign that the body is striving to eliminate toxins and return to its natural state of balance or homeostasis.*

✒ *In addition to being as natural and gentle as possible, all treatments should take into account the mental, emotional, and social aspects of a person as well as the physical.*

Eating a healthy diet to fuel the body properly is one of the cornerstones of naturopathy.

Naturopaths hold that infections seldom occur if the body is looked after in the way nature intended and that the body will cure itself of anything as long as it takes in only pure air and water, is kept clean, and given the right food and healthy activity. But they also believe that illness is natural and that methods of cure should follow the same natural principles.

So, far from from being suppressed, symptoms of illness should be encouraged to come out and the body helped to fight back and restore its proper balance, or homeostasis.

Naturopaths routinely prescribe brief periods of fasting to help conquer simple infections such as influenza. They also pay a great deal of attention to the health of the bowels (where nutrients are absorbed into the bloodstream). The diet prescribed in the treatment involves cutting out or reducing alcohol, eating "whole" foods, and also severely restricting intake of fats, salt, and sugar.

Because of the theory that bacterial toxins in the gut may play a part in the cause of many illnesses, most naturopaths encourage special diets to clear the gut and eliminate the overgrowth of "unfriendly" bacteria in the intestines that can contribute to toxicity, allergy, and poor immunity. Some even use a treatment for washing the gut clean known as colonic irrigation, or colon hydrotherapy *(see box on page 27)*.

Breathing

Good breathing is essential to relaxation, a fact that is becoming increasingly recognized in both the complementary and orthodox medical professions. Breathing properly can ease tension and promote calmness, which has an extremely important effect on the way our bodies function. When we are stressed or anxious, we breathe more rapidly, using only the upper part of the chest. This offers the quickest boost of oxygen to the system, but in the long run is not effective. When we are tired or depressed, we breathe more deeply, exhaling heavily and sighing.

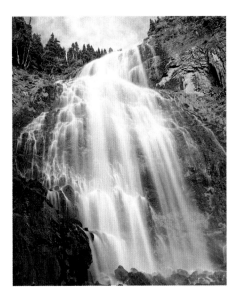

The invigorating air around a waterfall is charged with negative ions, which are thought to be beneficial to the body.

believed to have antiseptic properties. But breathing clean air on its own is not enough: how you breathe is also considered vitally important.

The correct way to breathe is using the diaphragm, a muscle separating the chest from the abdomen. Contractions and relaxations of the diaphragm force the flow of air in and out of the lungs. Diaphragmatic breathing is more relaxing and more efficient since the lungs are able to fill and empty completely. In turn, the body is able to work more effectively since it has a good quality supply of oxygen with which to do so. When we

Naturopaths believe breathing clean air is essential to health because clean air oxygenates the blood and makes the tissues function more efficiently. Air is also breathe from the chest, as we do in times of tension, fear, or anxiety, waste products build up in the lungs, leading to increasingly less efficient breathing and a feeling of tiredness and lethargy. Most practitioners will offer advice on breathing efficiently, and many therapies are focused around it, including Relaxation, Alexander Technique, Yoga, and Meditation.

Practitioners encourage long deep breaths that expand the rib cage, and also the use of air baths and ionizers to improve the quality of air for patients with respiratory conditions.

AIR PURIFIERS

A wide range of electrical devices is available to help people deal with the poor quality of air around them. In general they work by drawing air in, filtering out impurities such as dust, airborne fungi, and water and returning the clean air to the atmosphere.

Extremes of damp and dry air can both cause breathing problems, so a device called a dehumidifier draws the moisture out of air that is too damp while a humidifier puts moisture back into air that is too dry.

But the most popular devices among naturopaths are those that change the "ionization" of the air. Ions are electrically charged particles in the atmosphere. Positive ions are draining, and negative energizing. Clean, healthy air like that high up in the mountains or near waterfalls is highly charged with negative ions, and these are believed to have a beneficial effect on the central nervous system, metabolism, and many more aspects of health.

In the United States research has shown that asthmatic infants can benefit enormously from breathing ionized air and the Food and Drugs Administration (FDA) has approved the use of electrical ionizers in the treatment of allergies, hay fever, and respiratory conditions.

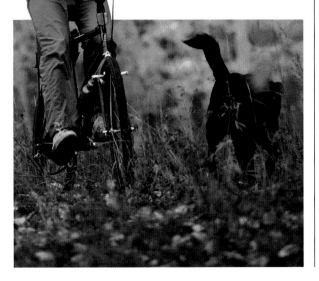

Exercise encourages the lungs to work to their full capacity, so improving the supply of oxygen to the bloodstream .

Complete Therapeutic Systems

Diagnosis and Therapy Systems

Hydrotherapy

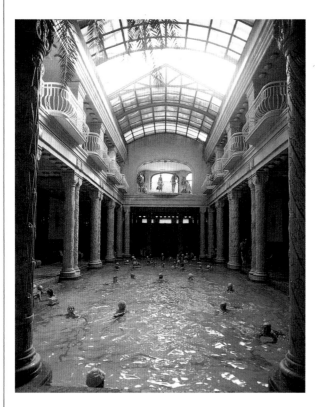

The famous Gelert baths in Budapest, one of the many ornate hydrotherapy establishments in Hungary.

Hydrotherapy – water therapy – is the use of water to promote healing. It is one of the oldest, simplest, and most effective of all the natural therapies. Water treatments include taking natural spring waters internally for their beneficial mineral content, and external treatments such as bathing, douches, and taking exercise in water.

Water cures originated in the use of natural spring water, often minerally rich, and sometimes also naturally warm to hot or very cold, and spas or watering places where people went to "take the cure" became popular all over Europe from the early 19th century. Many European spas were established during the time of the Roman occupation and are still in use. However, ordinary water is also used in hydrotherapy today. Water of either extreme of temperature is used, or can be used alternately. Hot water first stimulates and then relaxes, while cold water invigorates. Alternating hot and cold water stimulates blood and lymph circulation, relieves congestion, and tones tissues.

Through a variety of techniques, naturopaths use the therapy to improve circulation, stimulate the vital force, ease pain, reduce fever, relax the nervous system, and empty the bowels. Water therapy also contributes to encouraging the efficient elimination of wastes through the skin.

BATHS
The various forms of baths include arm and foot baths, sitz baths, and whole-body immersion. Special baths include Turkish baths, spa baths, sea-water baths (or thalassotherapy), saunas, and various baths containing herbs (such as moor peat), minerals (Dead Sea or Epsom salts are examples), and other nutrients (Karwendel oils) for specific ailments or cleansing. Massage is often recommended, to be given in conjunction with the bath.

Sitz baths are hip baths used as a tonic or in the treatment of abdominal or pelvic disorders. The baths comprise two "bowls": you sit in one containing hot water and place your feet in cold water and vice versa. Alternatively, some naturopaths advocate transferring from hot to cold every two minutes, using one sitz bath at a time. Sitz baths may be used to treat liver or kidney problems, constipation, and piles. The purpose of the bath is to relieve tissue congestion and improve blood and lymph circulation in the pelvic area.

DOUCHES
Douches or showers were first used by the naturopath Vincent Preissnitz, who developed hydrotherapy in the 19th century. Cold water was poured over the patient with great force while he or she was also hosed with jets of water. Today, douches involve the use of hot and cold water sprays on specific areas of the body. When possible a strong jet of water is used, although treatment is adjusted to suit the individual. In what is known as the "Scottish douche" the jets are directed at the spine to stimulate the nervous system. Other examples are the Blitz jet-douche and needle shower.

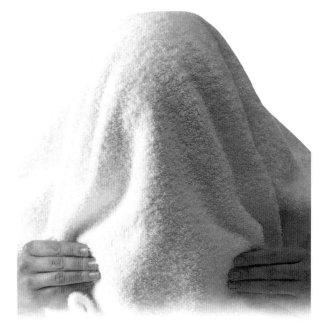

Steam inhalation is a form of home hydrotherapy that can be used to relieve catarrh, sore throats, and other minor respiratory problems, or simply to clear and rejuvenate tired skin.

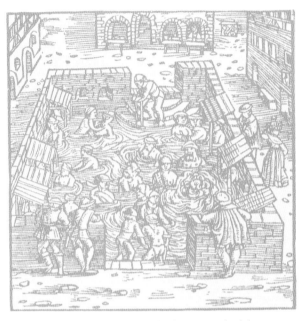

The beneficial effect of water has been recognized since Greek and Roman times. Here, a group of medieval health seekers enjoy a communal therapy session.

COMPRESSES

Compresses are either large pieces of absorbent cotton, lint, or, sometimes, small towels that are soaked in either hot or cold water and applied to a particular part of the body. For example, for a painful and inflamed joint a cold compress will be used. The joint will then be wrapped in a thicker piece of dry fabric, which helps to retain the heat generated by the compress and so ease the pain and inflammation. Compresses can be made using infusions or pastes made from herbal remedies such as arnica, comfrey, marshmallow, or St. John's wort.

Fomentations, which involve the application of hot and cold towels, are used to stimulate circulation, ease pain, and relieve lung congestion.

"Packs" often consist of whole body, trunk, or abdominal wraps, used to reduce fever and encourage elimination of toxins through the skin.

ENEMAS

Enemas involve the use of water internally to cleanse the lower bowel of impacted feces.

This is a practice often recommended by naturopaths as a means of removing a buildup of harmful toxins from the bowel. A catheter is used to pass water at body temperature into the rectum. It is held for five to ten minutes before being released, taking the toxins with it.

WALKING IN WATER

Nineteenth-century hydrotherapists advocated walking barefoot in dew or snow every morning. This may be impractical today, but walking in cold water baths about 14in/35cm deep is part of the regime in many modern hydrotherapy clinics and is said to have a general restorative effect. People with circulatory problems or diabetes should probably avoid this treatment unless under medical supervision.

COLONIC IRRIGATION

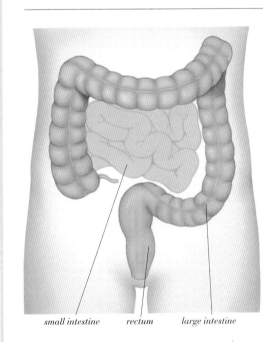

small intestine   rectum   large intestine

The anus, rectum, and colon (large intestine) are flushed out during a colonic irrigation session.

Colonic irrigation, or colonic hydrotherapy, is a way of flushing out toxic waste and impacted feces from farther up the bowel, in the colon. It is not the same as an enema. Water is kept at body temperature and flushed through a tube into the rectum. A second tube carries the water and colonic debris out of the body.

The procedure is dangerous and not without side effects, and should only be carried out by a highly trained practitioner who follows scrupulous hygiene procedures. Because it flushes good as well as bad bacteria out of the bowel, acidophilus and bifidus supplements are essential afterward to repopulate the gut with the bacteria it must have to stay healthy.

Because of the dangers involved in colonic irrigation, many practitioners disagree with the practice, while others use colonics only in special circumstances. A better, safer, and cheaper method is claimed to be colonic cleansing. This uses supplements and special fibers (such as psyllium husks) taken by mouth to achieve the same result.

Diagnosis and Therapy Systems

Food and Diet

Naturopathy encourages us to take responsibility for our own health by encouraging sensible diet and lifestyle management. This is a principle with which few conventional medical practitioners now argue. Diet is becoming rapidly and widely accepted as much of the basis of good health.

In naturopathic terms a good diet is a wholefood one comprising "live" foods – that is, foods that have not been processed or refined and are mostly organic. Such foods, believe naturopaths, fuel vitality and stimulate the vital force. Diets must also provide the necessary materials or "nutrients" on which the body relies for good health.

Many practitioners base their dietary recommendations on those devised by Lindlahr. He recommended the 60/20/20 diet, in which 60 percent of the diet was to be made up of raw foods, 20 percent was protein (preferably plant), and 20 percent complex carbohydrates. Tea, coffee, and alcohol, refined, processed, fatty, or salted foods should be avoided.

Naturopaths frequently also advise against drinking too much water, believing that the liquids best suited to the body are those that we ingest as part of fresh foods, supplemented by juice extracted from fresh fruit and vegetables.

But though practitioners of most traditions now agree that a balanced diet is essential, opinions differ about what exactly a balanced diet is. Some practitioners believe a vegetarian diet (one that excludes all meat) is necessary to be healthy, while others insist on cutting out all animal produce, including milk and eggs (veganism).

Macrobiotics, food combining, and nutritional supplementation can also form part of a naturopath's dietary recommendations, as do elimination diets and those tailored to specific needs. The prescribing of special diets and food supplements such as vitamins and minerals, which began in the United States in the 1950s, has now spawned its own therapy: nutritional therapy or nutritional medicine (*see page 74*).

ELIMINATION DIETS

Such diets are often used in diagnosing food allergies or intolerances. All suspect substances, which often include wheat and dairy produce, are eliminated from the diet to see how a person fares without them. They are then reintroduced, one at a time, to determine which particular substance(s) cause a reaction.

MACROBIOTICS

Macrobiotics, developed by the Japanese Michio Kushi, is based on the principle that ideally we should eat locally grown wholegrains, seeds, and plant foods.

Foods are divided into two groups, according to the Oriental principles of yin and yang. Yin foods are those that grow above ground, usually in hot countries, have a high water content, are soft, juicy, and cooling. Warming yang foods grow in a cold wet environment and tend to be made up of roots, stems, and seeds.

The object is to eat according to your individual needs and environment in order to maintain balance in the body. For example, when it is hot we should eat more cooling (yin) foods (*see page 75*).

THE HAY DIET

This food-combining regime was devised by the American Dr. William Hay from principles laid down by various experts including Lindlahr and Shelton. There are now several other versions of food combining, which all follow more or less the same principles: not to mix foods that clash and to avoid refined or processed foods.

Hay classified foods into three main groups:
* alkaline-forming foods
* concentrated proteins
* concentrated carbohydrates.

Proteins and carbohydrates are both acid-forming, but each requires a different digestive environment and should never be eaten at the same meal. You can eat alkaline-forming foods with either proteins or carbohydrates, in a ratio of four times alkaline foods to one acid in order to maintain the balance of alkaline and acid mineral salts in the body.

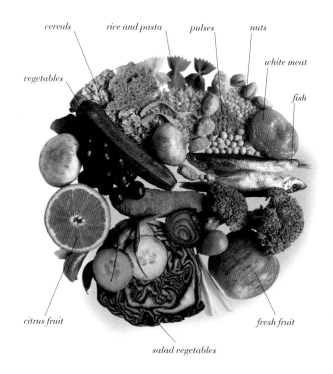

cereals *rice and pasta* *pulses* *nuts* *white meat* *fish* *vegetables* *citrus fruit* *fresh fruit* *salad vegetables*

Naturopaths recommend a balanced diet of which the majority (60 percent) is in raw form, with the rest being divided up equally between protein and complex carbohydrate.

Fasting

Fasting means not eating solid food for a specified period of time. It does not mean starving completely or going thirsty. Liquids must always be taken regularly during any fast.

Fasts can be of any length and they serve several purposes. Naturopaths believe they:
✻ cleanse the system of poisons accumulated from bad eating habits, a poor environment, and suppressed or repressed emotions
✻ enhance immune functioning and speed up healing
✻ give the digestive system a well-earned and often much-needed rest.

Fasting is particularly beneficial in the treatment of fevers and acute problems such as skin rashes or digestive upsets. Naturopaths also recommend fasting one or two days a month regularly as an important part of preventive healthcare – often advising timing the best moment by using a biorhythm reading *(see box, right)*.

Short fasts, lasting no longer than 48 hours, can be safely carried out by most healthy adults without supervision. However, strict supervision is necessary for fasts lasting longer than three days and for those undertaken by the chronically ill. There have been supervised fasts that have lasted for 21 days and more.

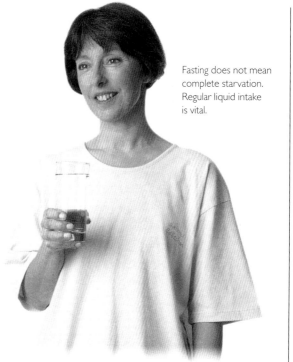

Fasting does not mean complete starvation. Regular liquid intake is vital.

A water fast can be enlivened by a squeeze of fresh lemon juice.

Fasts aimed at correcting specific conditions can sometimes seem extreme. Examples are
✻ the Guelpa fast – this is a three-day saline fast, often prescribed for rheumatic conditions
✻ the Schroth cure – also used in the treatment of rheumatism, this method alternates dry days with liquid days over a period of two or three weeks.

Other types of fasts include
✻ water fasts (in which nothing is eaten and only water is drunk)
✻ citrus mono diets (where you eat only oranges and drink their juice and water)
✻ other fruit mono diets (such as a grape fast)
✻ vegetable juice fasts.

The benefits of fasting are said to be enhanced by several processes such as hydrotherapy, deep breathing, and gentle forms of exercise.

CAUTIONS AND CONTRAINDICATIONS

Fasting for up to two days is safe. However fasts should not be undertaken except under medical advice by pregnant women, young children, and people who are seriously ill. Fasting should not be used to lose weight.

BIORHYTHMS

days of the month

emotional   *intellectual*   *physical*

According to the theory of biorhythms, which many naturopaths follow, our physical, mental, and emotional health are governed by cycles.

⁊ THE PHYSICAL CYCLE. *This lasts 23 days and governs vitality, immunity, confidence, strength, endurance, sex drive, and the ability to recover from illness.*

⁊ THE EMOTIONAL CYCLE. *This lasts 28 days and controls moods, emotions, creative abilities, and sensitivity.*

⁊ THE INTELLECTUAL CYCLE. *This takes 33 days to complete and it governs the ability to reason, learn, make decisions, and remember facts.*

These cycles can be charted on a graph, which some naturopaths use to help determine "critical" stages when you will be more likely to be accident-prone, depressed, or ill. Most charts are produced by computer these days.

Complete Therapeutic Systems

Oriental Systems

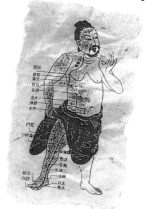

Oriental systems of medicine are based on the idea of life force flowing through the body along paths called the meridians.

TRADITIONAL Chinese Medicine has existed for at least 2,000 years. The earliest medical text, the *Huangdi Neijing* or "Yellow Emperor's Canon of Internal Medicine" is thought to have been written around 500–300 B.C. and is still used today.

Chinese medicine consists of acupuncture, moxibustion, and herbal medicine as well as acupressure massage, cupping, therapeutic exercises, and advice on diet and lifestyle. It is based on the principle of internal balance and harmony. When there is good balance between all the internal organs, the body and mind, and the external environment, there is good health. When this state of harmony and balance breaks down, there is disease.

VITAL ENERGY

The Chinese have a concept of universal energy or "life force." This vital energy known as chi (pronounced chee) or qi is said to be the basis of all life. In the human body the chi circulates through the body via 14 major energetic pathways known as "meridians." The meridians cannot be seen by the naked eye, but modern science has shown that their existence can be detected electrically. Most of the meridians connect to one of the major internal organs, and the chi is said to power the organ and enable it to function effectively.

YIN AND YANG AND THE FIVE ELEMENTS

The chi is regulated by the interdependent forces of yin and yang, which govern all living things. Yin qualities are typically coldness, weakness, hollowness, and dark, while the opposite yang qualities are heat, strength, solidity, and light. The person's constitution or the nature of the disease may be described in terms of the yin/yang balance. For example, a person with a high fever, bright red cheeks, and an intense headache would be someone with an excess of yang, while someone with symptoms of chronic fatigue, pallor, and cold limbs would have an excess of yin. Treatment aims to restore the yin/yang balance.

The body is also said to be made up of five basic elements, Wind, Water, Earth, Fire, and Metal. All five elements must exist in good balance in the body. If one element predominates the others will become unbalanced and disease will result. The elements are affected by the seasons, the weather, diet, and even emotional state, and all these have to be considered in diagnosis and treatment.

OTHER ORIENTAL SYSTEMS

There are many similarities between Chinese medicine and Ayurvedic medicine practiced in India *(see Ayurveda, page 34)*, partly due to the influence of Buddhism on both. But the practice of Chinese medicine itself spread with Chinese civilization to Korea, Japan, and Vietnam, and practice and theory are very similar in all these countries. In Tibet there is a blend of Chinese and Ayurvedic systems.

The yin/yang symbol of united opposites, each containing a seed of the other, represents the importance of wholeness in Eastern traditions.

CUPPING

Cupping has been used in China since the third century B.C. It involves lighting a match in a small, rounded "cup," made of glass, bamboo, metal, or pottery, and then removing it quickly and applying the cup to the skin. The flame creates a vacuum, and the cup sticks tightly to the skin. Several cups may be applied at any one time to a particular part of the body such as the back.

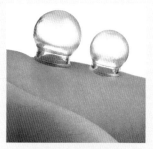

Cupping is slightly uncomfortable but not painful.

The jars are left in position for 10 to 15 minutes while the vacuum inside the cup produces strong suction on the skin and increases the blood flow and circulation. The cup is released by pressing the skin next to the edge of the cup so that the vacuum is broken.

Cupping is particularly helpful for conditions such as rheumatism, lumbago, and stiff neck and shoulders as it increases circulation and the mobility of affected areas.

Acupuncture

There are over 350 acupoints on the meridians of the body. Selected points are stimulated by inserting fine acupuncture needles in order to improve the flow of chi or qi in the meridians and to restore balance and healthy functioning to the internal organs of the body.

Treatment points are selected on the basis of pulse and tongue diagnosis, examination, and questioning *(see pages 18–19 on Oriental Diagnosis, and Acupuncture, page 90)* and categorized according to their effects on specific body systems and organs. The insertion of the needles is quick and virtually painless and often a comfortable and relaxed feeling follows.

Nobody knows exactly how acupuncture works but a growing body of research has shown acupuncture to be effective for a wide range of ailments including pain and joint problems, specific organ imbalances, mental and emotional problems, and childhood illnesses.

Increasing numbers of Western medically trained doctors and nurses are now studying and practicing acupuncture, while more people every year embark on full-time training in acupuncture as a career.

Acupuncture is economical and effective for both treating and preventing disease and has an important role to play in Western healthcare.

ACUPRESSURE

Acupressure involves the application of fingertip or nail pressure to acupuncture points on the body in order to remove blockages or pain and enhance the flow of chi. In Chinese medicine acupressure may be used in its own right or incorporated into an acupuncture treatment.

Typically the middle or index fingers or the thumbs are used, but sometimes, as in shiatsu *(see pages 96–7)*, the knuckles, elbows, or knees may be used to apply firmer pressure to large areas of the body.

Acupressure is particularly suitable for those who are anxious about acupuncture needles. It can also be easily learned and safely applied as a self-help technique. However, since its application is less direct and specific than an acupuncture needle, the results are likewise often slower and less specific. *(See also Acupressure, page 94.)*

MOXIBUSTION

Moxibustion methods include the burning of small cones directly on the skin over a specific acupuncture point and holding burning moxa near the skin. The skin itself is never burned. In the heated needle technique, copper coil-handled needles are positioned, small disks of paper slipped over them to catch falling ash, and moxa cones lit on the heads of the needles.

Moxibustion is the application of heat to specific points on the body in order to treat diseases and restore the smooth flow of chi in the meridians. Generally the heat is obtained by burning dried mugwort leaves (*Artemesia vulgaris,* known as moxa) either directly or indirectly on the skin.

The direct method involves rolling the dried moxa wool into small cones and placing them directly onto the skin. The tips of the cones are set alight but extinguished once heat is felt. With the indirect method prerolled moxa sticks are lit and held close to the skin until heat is felt. Sometimes a handful of moxa is lit in a specially designed box that is placed on the back in order to warm a larger area such as the kidneys. Moxa may also be placed on a slice of ginger or garlic, or on salt for more specific effects. Ginger helps to promote circulation while garlic has a strong antiseptic effect.

Moxa is widely used for conditions such as stiff neck, cold, weak back, frozen shoulder, and fatigue and has an invigorating and warming effect.

The size of acupuncture needles varies according to the area of the body to be treated and what effect the acupuncturist is aiming for – stimulation or calming.

Chinese Herbalism

The Chinese herbal tradition is believed to date back some 4,000 years to the Emperor Shen Nong (or Chi'en Nung). He is said to have described over 300 medicinal plants and their uses in a book called the *Pen Tsao*. Although versions of several ancient pharmacopoeia still exist today, the main surviving text on herbalism is the book by the physician Li Shih-chen describing almost 2,000 herbs and 10,000 herbal remedies, and written in the 16th century.

As well as the herbalism of trained physicians, there is also a folk tradition of herbal medicine in China. Many families had their own remedies, which were passed from generation to generation.

Traditional medicine came under question in the 20th century, but was reinstated under the communist regime. The barefoot doctors in the country districts were skilled in administering herbal prescriptions, the ingredients of which they had usually gathered and prepared themselves. Today, Chinese herbalism is very much an orthodox form of therapy and preventive treatment in China, and it is increasingly practiced in the West.

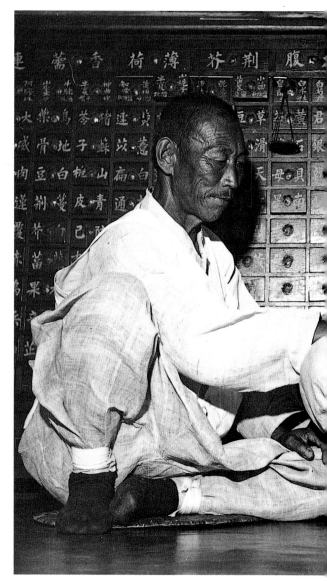

Not all Chinese herbal remedies come from plants; *ge jie* is made from the dried skin of a gecko.

The so-called raw ingredients of herbal preparations are usually dried materials. They are often prescribed as "soups," decoctions, or teas but may be taken in their raw form or processed into pills, powders, ointments, liquid tonics, or teas. They are classified according to their properties, such as "warming" and "cooling," and by their taste. The majority are of plant origin but a few are derived from minerals or from animal sources.

Usually the herbs are combined into formulas that are often adapted to suit changing circumstances as the client progresses. The careful adjustment of the remedy to suit the individual client is characteristic of Chinese medicine. Chinese herbalism can be used for a wide range of ailments, including asthma, skin diseases, menstrual problems, digestive disturbances, and migraine, and is effective when used on its own or in conjunction with another therapy such as acupuncture.

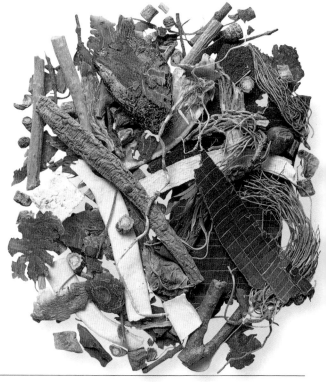

Chinese herbs are often prepared in combinations called formulas. Specific formulas can be tailored by a Chinese herbalist to suit particular conditions.

Japanese Medicine

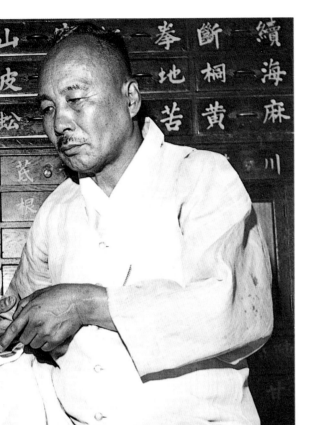

A Chinese doctor diagnoses his patient and prescribes the appropriate remedy.

Chinese medicine was introduced to the imperial court of Japan in the 5th century A.D. by Korean physicians. Monks and traveling physicians from Korea and China introduced Chinese ideas more generally during the 5th and 6th centuries. Medical works on acupuncture and moxibustion, with detailed diagrams, were made known in Japan by the Chinese doctor Zhi Cong around A.D. 560, and from the early 7th century Chinese medicine began to be adopted systematically under the influence of two Buddhist monks who had spent many years in China.

A Japanese adaptation of Chinese medicine still exists today. However, there are several distinctive features in Japanese medical practice.

A strong tradition of blind practitioners has resulted in very well-developed palpation techniques of diagnosis and treatment, such as abdominal palpation (*see Oriental Diagnosis, pages 18–19*); shiatsu, which is a specifically Japanese form of acupressure massage, has also developed.

Japan also has a strong herbal tradition, which has close links with Chinese herbal medicine but tends to use smaller amounts of more refined ingredients and also has different formulas of its own. (*See Herbal Medicine, pages 72–3.*) There are also a number of specifically Japanese manipulative and bone-setting therapies. Folk remedies, spa baths, and spiritual medicine in the form of prayers and talismans from shrines and temples are also popular.

The Japanese adaptation of Chinese medicine is known as kanpo, and the main foundations of present practice date back to the 16th and 17th centuries.

Japan was also exposed to Western influence at this time, when Christian missionaries began to arrive. Just as Buddhist monks had once cared for the sick, now Jesuits, followed by Dominicans and Franciscans, did the same. This type of medicine came to be known as "cosmopolitan" medicine.

During the 18th century, when the Dutch and Chinese were the only nations allowed to trade with Japan, Western understanding of anatomy was introduced, and at the same time many Oriental notions were introduced from Japan to Europe. Acupuncture and moxibustion became known for the first time in the West in this way.

"Cosmopolitan" medicine now officially dominates in Japan, but kanpo is also popular. This term is now often used to denote herbalism, but the whole range of Chinese medicine is practiced.

In the Japanese tradition, medical knowledge was passed on through itinerant monks.

Ayurveda

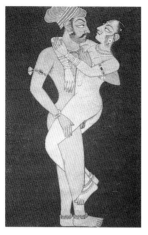

In Eastern traditions, sex is a healing technique that promotes the flow of energy.

Ayurveda, meaning the "Science of Life," is said to be the oldest and most complete medical system in the world and dates back to c.3000 B.C. Its roots are in ancient Indian civilization and Hindu philosophy, and it has been an important influence on the development of all the other Oriental medical systems. The original source of Ayurveda is the holy scriptures of the *Vedas* and the texts known as the *Samhitas*, which give a treatise on healthcare and describe medical procedures, including surgery and a form of massage of vital energy points (similar to Chinese acupressure).

Ayurveda has much in common with Chinese medicine. The human being is viewed as a microcosm of the universe, and both the body and the universe can be

Yoga is an important part of the Ayurvedic tradition, founded on the concept of balanced energy flow within the body.

seen partly in terms of five elements. In Ayurveda these are space or ether, air, fire, water, and earth, and they correspond with the five cognitive senses: hearing, touch, sight, taste, and smell, and also with five "senses" of action.

The concepts of life force or energy and balance within the body are important in Ayurvedic as in Chinese medicine. In Ayurvedic medicine, the life force is prana, similar to the Chinese chi, or qi. As in Chinese medicine, the functioning of the body is controlled by immaterial forces, linked to physical substances.

These substances are the three basic forces or doshas that exist in all things:
* Pitta, the force of heat and energy, linked with the sun, that controls digestion and all biochemical processes in the body
* Kapha, the force of water and tides, influenced by the moon, the stabilizing influence that controls fluid metabolism in the body
* Vata, linked to the wind, the force that controls movement and the functioning of the nervous system in the body.

When "not abnormal" these three forces ensure that the body is healthy, but when they are "abnormal" or unbalanced, disease follows.

Ayurveda emphasizes equilibrium – balance of mind, body, and spirit and balanced adaptation to external forces – and it focuses on keeping a person healthy rather than on disease itself.

The cure of a sick patient involves purification and palliation and is tailored to the nature and strength of the disease and of the patient. The first stage is generally control of diet, and fasting, combined with practices such as meditation, yoga (*see Yoga, pages 61–5*) and chanting, as well as following advice on posture, sleep, and other lifestyle matters. This alone may effect a cure, but herbal medication may also be required to treat excesses with their opposites (for example, cooling heat symptoms and warming cold symptoms) in order to restore balance.

For stronger disease, stronger treatment is then required, and this is purification, with purges, emetics, or enemas, and perhaps also medication to drain or nourish the body, depending on whether the disease is wet or dry. When the disease has been eliminated a period of palliation, with rest and careful diet, follows. Finally the patient is given rejuvenation therapy to restore full strength. Advice is given on lifestyle, exercise, diet, hygiene, and daily habits.

Ayurveda is used all over India and in many developing countries and is recognized by the World Health Organization.

Tibetan Medicine

Tibetan medical tradition is long established, and, because Tibet was not subjected to any European dominance in the age of empire, has been able to remain quite free of Western influence. Nevertheless, it is relatively recent in origin, as compared to Chinese or Indian medicine, and is believed to date back to about the 7th century A.D. The Tibetan ruler, King Songtsen Gampo, who introduced an Indian-derived script to his country, is said also to have introduced medicine, summoning to his court physicians from China, from India, and from Iran.

Tibetan medicine is based on a unique synthesis of Indian and Chinese traditional medicine and Tibetan Buddhism, with elements of Arabic medicine. As with the Ayurvedic and Chinese systems, it is holistic and takes into account such factors as diet, lifestyle, environment, weather, attitudes, and emotions alongside any symptoms of disease. The theory of meridians or energy channels is particularly highly developed. There is also a strong folk and religious tradition relating to healing, which runs parallel to the more orthodox medical tradition.

In Tibetan medicine disease is considered to be the result of an imbalance in the three "humors" that exist in all living things and that control organ function in the body. They are

❀ wind, relating to respiration and movement
❀ bile, relating to digestion, complexion, and the temperament
❀ phlegm, relating to sleep, joint mobility, and skin elasticity.

One root of disease is considered to be ignorance of the true nature of reality. As a result of this we fall prey to conflicting desires and emotions and these produce three types of mental state: attachment, aversion, and confusion, otherwise known as "the three poisons," which in turn lead to imbalance and disease.

Other causes of imbalance are factors such as the environment, diet, conduct in life, seasonal climatic influences, poison, and trauma, which act on the humors by their similar or contrary natures, causing excess or deficiency.

This theory differs from Ayurvedic theories in that the "three poisons" are said to develop within the growing fetus, generating phlegm, bile, and wind.

In Tibet itself, medicine is still closely linked to religion and magic. Prayers and

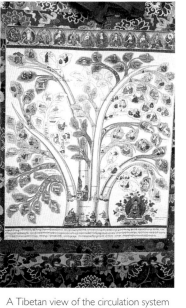

A Tibetan view of the circulation system showing the veins and arteries laid out like the branches of a tree.

rituals to protect from evil and prevent misfortune play their part in maintaining and curing disease, and this aspect is not entirely separate from medical practice.

Diagnosis is based on pulse-taking, urine analysis (which is exceptionally highly developed and which may stem from medieval European medicine, as introduced by the Persians), tongue diagnosis, and observations (see *Oriental Diagnosis, pages 18–19*). Treatments, which aim to restore the balance of the humors, include herbal medicine, accessory therapies (massage, moxibustion, acupuncture, dietary and behavioral advice, religious rituals, and purification techniques).

Tibetan medicine is practiced throughout Tibet, India, Ladakh, Nepal, and Bhutan and is now becoming more widely available through Tibetan physicians living in Western countries.

Ritual prayers and chanting are a significant part of the healing practice, and medicine is indissoluble from religion. Many lamas (monks) are also doctors.

Diagnosis and Therapy Systems

Traditional Arabic Medicine

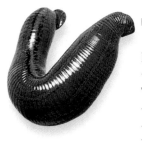

The leech, a blood-sucking worm, was used to "bleed" patients in medieval medicine and is also part of the Unani tradition.

Traditional Arabic or Islamic medicine became known in India, where it is widely practiced, as Unani-Tibb. "Tibb" is an Arabic word meaning "medicine," while "Unani" is thought to be derived from "Ionian" (meaning Greek) – acknowledging the influence of the early Greek healing traditions on this system of medicine.

The system dates back to the 7th century, when the Arab-Islamic world adopted the traditions of Europe as it expanded into areas that had been part of the Greco-Roman empires. Medical practice and theory were then dominated by the works of the Greek physican Galen (A.D. 130–200) who studied anatomy and made use of numerous drugs.

The Muslims who invaded India in the 11th century brought their medicine with them, and the system is prominent today, particularly among Muslims, in India and its surrounding countries. It owes most to the work of the 10th-century Persian physician Ibn Sina, known in the West as Avicenna. A follower of Galen, he considered the physical, emotional, and spiritual aspects of health and developed a system of botanical medicine and dietetics for health.

Unani-Tibb has been influenced by Ayurvedic medicine, as well as influencing it. It is a holistic system that treats the imbalances that lead to disease and encourages the patient to adopt a balanced way of life. It incorporates the following concepts:

❋ four elements, namely, earth and water (heavy) and fire and air (light)
❋ nine temperaments, one equable (balanced) and eight nonequable and relating to hot, cold, wet, and dry
❋ four humors, as in ancient Greek medicine – blood, phlegm, yellow bile, and black bile – semigaseous vapors that maintain body fluids and balance digestion.

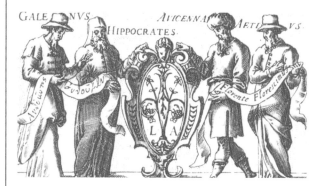

Avicenna (second from the right), the greatest known Arabic physician, author of many important medical tracts, including a medical poem, *Al Arjuza fi l tibb.*

UNANI PHILOSOPHY

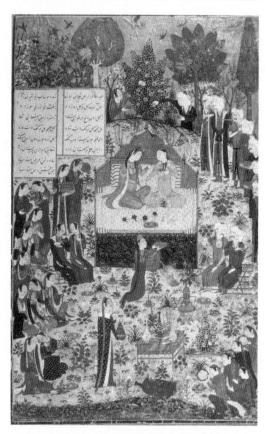

Gardens were not mere luxuries in a desert country but a source of the medicinal herbs that made up many of the remedies in Arabic medicine.

Health is considered to be the body's natural state, but each person has unique predisposing factors, which react within a matrix of external factors to produce the imbalance of the humors that enables a disease to take root.

Diagnosis is formed by pulse and urine analysis, and by examining six external factors: climate, food and drink, physical activity and rest, sleep, emotional factors, and excretion. Modern techniques such as X-rays and ultrasound have been adopted in recent times. Treatment stresses dietary change and uses herbal medicines but also frequently incorporates various forms of hydrotherapy, including steam baths. Prayers may also be recommended.

This system of medicine treatment is often hospital-based, and through it, hospitals were established throughout the Islamic world from as early as the 8th century.

Shamanism

PREHISTORIC paintings on walls in caves in Europe show that shamanism was practiced at least 20,000 years ago. The word comes from Siberia, from the language of the Evenk peoples who hunted and herded reindeer for a living. However, shamanism has been found in most tribal cultures in every continent, from Alaska to Borneo. Witch doctors or sangomas (Africa), medicine men (North America), yogis or holy men (India), and witches and wizards (Europe) are all shamans who follow more or less the same practices everywhere.

The essence of shamanism is the ability of the shaman to enter a trance or dream state of altered consciousness (and sometimes to help the sufferer into the same state). Shamans claim this takes them into the spirit world where they can use their ability to control the spirits to make changes that affect the physical world. In a trance state, they are able to separate their souls from their bodies and fly to any part of the cosmos to seek the cure, or the reasons for the illness, and so cure the patient. They also use herbal medicine and cleansing rituals. Traditionally shamans were not only highly skilled at healing the sick but had the ability to foretell the future, interpret dreams, and ward off evil spirits. In traditional hunting societies, they were able to seek out the souls of prey animals and lead the tribe to the best hunting grounds.

Shamans in the traditional hunting societies were usually men and were held in the highest regard, often having a status equal to that of a chief or leader. Genghis Khan, leader of the Mongol hordes, was a shaman. In the more agrarian societies of Africa, India, and Asia, many shamans were women, and in Korea, all shamans are female.

SHAMANISM TECHNIQUES

The techniques used by a shaman to bring about a state of altered consciousness include drumming, rattling, chanting, dancing, and the taking of natural hallucinogenic drugs. Drums are a feature of the northern shamanic traditions, whereas rattles are significant in South America, as are hallucinogenic plants. In Peru, shamans are known as *vegetalistas* because of their skilled use of dangerous plants. Through these means, the shaman claims to be able to move between the real and the spirit worlds at will. He may go into a deep trance state or more dramatically allow himself to be temporarily taken over by the spirits that he has summoned. However, a shaman always controls and summons the spirits; he is not possessed by them.

During their rituals many shamans call on the help of the essential spirit of animals or sacred objects to which they feel a special connection. By harnessing the energy of their guardian spirits, the shaman divines what the problem is – whether physical, spiritual, or emotional – and what remedy is needed to treat it.

Contemporary or neo-shamanism uses many traditional techniques but emphasizes a direct connection to a spirit guide rather than using a shaman as an intermediary. New forms of so-called shamanism, which are popular in many New Age groups, such as "Trance Dance," have little connection to real shamanism.

A Siberian shaman in full ritual dress, dancing and holding his large drum.

Shamanic rattles are used to call up the spirits. This example is sacred to the frog spirit.

CAUTIONS AND CONTRAINDICATIONS

Because of the profound emotional states that can be entered into during some rituals, always look into the background and credentials of anyone you consult and speak to people they have treated before agreeing to treatment yourself.

Individual Therapies

PHYSICAL THERAPIES • Bodywork

OVER THE last centuries, elaborate systems to "work" the body to prevent and treat disease and illness have developed. Bodywork or physical manipulation used in therapy is usually described as being a manipulative technique. This is any system of treatment in which the practitioner uses his or her hands to bring about beneficial changes either in the client's muscles and skeleton, or, through them, in other parts of the body. From here a whole new philosophy of physical medicine was developed to integrate the body structurally, and through touch, to evoke muscular relaxation.

ANCIENT TRADITIONS

All the ancient civilizations were well acquainted with bodywork: the Indians, Japanese, Chinese, Greeks, Egyptians, and the native peoples of both North and South America, all practiced manipulation, and Hippocrates described spinal manipulation in his work called the *Corpus Hippocrateum*.

In Europe, during the Middle Ages, manipulation, together with massage, became most closely identified with a group of healers known as "bone-setters." Such exponents of traditional forms of therapy were found worldwide, and they remained popular until modern conventional medicine came into its own in the 19th century. At that time, the new medical practitioners poured scorn on the methods and practices of bone-setters, and the therapy all but died out. In fact, it almost certainly would have died, had it not been for two men living in North America.

In the mid-1870s, Andrew Taylor Still (1828–1917), an American doctor dissatisfied with contemporary trends in medicine, developed a new form of manipulation, which he called "Osteopathy." Osteopathy brought the practice of bone-setting into the age of science, training practitioners at formal schools where anatomy and physiology were taught in great detail.

In 1895, Daniel David Palmer (1845–1913), a Canadian magnetic healer, discovered that "displacement of any part of the skeletal frame may press against nerves, which are the channels of communication, intensifying or decreasing their carrying capacity, creating either too much or not enough functioning, an aberration known as disease." He called his method of

manipulation "adjustment," and this method led to the establishment of a form of therapy known as chiropractic. Less than a century later, both therapies are considered to be almost mainstream.

Further innovations in manipulative methods occurred later in the 20th century, mostly after World War II, and almost all are based on osteopathic and chiropractic theory. Ida Rolf, for example, a European who traveled to the United States before the war, devised a method that concentrated on relaxing deeper soft tissues of the body, thereby "expanding the body." She believed that when the body was realigned so that physical structures were in a straight vertical line, the earth's field of gravity could properly support the body's own energy field, establishing physical and psychological well-being.

Marion Rosen, also an American, introduced bodywork that incorporated a sense of touch to integrate the body with what she called the "psyche," or the soul. In Australia, an industrial chemist named Tom Bowen introduced a unique concept of having periods of rest between a series of moves within a treatment session.

MODERN METHODS

Manipulation today consists of many different procedures, each of which may constitute a full therapy in itself. Accordingly, there are massage therapists who specialize to the extent of administering massage only.

The skeleton, the underlying framework that holds the whole body up.

Acupressure and shiatsu utilize energy points; myotherapy involves pressure on deep trigger points. Then there are physical therapists who combine massage and articulation. Some practitioners specialize in adjusting only specific joints in the body, and as the methodologies are refined, there is an increasing amount of overlap between the therapies.

Manipulation is gaining credence not only because there is a demand for it but also because it has been shown to benefit a large number of people.

Chiropractic • 1

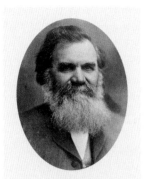

Daniel David Palmer (1845–1913), the founder of chiropractic

Chiropractic – a term that derives from two ancient Greek words meaning "manually effective" – is technically described as "the diagnosis, treatment, and rehabilitation of conditions that affect the neuro-musculoskeletal system." Through a series of special examination and manipulative techniques, chiropractors can diagnose and treat numerous disorders associated with the nerves, muscles, bones, and joints of the body. The emphasis chiropractors put on the spine has led many people to believe that the therapy is useful only for treating back pain. In fact, skilled therapists can treat almost every structural problem from headaches to ankle problems.

In 1895, Daniel David Palmer, the founder of chiropractic, treated his office janitor for deafness by realigning some small bones in his spine. Fascinated by this discovery, Palmer moved from his native Canada to Davenport, Iowa, where he developed the principles upon which chiropractic is based.

In particular, he devoted considerable attention to the spine, noting that it is integral to all three functional elements of the human body: it surrounds and protects the spinal cord, a major factor in the nervous system; it supports a great number of individual muscles; and in that it actually consists of an entire series of linked bones, it also therefore has virtually as many joints. Palmer believed that any damage, disease, or structural change of the spine can affect the health of the rest of the body, and that through manipulation, chiropractors can not only improve structural problems such as sciatica or the effects of injury but also help with conditions such as asthma, which can be helped by easing tension in the chest muscles.

He then went on to develop the use of spinal adjustment to treat disease, discovering that by gently moving back into place those bones that appeared to be misaligned he could reduce many of his patients' symptoms without recourse to drugs or surgery. Daniel Palmer established his first chiropractic school in Davenport in 1895. In the same year, W.C. Roentgen invented the X-ray machine, which early chiropractors found useful for making accurate spinal assessments. In 1907, Bartlet Joshua Palmer took over his father's fledgling infirmary. His name is now primarily associated in the United States with those chiropractors who use chiropractic as their sole therapy for ailments.

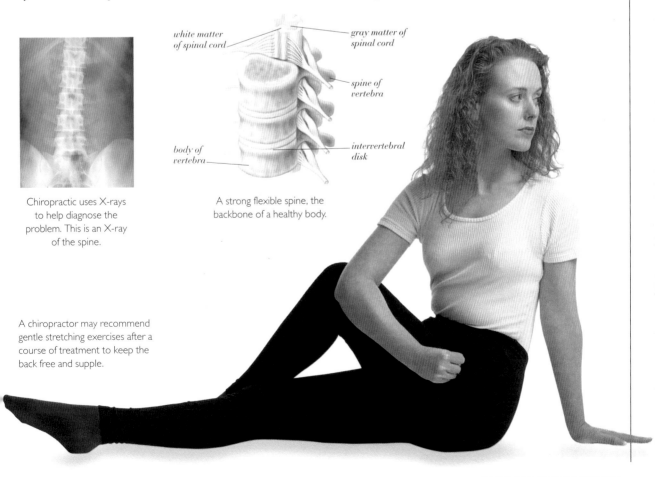

Chiropractic uses X-rays to help diagnose the problem. This is an X-ray of the spine.

white matter of spinal cord

gray matter of spinal cord

spine of vertebra

body of vertebra

intervertebral disk

A strong flexible spine, the backbone of a healthy body.

A chiropractor may recommend gentle stretching exercises after a course of treatment to keep the back free and supple.

Chiropractic • 2

Chiropractors regard the body's nervous system as fundamental to health. Pain and disease are the result of undue pressure on the nervous system by mechanical, chemical, or psychological factors. Restoration to health and maintenance of health thereafter depend on the normal functioning of the nervous system. Because the nervous system is so well integrated with muscles and bones in the body, diagnosis and assessment of a patient's neuro-musculoskeletal condition is undertaken from the biomechanical standpoint: the mobility of each of the patient's joints is monitored to establish the range of movement in each vertebral or joint segment. It is the joints, after all – especially those of the spine – that are subject to the most stress and strain in everyday life.

Injured joints lose some of their inherent flexibility when they repair, placing more stress on adjacent structures (such as the soft intervertebral disks, ligaments, and nerves). Initially, the body is able to compensate for these regions of stiffness, but as further stress occurs, this ability to compensate decreases to such an extent that an even worse injury may result.

Treatment accordingly comprises very precise adjustments to the spinal segments or to individual vertebrae to restore flexibility to stiff and painful joints, to lessen stress on neighboring joints and any other structures that have become swollen and inflamed, and to reduce the reactive muscle spasm (tension) and pain.

Trauma elsewhere in the body may require further, different forms of adjustment but with exactly the same goals. In such a case, the chiropractor again locates the area of diminished flexibility and assesses the effects on the surrounding musculoskeletal structures. Because chiropractic focuses on improving the movement at individual body joints that often have been stiff and inflexible for some time, a few sessions of therapy and associated exercises may be required before a patient is able to move with genuine flexibility, and for the muscles to regain a measure of healthy support.

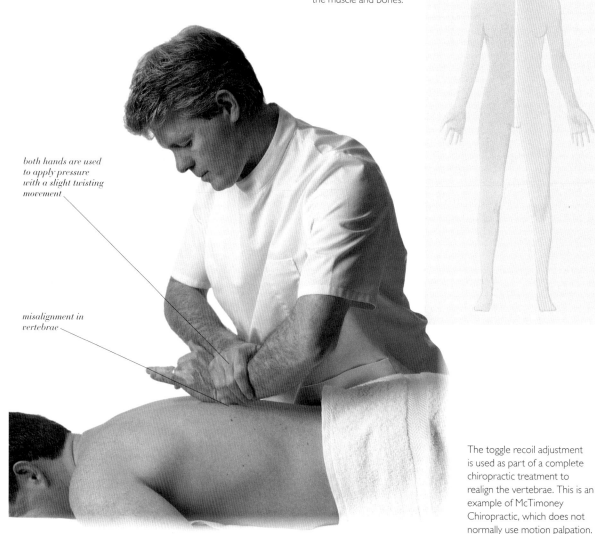

Chiropractic places great emphasis on the health of the nervous system. Diagnosis involves assessment of the nerves as well as the muscle and bones.

both hands are used to apply pressure with a slight twisting movement

misalignment in vertebrae

The toggle recoil adjustment is used as part of a complete chiropractic treatment to realign the vertebrae. This is an example of McTimoney Chiropractic, which does not normally use motion palpation.

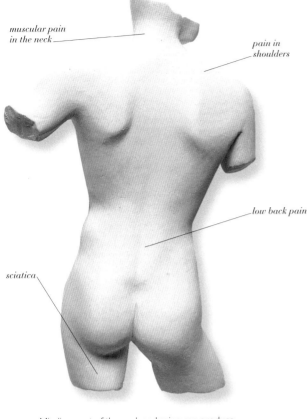

muscular pain
in the neck

pain in
shoulders

low back pain

sciatica

Misalignment of the neck and spine can produce
referred pain elsewhere in the body.

WHAT CAN CHIROPRACTIC TREAT?

Chiropractic treatment can benefit many conditions but is most useful for:

- *back pain (including the back pain of pregnancy)*
- *general pain resulting from pressure or injury on the neuro-musculoskeletal system*
- *sciatica (see page 191)*
- *muscular pain in the neck, shoulder, or upper arm*
- *aches and pains from sporting activity*
- *muscle strains and joint sprains*
- *headaches*
- *stiffness and other forms of impaired movement in the arms or legs*
- *asthma and other internal disorders under some circumstances.*

A chiropractor should not, on the other hand, be asked to treat

- *any disorder arising from weakness or disease of the bones themselves (such as osteoporosis, rheumatoid arthritis, and other conditions – such as bone cancer – that actively alter bone tissue)*
- *conditions that arise as a result of severe pressure on the spinal cord (such as, for example, in a broken back, a tumor, or lesion)*
- *conditions that arise as a result of a severe disturbance of the blood circulation.*

ELEMENTS OF THERAPY

DIAGNOSIS Where it is necessary, considerable use of X-rays is made in order to gain information about the client's underlying bone structure, and to rule out non-mechanical problems (such as organic disease or deformity). Chiropractors also diagnose problems through observation and palpation (hands-on examination). X-rays are used to pinpoint the area of damage, assess its extent, and decide if chiropractic treatment is suitable. X-rays are taken in a weight-bearing position, so that the practitioner can see what the spine looks like under normal conditions. If the examination reveals a "subluxation," then the chiropractor will undertake treatment. "Subluxation" is the term used for defective joint movement and its effect on the nervous system and surrounding structures.

TREATMENT Chiropractors tend to concentrate on localized problem areas, if possible, rather than undertaking generalized stretching, loosening, and massage procedures. They aim to restore the spine and musculo-skeletal system to normal function by using a variety of special chiropractic manipulative techniques. Mobilization involves moving a joint as far as it will comfortably go within its normal range of movement, and manipulation shifts it further with any one of a number of different techniques. Where manipulation is involved, the chiropractor will use the correct amount of force at the correct speed to thrust into the spinal joint to the correct depth. There are around 150 different chiropractic techniques.

METHOD Adjustments involve direct manual contact, predominantly in movements described as "high velocity low amplitude" – that is, rapid but short. (Outside the United States, such quick, brief movements are alternatively described as "short lever" actions.) Patients are treated according to their specific problem, age, build, general health, and pain levels. Ice treatments may also be used to reduce pain and swelling. Applied kinesiology, which was originated by American chiropractor Dr. George Goodheart, is also part of some chiropractors' treatment.

> **CAUTIONS AND CONTRAINDICATIONS**
>
> Chiropractic is not suitable for broken or fractured bones or for people with bone disease, such as cancer of the bone.

Osteopathy

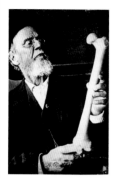

Andrew Taylor Still (1828–1917), the founder of osteopathy.

Osteopathy is a manipulative therapy that works on the body's structure (the skeleton, muscles, ligaments, and connective tissue) to relieve pain, improve mobility, and restore all-round health. Osteopaths believe that we function as a complete working system – our body structure, organs, systems, mind, and emotions are all interrelated and mutually interdependent. Because of this, problems that affect one part of the structural body upset the balance of the body generally, and also the emotions. Similarly, internal problems can reveal themselves in the body's structure as it adapts to accommodate pain, discomfort, or disease.

In Britain over 5 million people a year visit an osteopath, many of them now referred by a doctor. In the United States, where osteopaths are also medically trained doctors, the figure is in excess of 100 million.

Osteopathy was devised in 1874 by Andrew Taylor Still. He trained as an engineer before receiving formal medical training at Kansas City School of Physicians and Surgeons, after which he worked as an army surgeon. He was unhappy with the often brutal medicine of his day, and he felt that stimulating the body's natural powers of self-healing would be preferable. He was interested in the body as a machine and became aware that many illnesses were the result of a misalignment of the body's structures. Manipulation could restore the balance and cure illness, he believed.

His philosophy was that "structure governs function," a belief that remains one of the basic principles of modern osteopathy. He claimed that tension in muscles and misaligned bones places unnecessary strain on the body as a whole. The initial strain can be caused by any number of factors, such as physical injury, or habitual poor posture, or by destructive emotions such as anxiety and fear. Adjusting the framework of the body would relieve that strain and enable all the systems to run smoothly so that the body would heal itself.

MODERN THERAPY

Osteopaths regard the body as a unit, a whole being made up of contributory parts. An abnormality in the structure or reaction of one part exerts an abnormal influence on all the other parts, which in turn affects the whole body. The normal, healthy body contains within itself all the necessary mechanisms for its own defense against injury and infection, and for restoration to normality following trauma. This defense and restoration take place best if the body is maintained in optimum condition, when there is maximum structural mobility and flexibility.

Osteopathy is therefore aimed at encouraging the body's internal mechanisms to focus on their own self-corrective function on the imbalance. The osteopath's aim is to correct the dysfunction so that the body is then in a fit state to heal itself. Osteopathic treatment is concerned as much with maintenance as with cure. A regular checkup enables the osteopath to detect and restore areas of dysfunction before they manifest as disease.

> ### CAUTIONS AND CONTRAINDICATIONS
>
> Osteopathy should not be used to treat any disorder arising from weakness or disease of the bones themselves (osteoporosis, rheumatoid arthritis, and other conditions – such as bone cancer – that actively alter bone tissue); conditions arising from severe pressure on the spinal cord (as, for example, in a broken back, a tumor, or a lesion); conditions arising from a severe disturbance of the blood circulation.

Osteopathy can help in acute cases such as a sports injury. Here the McMurray's maneuver is used to replace the medial meniscus of the knee joint.

knee joint

quick snap action replaces joint

injured sports person treated at side of field

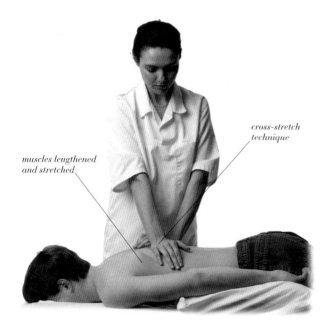

A cross-stretch technique is used to lengthen
the postural muscles of the back and release tension.

*muscles lengthened
and stretched*

*cross-stretch
technique*

Osteopathy employs a wide range of manipulative techniques, varying according to the part of the body being treated. Tight muscles will be relaxed in order that fluids may flow freely, allowing blood to carry nutrients and oxygen to where they are needed, and allowing the waste products in the lymphatic fluid to drain away. Some regions may require gentle, slow, low-velocity touch, while soft tissues and some joints may need flexing or massage. Joints with reduced mobility may require joint mobilization therapy. At all times, however, it is the entire body that is undergoing treatment. The local body area, which is subject to the presenting complaint, naturally receives close attention, but the osteopath also minutely examines the rest of the body for other factors that may predispose or contribute to the complaint.

ELEMENTS OF THERAPY

DIAGNOSIS Diagnosis is made by the practitioner asking numerous questions and listening to the responses. He or she will then assess body framework and posture, evaluating the way the body functions before checking parts such as the spine, hips, and legs. Joints will be tested to establish how well and with what ease they move, and the osteopath will palpate the tissue as it moves. This is known as active movement testing.

There will also be passive movement testing, which means feeling the body's response to the movements of sitting, standing, walking, and so on. The way in which movement is restricted can reveal the cause of a problem. The main physical examination is carried out by means of palpation (touch) and movement, and joint testing, but sometimes it may be necessary for further tests or X-rays at a hospital.

TREATMENT There is a wide range of techniques used. However, some osteopaths favor one or more particular forms of treatment. The techniques and the amount of pressure used will be adapted by the practitioner to suit particular conditions.

Manipulative techniques used by the osteopath involve both direct contact and indirect contact and, therefore, include long-lever and short-lever actions. Osteopaths use many techniques depending on the state and also the position of the muscles being treated, and each one is carefully calculated and executed with engineering precision.

WHAT CAN OSTEOPATHY TREAT?

Osteopathic techniques can be adapted to treat almost anyone of any age or level of health. An osteopath may be asked to treat a patient who is complaining of:

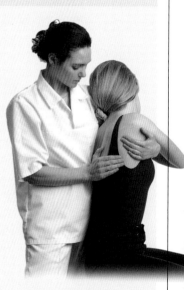

A dorsal sitting technique is used to release tension in the upper back through rotation.

- *back pain (including backache felt during pregnancy)*
- *sciatica*
- *muscular pain in the neck, shoulder, or upper arm*
- *joint pain from arthritis*
- *sprains and strains at the elbow, wrist, knee, or ankle*
- *headache*
- *painful sinuses*
- *reduced jaw mobility*
- *postural stress from occupational disposition*
- *recurrent strain injuries*
- *some digestive and respiratory difficulties*
- *some gynecological problems*
- *aches and pains in the body framework, resulting from a disorder of the body, including chronic illness*
- *aches and pains following childbirth.*

Cranial Osteopathy

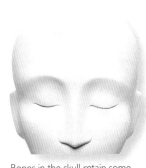

Bones in the skull retain some capacity for movement throughout life.

Cranial osteopathy is a specialist technique used to manipulate the bones of the skull with a touch so light that many people can barely feel it. Advocates claim it is based on sound anatomical and physiological knowledge combined with palpatory skills that are finely tuned and extremely sensitive qualities of touch.

It was developed in the 1930s by American osteopath William Garner Sutherland, a disciple of Andrew Still. His osteopathic training taught him that the bones of the skull, which are separate at birth, grow together into a fixed structure and are immovable, but he noticed that these bones retained some potential for movement even in adulthood. If they could move, they could also be susceptible to dysfunction. With experimentation on himself and others, he discovered that compressing his skull could have severe mental and physical effects. He discovered that the cerebrospinal fluid that surrounds the brain and the spinal cord fluid had rhythms, which he called "the breath of life," because the rhythms appeared to be influenced by the rate and depth of breathing. By gently manipulating the skull he found he could alter the rhythm of this fluid flow.

As the bones of the skull are moving normally, the cranial rhythm remains balanced, but any disturbance to the cranial bones can disturb the normal motion of the bones and the cranial rhythm, which, in turn, affects function in other areas of the body. An example of this is the birth process, when the bones of the skull can become disturbed, causing unresolved strain within the cranium. And it is this dysfunction that causes disease and ill-health.

ELEMENTS OF THERAPY

Therapy comprises gentle manipulations using fine, sensitive touch applied directionally, mostly at the cranium and the sacrum, but also elsewhere. The idea is to resolve any compression or distortion of the cranial bones, especially if any part of the rest of the body is deemed to be affected by such compression or distortion.

CAUTIONS AND CONTRAINDICATIONS

Cranial osteopathy should not be used to treat anyone who may be suffering from raised intercranial pressure, or patients with severe psychological disturbances.

CRANIOSACRAL TECHNIQUES

In any craniosacral therapy, the practitioner begins by working the whole body to tune into the network of connective tissues. The four positions shown below

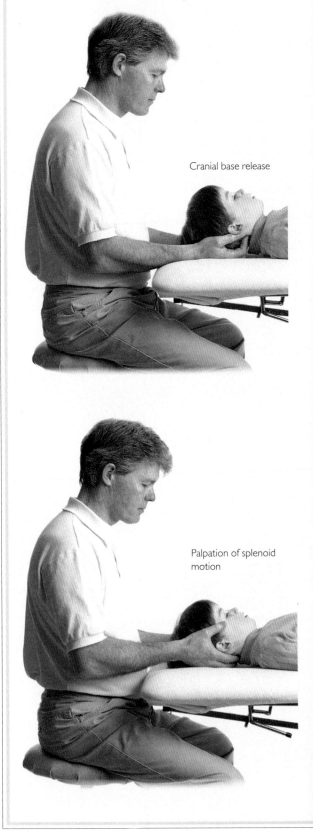

Cranial base release

Palpation of splenoid motion

improve the movement of the cranial bones. There is no set sequence, and the practitioner works as the movement of the bones dictates. Each position is held while the practitioner applies very light pressure.

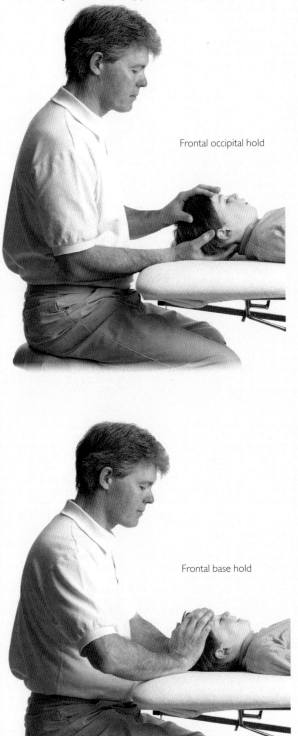

Frontal occipital hold

Frontal base hold

WHAT CAN CRANIAL OSTEOPATHY TREAT?

Treatment is extremely gentle, and when given by a fully qualified osteopath, it is perfectly safe for almost everyone, from newborn babies to the elderly.

Cranial osteopathy is the backbone of pediatric osteopathy. A cranial osteopath might be asked to treat the following:

- reduced capacity for self-healing (an immune system problem, perhaps)
- the symptoms of a direct trauma to the head or pelvis
- headaches
- painful sinuses
- reduced jaw mobility
- tinnitus
- residual effects of meningitis
- pain or strain created by childbirth
- some digestive and gynecological disorders.

Cranial osteopathy is particularly useful in treating patients who are hypersensitive to direct manipulation at the site of their presenting complaint. Hyperactivity in children, feeding problems in infants, and such problems as colic, poor coordination, sleep problems, learning difficulties, and glue ear may respond to treatment.

CRANIOSACRAL THERAPY (CST)

Craniosacral therapy is a recently established form of cranial osteopathy based on Dr. Sutherland's work but developed and popularized by John E. Upledger. Still evolving, this therapy retains several authoritative models as promulgated by a number of individual teachers. Upledger himself has evolved a model intended to promote "somatoemotional release." Others with backgrounds in chiropractic have evolved additional sacro-occipital techniques suggestive of a more mechanical approach.

Basically, the aim of the therapy is virtually the same as that of cranial osteopathy. The treatment comprises a sequence of movements that are not dictated by symptoms: it aims instead to improve the overall functioning of the cranial system and the membrane structures of the body. Practitioners are required to have some training, but they do not necessarily have to have medical qualifications.

Individual Therapies

Rolfing

Rolfing is named after its founder, Dr. Ida Rolf (1896–1979), an American biochemist whose therapy was intended to integrate manipulative forms of treatment with bio-energetics (the study of energy in living systems). Rolf recognized that when we are well aligned, gravity can flow through us, allowing us to move easily. A poorly aligned body is pulled down by gravity and must struggle to keep its balance, trying to compensate for misalignment in one area by making changes in another, until the entire structure is weakened. The aim of the rolfer is to realign body structure, restoring it to balance.

Rolfing relies predominantly on deep massage of the muscles and connective tissues (fascias). It does not focus on any specific area of symptoms but rather on manipulating the connective tissue to allow the body to return to a state of balance. When the body is balanced, the mind, nervous system, and all the organs and tissues to which it relates, function more efficiently and our innate healing system can work at its optimum.

ELEMENTS OF THERAPY

A full course of rolfing involves ten treatments, lasting about an hour each. Each session features a different part of the body, but is meant to fuse it with the parts that have been treated earlier, ultimately leading to complete integration.

Tension in the fascial network is returned to normal by deep, slow pressure, allowing it to lengthen and separate where it has been shortened and compacted.

Movement and psychology have become part of the training, and practitioners do not simply use deep manual pressure to stimulate changes. Emotional and physical problems may surface during treatment.

WHAT CAN ROLFING TREAT?

Rolfing may be used to treat any of the following:

- *musculoskeletal pain resulting from mechanical stress*
- *poor posture (caused by physical and psychological factors)*
- *breathing difficulties.*

CAUTIONS AND CONTRAINDICATIONS

Rolfing should not be used to treat any disorder arising from weakness or disease of the underlying bones themselves (such osteoporosis, fracture, and other conditions); a patient suffering from acute skin inflammation; sufferers of organic or inflammatory diseases such as cancer or rheumatoid arthritis.

Myotherapy

Throughout life – thanks to the exigencies of birth, active childhood, and the traumas, diseases, and occupational stresses of adulthood – our muscles tend to accumulate tender, irritable spots (trigger points). The ancient Chinese were aware of them 3,000 years ago, but it has taken Western physicians until the 20th century to come up with a successful therapy to relieve trigger points.

Dr. Janet Travell devised Trigger Point Injection Therapy (TPIT) during the 1940s, after she had published her study of muscular pain caused by trigger points. Later, the physical fitness expert Bonnie Prudden adapted this standard medical procedure so that it could be applied manually, using the pressure of thumbs, hands, or an elbow.

Firm pressure is applied to painful trigger points of the back.

ELEMENTS OF THERAPY

The client lies on a table for the myotherapy session. Sustained, firm pressure is applied for about seven seconds at a time to the highly irritable spots in abnormally taut bands of muscle. Once the trigger points have been relieved and the muscles released, the client is encouraged to undertake some passive stretching exercises to retain the flexibility created during the course of the lesson.

CAUTIONS AND CONTRAINDICATIONS

Myotherapy should not be used to treat sufferers from organic disease; people who bruise easily; or patients with a low pain threshold.

Bonnie Prudden certified myotherapists accept only clients who have been referred to them by medically qualified physicians.

WHAT CAN MYOTHERAPY TREAT?

Myotherapy can be an appropriate treatment for:

- *chronic recurrent pain of musculoskeletal origin.*

Physical Therapies

Rosen Technique

This form of therapy is named after Marion Rosen, a German-born physiotherapist who completed her training in Sweden before moving to San Francisco, California. Her approach combines massage, breathing exercises, and relaxation techniques with aspects of psychoanalysis. Although she strongly encouraged her clients to verbalize their sensations and emotions while considering their problems (after noting that clients who openly talked about events concerning the moment of injury tended to recover more quickly), she taught no specific procedure: practitioners are trained to act on their own observation and intuition.

> **CAUTIONS AND CONTRAINDICATIONS**
>
> There are no known contraindications to the Bowen and Rosen methods, but it is advised that you consult your physician before undertaking any complementary therapy.

WHAT CAN THE ROSEN TECHNIQUE TREAT?

The Rosen technique is useful on its own and in conjunction with psychotherapy and can treat

- conditions related to aging, including dementia and joint immobility
- body tension
- addictions
- general injuries to the soft tissues
- circulatory problems
- chronic health conditions.

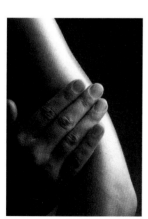
Light, gentle touching is the essence of the Rosen technique.

ELEMENTS OF THERAPY

The Rosen technique involves a light, gentle touching, particularly on areas of the body that are regarded as "holding breath" and therefore static. Such areas are apprehended as retaining uncomfortable memories that, by means of verbalizing and breath control, can be released. As a result of this, habitual body tension is also released. Some psychiatrists have found the Rosen method to be a useful adjunct to their own therapies.

Bowen Technique

Tom Bowen, an industrial chemist working in Victoria, Australia, between the 1950s and 1970s, devised a program of linked manual maneuvers that together comprise an individual form of therapy. In 1974 he invited osteopath and natural therapist Oswald Rentsch to study and document the method. Following Bowen's death in 1982, Oswald and Elaine Rentsch have trained people in the technique all over the world.

ELEMENTS OF THERAPY

The method consists of a series of "flicklike" maneuvers ("vibrational" movements) over muscles, tendons, and connective tissues, applied in precise sequence at specific points on the body. After the therapist has administered three or four of these movements, the client is left for between two and ten minutes for the body to "process" them before the next sequence of maneuvers is applied.

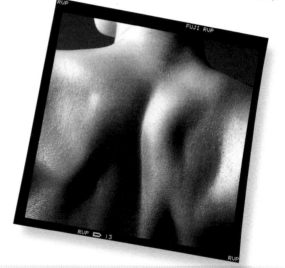
The vulnerable area of the back responds well to the Bowen technique.

WHAT CAN THE BOWEN TECHNIQUE TREAT?

The Bowen technique is helpful in many conditions, but is particularly useful for treating people suffering from:

- sprains and strains resulting from sports activity
- back pain
- neck pain
- virtually any pain of musculoskeletal origin, acute or chronic.

The technique is effective on clients of all ages.

Massage

Massage is one of the oldest forms of remedial therapy. First practiced in a structured way probably in China and Mesopotamia more than 5,000 years ago, the art of massage was already well known to the physicians of ancient Greece when Hippocrates, the "father of medicine," wrote in the 5th century B.C. that "the way to health is a scented bath and an oiled massage every day."

Most modern methods of massage derive mainly from Swedish massage as developed by Per Henrik Ling, a Swede who visited China during the 19th century. Ling was so greatly impressed by the massage techniques he observed when he was there that he synthesized his own form of therapy to incorporate these ancient Oriental skills.

Massage is an excellent way to relax mind and body, and so bring relief from everyday stresses and strains. It also helps to restore a sense of calmness and balance after any shock or trauma.

THE BENEFITS OF MASSAGE

Touching and stroking are not only important for adults, they also play a vital role in the healthy development of infants and young children. Those who care for babies born prematurely know that infants confined to incubators are more likely to thrive when gently stroked than when deprived of touch.

A regular body massage can enhance general health and vitality, while specialized methods can coax tension from muscles, ease stiff joints, promote healthy circulation of the blood, and stimulate lymphatic drainage to encourage the elimination of wastes from the body. Massage brings a healthy glow to dull skin and keeps the body feeling firm and supple.

Massage is effective for almost any condition and is particularly helpful for tension headaches, back pain, hyperactivity, and also insomnia.

TYPES OF MASSAGE

SHIATSU An ancient form of pressure-point massage, shiatsu has been practiced for centuries in Japan. It is based on the principles of the Chinese discipline of acupuncture *(see page 90)* and applies pressure to key acupuncture points with the purpose of promoting the smooth flow of energy around the body.

THERAPEUTIC MASSAGE This comforting form of massage consists mostly of soothing strokes and rubbing and is now in wide use in both conventional and unconventional medicine for the relief of pain or physical discomfort. In recent years it has been shown to encourage recovery after a heart attack and to ease the suffering of patients with some types of cancer.

REFLEXOLOGY This is a specialized massage for the hands and feet; it is used for both diagnosing and correcting imbalances in the body *(see pages 52–3)*.

SPORTS MASSAGE This form of therapy features deep tissue massage that aims to ease stiff joints, relax tense muscles, and restore suppleness.

BABY MASSAGE By no means solely used on babies, baby massage relies on specially gentle strokes for promoting general health and happiness.

BIODYNAMIC MASSAGE This therapy combines massage with elements of physical exercise and psychological development *(see box on page 106)*.

HOW TO GIVE A BASIC MASSAGE

Choose a quiet, warm room with subdued lighting. The person who is to receive the massage will need a comfortable but firm surface (like a mattress, futon, or thick blanket) to lie on. Have a soft pillow handy to support the head, and one or more large bathtowels to cover those parts of the body not being massaged.

WHAT CAN MASSAGE TREAT?

Massage is an effective and wide-ranging therapeutic tool that works on a physical and psychological level. Conditions that respond best to massage are

- circulatory disorders
- heart disorders
- high blood pressure
- headaches
- hyperactivity
- insomnia
- back and neck pain

- stress and its related disorders
- anxiety and depression
- physical discomfort and pain in many parts of the musculoskeletal system.

CAUTIONS AND CONTRAINDICATIONS

Massage should not be performed on open wounds, cuts, or sores; sufferers from blood circulation disorders (such as phlebitis, thrombosis, or varicose veins); or on anyone with an abnormally high fever. Massage is not recommended during the early stages (the first trimester) of pregnancy. During the last trimester, however, gentle stroking can help to ease backache and promote relaxation, although it is important to avoid the more vigorous movements.

METHOD Massage should ideally be rhythmic and free-flowing. Different strokes should merge into one another. When giving a full body massage it is often a good idea to start with the face or back, in order to encourage relaxation, before moving on to the arms and legs. You can then include the stomach if desired. But there are no hard and fast rules: even a five-minute shoulder or face massage can be most relaxing.

MASSAGE TECHNIQUES

STROKING (EFFLEURAGE) Slow, stroking movements are the basic elements of all massage. They are usually performed with the hands close together and the thumbs about 1in/2.5cm apart. Long, sweeping movements are warming and relaxing. Brisk movements are invigorating, and stimulate the blood circulation and lymph flow.

KNEADING (PETRISSAGE) Use fingers and thumbs to squeeze and roll the flesh, as if kneading dough. This is ideal for shoulders, hips, and thighs. Kneading stretches and relaxes tense muscles and improves the circulation, so helping to pump nutrients to the tissues and drain away wastes. Light kneading tones up the skin and top layer of muscles; firm kneading has a beneficial effect on the deeper muscles.

FRICTION Small circular movements with the fingers, the pads of the thumbs, or the heel of the hand help to break up the tiny crystals that stick muscle fibers together. Rub firmly and energetically.

PERCUSSION (TAPOTEMENT) Brisk, bouncy hand movements involving chopping, hacking, and slapping motions are stimulating rather than relaxing and should be confined to fleshy, muscular areas such as the thighs and the buttocks. Do not use on bony areas, and never over broken veins. Keep your touch light and springy, the wrists loose and flexible. Use this therapy sparingly, in short, swift bursts. Avoid it altogether if the person massaged is feeling particularly sensitive.

KNUCKLING Curl your hands into loose fists, place the middle section of your fingers against the skin of the person to be massaged and use small circular strokes to create a rippling effect. Use on the shoulders, palms of the hands, and soles of the feet.

PRESSURING Using the pads of the thumbs or forefingers, apply deeper pressure to certain areas, such as around the shoulders or on both sides of the spine. This is ideal for paying persistent attention to very tense knotted muscles in order to encourage them to relax.

BASIC MASSAGE

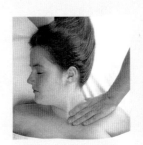

Turn the head to one side, support the head with one hand and stroke with smooth movements to promote relaxation.

Move down the large neck muscle with firm but careful pressure until you feel a tense point. Apply pressure for 15 to 60 seconds.

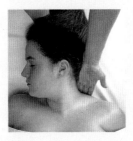

Knead with finger behind the shoulders to relax muscles and release deep contraction. This revitalizes tissue and improves circulation.

SPECIAL NOTE The latest research has shown that massage can be extremely beneficial in enabling people with cancer to relax and feel better. Although it is inadvisable to massage over the actual site of a cancer, gentle massage is acceptable as long as it causes no pain or discomfort *(see pages 140–1.)*

Effleurage on the back relaxes tension and promotes well-being. A thorough back massage lasts about 30 minutes.

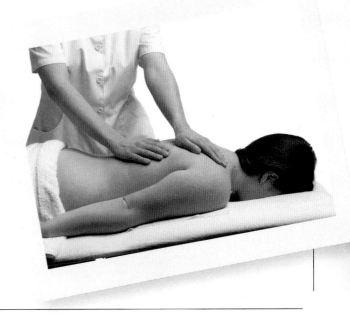

Individual Therapies

Aromatherapy

Aromatherapy is the use of essential oils from plants to enhance general health and appearance. The term was coined by its originator, the French chemist René-Maurice Gattefosse.

Aromatherapy is used for a wide variety of problems, ranging from anxiety and insomnia to acne, cellulite (fatty deposits beneath the skin), and aging skin.

THE BENEFITS OF AROMATHERAPY

Each essential oil has its own characteristic aroma and profile of therapeutic properties. Some oils are soothing and relaxing, others are stimulating and invigorating. Certain fragrances have an effect on a user's mental state: jasmine and neroli may lift depression, marjoram soothes anxiety, and peppermint can enhance mental concentration. But an even greater number of essential oils are physically therapeutic and possess antibacterial, antiseptic, or anti-inflammatory properties. These can be highly effective in relieving the symptoms of such common infections as colds and influenza.

HOW TO USE ESSENTIAL OILS

There are several ways to use essential oils to reap the full benefits of aromatherapy. Choose those oils with the properties that are most suited to the effect desired, and use them either singly or in combinations of no more than two or three at a time.

WHAT CAN AROMATHERAPY TREAT?

Like most complementary therapies, aromatherapy works on the whole body to improve general health and well-being. It is particularly effective for:

- *stress and anxiety-related problems*
- *muscular and rheumatic pains*
- *digestive disorders*
- *women's problems such as PMS, problems associated with the menopause, and postnatal illness*
- *skin conditions.*

On the skin essential oils are highly concentrated: always mix an essential oil with a carrier oil before applying it to the skin. Add one to three drops of essential oil to a teaspoonful of a vegetable oil such as almond, soybean, grapeseed, avocado, or wheat germ oil. Store larger quantities of unused oil in a bottle made of tinted glass and keep in a cool place. Apply the mixture directly onto the skin, rubbing it in gently.

Alternatively, use the aromatherapy oil in place of an ordinary massage oil.

To benefit directly from the aroma of an essential oil, add a few drops to a bowl of steaming hot water and position the bowl near enough for you to be able to inhale the vapor. Inexpensive vaporizers are also available.

Alternatively, place a few drops of essential oil onto a ball of dampened absorbent cotton and put the ball on a hot radiator. Another option is to put a few drops of essential oil into an atomizer of the type used to spray indoor plants (five drops to 1 cup/250ml of water) and spray around the room. This will freshen up stuffy rooms, creating an atmosphere conducive to study or to relaxation at home, or potentially keeping minor infections at bay in an office.

In the bath add five to ten drops of essential oils as the hot water is running. The benefits come from inhaling their vapors as well as absorbing the oils themselves through the skin.

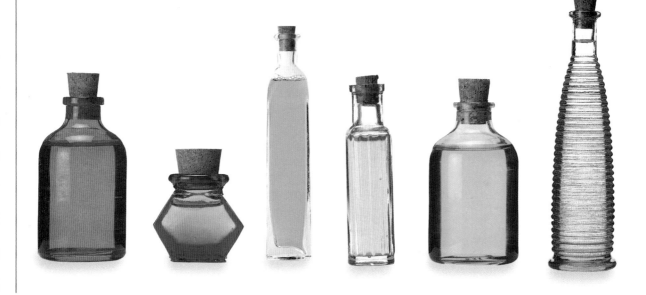

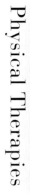

Physical Therapies

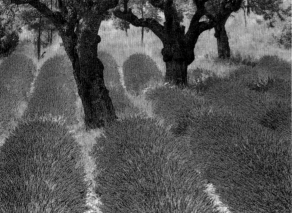

THE TEN MOST USEFUL ESSENTIAL OILS

KEY	OIL	EFFECT	USED FOR
❧	CAMOMILE	Calming	premenstrual tension/pain, indigestion, mildly antiallergic, allergic rhinitis/pollinosis (= hay fever), acne, eczema, and other sensitive skin conditions
❧	EUCALYPTUS	Antiseptic	premenstrual tension/pain, indigestion, mildly antiallergic, allergic rhinitis/pollinosis (= hay fever), acne, eczema, and other sensitive skin conditions
❧	GERANIUM	Mildly astringent	cuts, sores, fungal infections (e.g. athlete's foot), use as insect repellent, soothing skin problems, eczema, bruises, mildly diuretic, fluid retention, antidepressant, feeling run-down
❧	LAVENDER	Mildly analgesic	headache, other aches and pains, wounds, bruises, antiseptic, insect bites, oily skin, acne, swelling, calming insomnia, mild depression
❧	ROSE	Antiseptic	sore throat and sinus, congestion, swollen eyes, puffiness, some blood circulation problems (including broken capillaries), mildly sedative, insomnia, premenstrual tension/pain, antidepressant, menopausal symptoms in women, reduced libido, anorexia nervosa
❧	ROSEMARY	Mild stimulant	physical and mental fatigue, forgetfulness/absentmindedness, respiratory problems (including asthma), soothing rheumatic aches and pains, pain following violent exercise, mildly astringent use for greasy hair
❧	SANDALWOOD	Antiseptic	dry, cracked, or chapped skin, acne, calming relaxation during meditation, aphrodisiac
❧	MARJORAM	Mildly analgesic	menstrual pain, headache, sore throat, mildly sedative, insomnia, warming, improving blood circulation, some fungal infections (such as thrush), acne
❧	JASMINE	Antidepressant	depression, especially postnatal, (reputedly) strengthening contractions during labor, aphrodisiac
❧	NEROLI	Mildly sedative	insomnia, anxiety, nervous depression, mildly warming, improving blood circulation, acne, mildly analgesic, premenstrual tension/pain, backache

❧ **SPECIAL NOTE** Essential oils are obviously highly concentrated: applied directly to the skin they may sting or cause irritation. Before using an essential oil for the first time – especially if there is a personal history of allergic reactivity – a skin test under the supervision of a clinical ecologist or other qualified practitioner is strongly recommended.

You should never swallow essential oils except when directed to do so by a practitioner who is skilled in the internal medical use of oils. In some countries, essential oils that are to be taken internally in this way are available only on prescription from a physician. On the other hand, herbal decoctions and infusions (tisanes and teas) are readily and generally available.

CAUTIONS AND CONTRAINDICATIONS

Aromatherapy should be avoided altogether during a pregnancy with complications. During a normal healthy pregnancy it should be avoided during the first trimester and then used only under the supervision of a qualified aromatherapist. Lavender, geranium, Roman camomile, rose, and ylang-ylang essential oils are safe to use in a normal pregnancy when properly diluted.

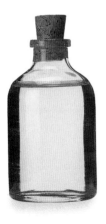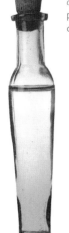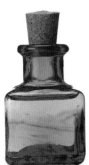

Essential oils have many different properties and can be combined in different ways.

Lavender *Lavandula angustifolia* (above) produces the most versatile of the therapeutic oils.

Reflexology

Reflexology may be described as a specialized form of massage of the feet and – less commonly – of the hands. Performed to detect and correct "imbalances" in the body that may be causing ill-health, it is, however, much more than simply massage.

The therapy has its roots in the practices of the healers of ancient Egypt, Greece, and possibly also of ancient China. Among the pictographs dating from around 2300 B.C. in the tomb of the Egyptian physician Ankhmahar at Saqqara, for instance, is one that portrays two attendants working on the hands and feet of two "patients." Reflexologists also claim that manipulation of the feet for healing purposes was common among the native peoples of both North and South America.

Alternative names for reflexology include reflex zone therapy and zone therapy. There are several variant forms or extensions of the therapy, including Morrel

Reflexology was considered a useful therapy by the ancient Egyptians.

reflexology. Perhaps the most widely divergent among them, however, are the Vacuflex system and the metamorphic technique *(see page 54).*

MODERN THERAPY

Modern reflexology stems mainly from the work early in the 20th century of two Americans, Dr. William Fitzgerald and Eunice Ingham. It was Fitzgerald who first proposed the theory that the body is divided into ten equal zones that extend the length of the body from head to toe, and that stimulation of an area of the foot in one zone affects other parts of the body in the same zone.

This work was continued by Eunice Ingham, who developed a "body-chart" which, she claimed, showed how the entire body was reflected in the soles and sides of both feet. In this way, for example, the big toe is intimately connected to the head, and the ball of the foot reflects the thyroid area *(see diagram below).*

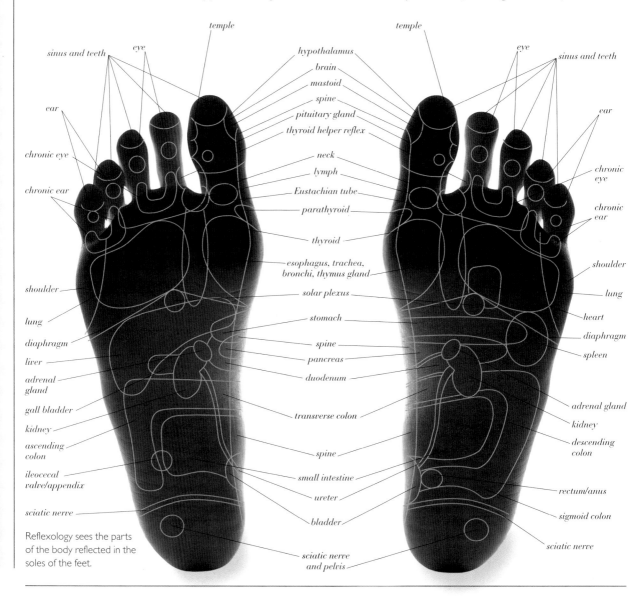

Reflexology sees the parts of the body reflected in the soles of the feet.

HOW TO DO BASIC REFLEXOLOGY

The setting should be peaceful. The therapist takes a case history of past and present health and current lifestyle. The treatment itself as it progresses should reveal any other problems. The therapy can be quite safely and effectively practiced by a nontherapist if a trained professional is not available.

The person who is to receive the therapy should be seated in a comfortable position, barefoot and with the legs supported.

METHOD Clean and dry both feet thoroughly before checking them for corns, calluses, swelling, deformities, and anything else that might be painful to the touch. Relax the feet by stroking them as you talk. Starting with the toes, work down the length of each foot to the heel, including the top and sides. Both feet should be worked on simultaneously. A full reflexology session usually lasts between 45 and 60 minutes. Most therapists agree that for best results a number of treatments are essential, and should take place on a regular weekly or, at most, twice-weekly basis.

SELF-HELP To do reflexology on one's own feet is extremely difficult, but shoes, mats, rollers, and brushes that stimulate the reflexes are widely available as a method of self-help.

While in self-treatment you do not benefit from a transfer of energy from the reflexologist to the person being massaged, it is very useful as preventive therapy and in times of emergency.

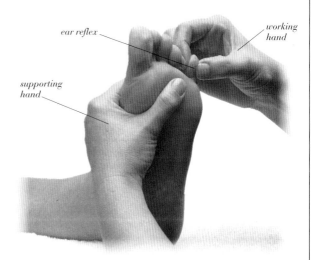

ear reflex   *working hand*

supporting hand

The reflexologist supports the foot in a firm but gentle grip while stimulating the reflexes of the foot; here the ear reflex on the fifth toe is gently worked while the patient relaxes.

ELEMENTS OF THERAPY

APPLYING PRESSURE Therapists use a variety of ways to put pressure on the reflex points, including rubbing, rotating, and caterpillarlike movements, but all usually begin with firm but quite gentle stroking movements over the entire feet. In the West, fingers and thumbs are used, whereas Oriental practitioners tend to use sharpened sticks or similar objects. In Vacuflex (*see page 54*), a vacuum pump and pads are used.

EFFECTS The person being treated will experience a variety of sensations as different areas of the feet are worked on. Any feeling of pain or discomfort when a "congested" area is being treated is usually brief and soon goes, leaving a feeling of release that can often be felt almost at once. Most people report a feeling of lightness and relaxation, with renewed energy, immediately after a session of treatment. This may occasionally be followed by further reactions – known technically as cleansing reactions – as the treatment takes effect: they may include headaches, a running nose, a mild rash on the skin, and a strong urge to urinate.

WHAT CAN REFLEXOLOGY TREAT?

Reflexology is a good all-round therapy for people of any age. It is, however, most useful for conditions such as:

- digestive problems
- menstrual irregularities
- stress and stress-related disorders
- fatigue
- aches and pains
- inflammatory skin conditions
- pregnancy problems
- chronic conditions affecting the elderly and children, such as dementia in the elderly, and glue ear and colic in children.

CAUTIONS AND CONTRAINDICATIONS

In her famous book *Stories the Feet Can Tell*, Eunice Ingham suggested that the only condition for which reflexology should not be used is thrombosis (blood-clotting within the veins). Other opinions vary: some reflexologists see the therapy solely as a means of preventing diseases and disorders before they occur; others insist that it is a highly effective way to treat a wide variety of existing conditions.

Though apparently effective, little definitive scientific research has so far been carried out into the therapy.

Vacuflex and the Metamorphic Technique

The Vacuflex Reflexology System (known as VRS) was devised and developed during the 1970s by Inge Dougans, a Danish reflexologist who came to believe that reflexology achieved its effects by means of treating the "energy meridians" defined by Oriental medicine systems rather than Fitzgerald's carefully defined "zones."

ELEMENTS OF THERAPY

The system has provided a way of stimulating all the reflex areas at the same time at the beginning of each session. Special Vacuflex "boots" are worn for the first stage of treatment, inside which a vacuum is created. This allows the reflexologist to identify congested areas, which are then treated by a special vacuum method.

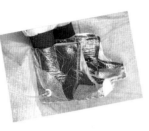

Vacuflex boots create a vacuum around the feet to squeeze the feet and stimulate the reflexes.

METAMORPHIC TECHNIQUE

The metamorphic technique was devised in the 1960s by British reflexologist Robert St. John, who at first called it "prenatal therapy."

Practitioners of the technique believe that disease and ill-health can often be traced back to problems before birth. By stimulating different reflex points – especially on the feet, but also on the hands and head – energies "blocked" during the nine-month prenatal period can be encouraged to unblock, and so allow the body's natural self-healing processes to function fully once again.

According to followers of the system, the vertical outline of reflex points in the foot corresponds to the vertical length of the head and the spine, seen from one side. But problems also run in a sequence from the head to the base of the spine (and thus also from toe to heel) according to the moment during the prenatal period at which each event happened.

Little scientific research has been carried out to date to verify or support these theories. Good results have nonetheless been reported in a number of conditions.

❧ **FIRST STAGE** Special boots made of felt are fitted around the feet, and the air inside is withdrawn by a vacuum pump. This squeezes the feet firmly so that all the reflexes of the feet are stimulated at the same time. The pressure is adjusted for each individual. After about five minutes, the therapist removes the boots and quickly examines and notes the resulting areas of discoloration on the feet on the principle that they reveal areas of "congestion" and ill-health in the body. The marks generally remain visible for only 20 to 30 seconds. The progress of treatment is said to be evident in the change of the depth or area of discoloration at each session.

❧ **SECOND STAGE** The therapist then places silicon pads of different sizes and in different combinations on specific reflex points along the "meridians" or "energy pathways" on the feet, legs, hands, and arms. The pads stay in place by gentle suction. Although they remain on for only a few seconds, it is said to be long enough to stimulate the reflex points into activity.

Vacuflex therapists claim that through wide use in a number of countries this has been shown to be highly effective in treating an extensive range of disorders.

When the boots are removed the skin on the soles of the feet shows up in different colors, indicating areas of congestion, for about half a minute, so diagnosis has to be done quickly.

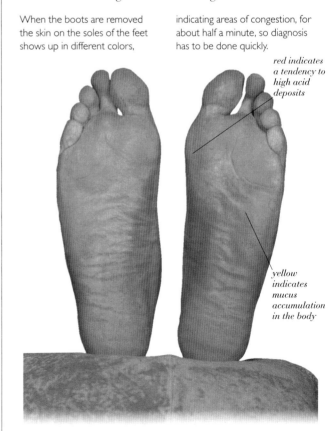

red indicates a tendency to high acid deposits

yellow indicates mucus accumulation in the body

Polarity Therapy

Polarity therapy was developed over the course of 50 years by Dr. Randolph Stone (1890–1983), an Austrian-born naturopath, chiropractor, and osteopath, who also took an interest in the theories and practice of Oriental medicine and in spirituality.

Polarity therapy is a holistic system of healing, based on Stone's belief that humans are predominantly spiritual beings whose health and happiness depend upon the free flow of energy within their bodies.

ELEMENTS OF THERAPY

The therapy is based on Ayurvedic principles. Energy steps down from the Source (the origin of all energy) in the form of a double helix. Within the body, where the helix crosses over itself, a spinning energy center is formed and is known as a "chakra." Each chakra has a different elemental quality: ether (throat – mid-cervical spine); air (mid-thoracic spine); fire (mid-lumbar spine, just behind the solar plexus); water (lumbosacral junction – small of the back); and earth (near the end of the tailbone, just behind the rectum). It is a holistic therapy and works on physical, emotional, and mental levels.

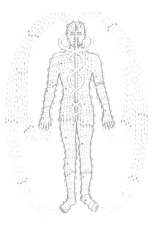

Polarity therapy is based on the concept of the energy flow between the five energy centers or chakras in the body.

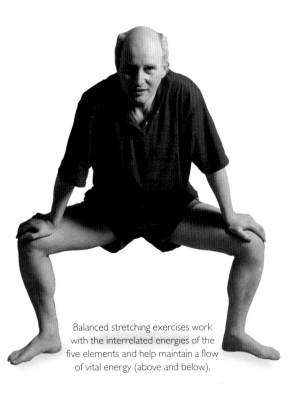

Balanced stretching exercises work with the interrelated energies of the five elements and help maintain a flow of vital energy (above and below).

There are four aspects of Polarity therapy: therapeutic bodywork, using three levels of touch; awareness/ counseling skills; health building and/ or cleansing diets and procedures; and there are also gentle polarity stretching exercises. Clients take responsibility for their own health.

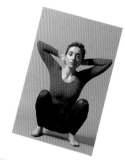

WHAT CAN POLARITY THERAPY TREAT?

Polarity therapy is not designed to treat specific symptoms, but to encourage healing and good health through the release of energy. It can, however, have a dramatic effect on overall health. The following conditions are examples which may respond to treatment:

- allergies
- back pain
- respiratory disorders
- ME
- migraine
- headache
- cardiovascular problems
- digestive disorders
- postnatal problems and issues arising perinatally
- both emotional and mental issues
- stress and stress-related illnesses.

ZERO BALANCING

Dr. Fritz Smith, an American acupuncturist, osteopath, and physician, developed zero balancing (ZB) in 1975, by combining Oriental and Western practices in the field of healthcare. Zero balancing attempts to achieve a balance between body energy and the musculoskeletal structure using finger pressure and sustained stretching exercises to release tension that has accumulated deep in the body. Creating a sense of stillness, it is said to be effective in the relief of stress, pain, and emotional difficulties.

CAUTIONS AND CONTRAINDICATIONS

There are no known contraindications to Polarity therapy and zero balancing if they are undertaken by a registered professional. Consult your physician before seeking treatment.

Individual Therapies

BALANCE AND MOVEMENT •Western Forms

CIVILIZATIONS throughout history and all over the world have known that the way we use or misuse our bodies affects our health. The link between habits and health has been taken for granted longest in Oriental countries, in which a wide range of methods to keep the body supple and strong has been established for hundreds of years. In the West it is really only since the early 20th century that a variety of techniques as wide-ranging as those in the East has developed.

At the same time we are all too aware that many of our aches and pains result from bad habits of posture and movement, contributing to a losing battle against gravity, and we may also suspect that it cannot be natural for our bodies (and minds) to become stiffer and more inflexible as we age.

Feldenkrais

Moshe Feldenkrais, who died aged 80 in 1984, was an engineer and physicist who worked on France's early atomic research program and on the British antisubmarine project during World War II. But it was the martial arts, and the body mechanics involved in them, that most fascinated him.

The recurrence of an old knee injury set him off on the research that was to be his life's work. Like Matthias Alexander, in healing himself he invented a method that not only helps treat people with serious physical problems (most notably, spasticity) but is also increasingly used by musicians, dancers, and sportspeople to improve their awareness and performance.

WHAT CAN FELDENKRAIS TREAT?

The gentle exercises are designed to improve posture, and through that many health problems may be resolved. In particular, Feldenkrais may be useful for:

- *victims of stroke and other conditions where there is a loss of control of movement*
- *people with spinal disorders*
- *people with musculoskeletal pain and injuries*
- *arthritis*
- *chronic pain.*

ELEMENTS OF THERAPY

FUNCTIONAL INTEGRATION This is the one-on-one application of the Feldenkrais method by a trained practitioner, usually in 45- to 60-minute sessions. The practitioner uses gentle manipulation and movements to encourage the body into new, easier ways of moving. In Feldenkrais terms, this feeds information directly into the nervous system with the result that the body effectively reprograms the brain.

AWARENESS THROUGH MOVEMENT In contrast to the comparatively passive approach of functional integration, awareness through movement is taught in group classes and comprises a series of directed movements for students to follow actively. It is not conventional exercise, however, because the object is for each student to stay attentive and tune in to precisely what the body is doing. Movements may be very slight, perhaps only lifting one foot a fraction off the floor. But even this may quickly bring a realization of unnecessary muscle tension, release from which can lead to a state of profound relaxation.

> **CAUTIONS AND CONTRAINDICATIONS**
>
> There are no known contraindications to the Feldenkrais method, although it is recommended that you consult your physician before undergoing treatment.

Feldenkrais teacher

functional integration movement

rollers to support body

One of the many possible maneuvers used in a functional integration lesson. The student comes to learn how to release chronic tension in muscles and how to move with more coordination.

The Alexander Technique

Probably the most widely known Western system of movement therapy, the Alexander Technique is a method of bringing the way we move under our conscious direction and avoiding a buildup of muscular tension.

F. Matthias Alexander, who was born in Tasmania in 1869, developed his theories in an effort to save his career when his voice began to be afflicted with such hoarseness that he had to cancel some of his performances as a reciter/actor. Noticing that when he began to recite in public he tended to contract muscles in his head and neck that apparently had little or nothing to do with his voice, he began by experimenting on himself. At first, inhibiting the muscular contractions proved almost impossible to achieve. However after ten years of research, practice, and study he had not only improved his voice, his breath control, his posture, and his acting "presence" but had derived an effective, non-verbal, hands-on technique that has been transforming people ever since.

Alexander's clientele rapidly expanded outside the theater to include famous scientists and physicians. In 1937, 19 doctors signed a letter published in the foremost British medical journal, the *Lancet*, calling on the profession to recognize that it was only possible for medical diagnoses to be complete if they took into account Alexander's idea that the way patients used their bodies affected how well or badly they functioned.

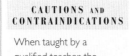

CAUTIONS AND CONTRAINDICATIONS

When taught by a qualified teacher, the Alexander Technique is safe for everyone, although it is recommended that you consult your physician before taking classes.

ELEMENTS OF THERAPY

❧ IDEOLOGICAL BASIS

Alexander said that if we constantly move in a way that we eventually discover is wrong and harmful, we should not try immediately to take some sort of opposing "corrective" action, and thereby possibly add insult to injury; instead we should find a way to STOP doing it wrongly and harmfully.

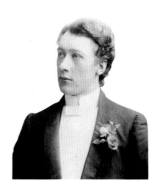

F. Matthias Alexander (1869–1955), founder of the Alexander Technique.

❧ METHODOLOGICAL BASIS

Alexander's basic discovery was what he called the "Primary Control Mechanism." When the head, neck, and spine are in a properly balanced relationship, so-called "antigravity reflexes" spring into play. A Tufts University group led by Professor Frank Pierce Jones developed what were then new photographic techniques to confirm the physical basis of Alexander's claim.

❧ METHOD

That the technique relies on hands-on guidance is fundamental. Alexander noticed early on in his experiments how difficult it is for us all to break bad postural habits – they are so deeply ingrained that the easiest and most balanced way of, say, standing up, may well actually feel "wrong" when first we are encouraged to do it. In a session that lasts between 30 and 60 minutes, an Alexander teacher uses hands to guide you as you repeat a simple task such as sitting down in a chair and standing up again.

WHAT CAN THE ALEXANDER TECHNIQUE TREAT?

The Alexander Technique does not set out to cure specific illnesses; however, many conditions are resolved through practice. In particular, the following appear to respond to the Technique:

❧ stress and stress-related disorders

❧ fatigue

❧ insomnia

❧ anxiety

❧ breathing disorders

❧ neck, back, and joint pain

❧ circulatory disorders

❧ anxiety and depression

❧ chronic muscle tension

❧ digestive disorders.

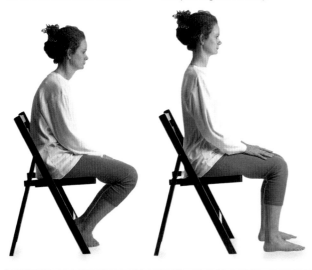

Before Alexander teaching, the body is out of balance, with curved shoulders, and feet not resting on the ground. After teaching, the body is in balance, the spine aligned correctly.

Hellerwork

Hellerwork is based on the bodywork methods of Ida Rolf *(see Rolfing, page 46)*, adding the elements of manipulation and movement coaching using video feedback. It also specifically involves dialogue between client and practitioner to explore the mind–body connection.

Designed to realign and balance the body systematically, therapy thus normally consists of a series of 11 sessions of deep-tissue bodywork and movement "education." Each session lasts for 90 minutes. Hellerwork practitioners claim that the method can relieve aches and pains, improve posture, dissipate tension, increase relaxation, extend overall flexibility and sporting ability, and enhance body awareness.

WHAT CAN HELLERWORK AND THE TRAGER APPROACH TREAT?

Hellerwork aims to prevent rather than treat health conditions by balancing the mind and body. Many conditions do, however, respond to regular treatment, including

- headaches
- aches and pains in the musculoskeletal system
- stress and related disorders.

The Trager approach is slightly more wide-ranging in its effect and can be used to treat

- problems affecting mobility
- musculoskeletal disorders
- neurological disorders, including sciatica
- asthma
- headaches and migraine
- high blood pressure.

CAUTIONS AND CONTRAINDICATIONS

Hellerwork and the Trager approach are suitable for most people, since the therapy is easily adaptable. However, it is not recommended in some types of cancer, where the manipulation may encourage the spread of the disease.

The Trager Approach

Trager psychophysical integration was created by Chicago physician Dr. Milton Trager to help victims of polio and other neuromuscular disorders. Having suffered as a weak teenager with a congenital back problem, Dr. Trager healed himself and thereafter spent 50 years developing and refining his system of movement reeducation before beginning to instruct and certify practitioners.

ELEMENTS OF THERAPY

The method is based on Dr. Trager's conviction that the body and mind are inextricable. The client is encouraged to relax deeply, to let go of conscious muscular control and allow the unconscious mind to choose the freer, less restrictive body movements demonstrated by the practitioner.

A typical Trager session lasts between 60 and 90 minutes. The client lies passively on a flat surface (the "table") and is gently but rhythmically manipulated to promote real flexibility of limb motion. Movements are carefully adapted to the individual client so that tension may be released without discomfort.

The method is especially suitable for people in pain – particularly back pain – and those with severe restriction of movement. Mobility may increase dramatically, even in one session.

Each session also includes instruction in Trager Mentastics, a form of light, mind-directed movements intended to keep the body open and pain-free. Clients can practice mentastics on their own as homework between sessions.

The Trager approach involves gentle bouncing movements to help release tension from the shoulders.

Trager logo "dancing cloud"

the relief of tension

Eastern Traditions

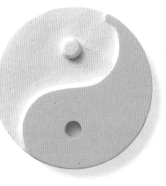

The yin/yang symbol is a perfect representation of the concept of balance in all aspects of life.

DRAWING on ancient traditions said to go back at least 3,000 years, Oriental movement and balance therapies aim to affect the flow of life energy, or chi. They encourage sensitivity and flexibility in the body while at the same time utilizing breath control and an inner focus to free up energy blockages and increase energy levels. T'ai chi and chi kung, for example, are practiced on a daily basis by hundreds of millions of people in China, where they also form part of normal hospital therapy.

WHAT CAN CHI KUNG TREAT?

Chi kung works to encourage the flow of energy within the body, placing emphasis on learning to feel and move it through gentle drills. A number of conditions respond to chi kung, including

- *chronic health problems, particularly those involving the immune system*
- *sexual problems (i.e. premature ejaculation)*
- *stress and stress-related disorders*
- *conditions exacerbated or caused by aging.*

Chi Kung

An ancient Chinese system for the development of internal energy, chi kung or qi gung (pronounced "chee goong") is, like t'ai chi *(see page 60)*, based on the principles of the Taoist religion as extended to Oriental medicine.

Unlike yoga *(see pages 61–5)*, chi kung puts less emphasis on stretching movements and postures, and more on learning how to feel and move energy inside the body. Some of the basic chi kung drills involve standing still for anything from minutes to hours at a time, sensing the movement of energy in the body.

Other chi kung exercises involve gentle, rhythmic swinging or stretching movements to generate and conserve energy, not to burn calories. The chi kung practitioner aims to avoid stress on joints and muscles and directs his or her awareness inside the body rather than concentrating on building up what the Chinese refer to as "external" strength in the form of tight, well-developed muscles.

As a result, chi kung practice develops enormous inner power in a pliable, flexible, relaxed body. An experienced practitioner can use the therapy not only for healing but also in a preventive capacity. Chi kung is one of the most effective of all Oriental methods for combating stress and is also becoming highly popular as a method of enhancing and managing sexual potential. Taoist "secrets" of how to conserve sexual energy are now receiving serious attention as an important part of resistance to the aging process.

The main difficulty with chi kung lies in finding a teacher who really knows how to develop internal chi power in students.

CAUTIONS AND CONTRAINDICATIONS

There are no known contraindications to chi kung, although it is advised that you consult your physician before taking classes.

internal chi power developed

Although chi kung involves physical activity, its aim is to develop and conserve the internal energy and integrate body and mind.

T'ai Chi Chuan

T'ai chi chuan, also known as t'ai chi, is an old Chinese system designed to develop chi within the body. It can be used to rejuvenate, to heal and prevent illness and injuries, and also to lead to spiritual enlightenment. Furthermore, t'ai chi's flowing, gentle movements can provide the basis of a devastating martial art.

T'ai chi seems to have developed from traditional chi kung practices a few centuries ago and is now one of the most popular Oriental movement arts in the West. Students learn a basic form or sequence of movements. A short form may take around 5 minutes to complete, a long form around 30 minutes or more. Although precision in the movements is important and breathing must be synchronized, t'ai chi is ultimately a moving form of meditation in which the practitioner "flows with" the direction of the energy in and around the body.

One stage of the classic t'ai chi sequence called the Five Elements.

WHAT CAN T'AI CHI TREAT?

T'ai chi can help with most stress-related problems and can also encourage healing and rehabilitation following injury, surgery, or serious illness such as heart attack or stroke. Other conditions that respond to regular practice include

- anxiety and depression
- muscular tension
- chronic ill-health
- high and low blood pressure and other circulation problems
- spinal problems and bone conditions.

Another part of the Five Elements sequence represents a strong tree moving in the wind.

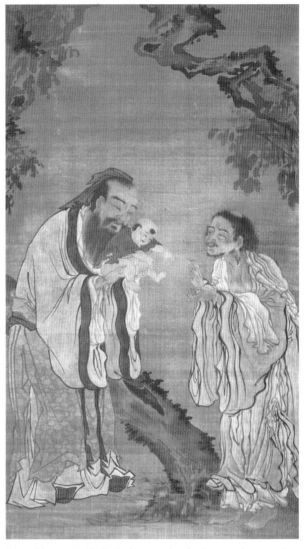

Prince Sakyamuni with Confucius and Lao Tzu, the founder of Taoism. Both t'ai chi and chi kung are based on the Taoist principles of perfect harmony between the yin and yang energies of the body and the smooth flow of the life force known as chi.

Like chi kung, t'ai chi is a "soft" internal art and results in a buildup of inner power within a flexible and responsive body. It develops balance, control, and an efficient posture. No straining or "external" (muscular) strength is required – yet old t'ai chi masters routinely defeat younger martial arts experts who have trained exclusively in "external" forms of karate and kung-fu.

Conventional medical examinations of t'ai chi students in China have proved that it has beneficial effects similar to those of Western aerobic exercise but without the stresses and strains. It is also renowned for its relaxing and calming effects, recommended particularly to relieve high blood pressure, anxiety, insomnia, and other stress-related conditions.

CAUTIONS AND CONTRAINDICATIONS

T'ai chi is perfectly safe for people of all ages and level of fitness, although it is advised that you consult your physician before taking classes.

Yoga

Nobody knows for sure how old yoga is, but recent archeological evidence suggests it may be as much as 5,000 years old. Many ancient statues show people in yoga postures, apparently meditating, which emphasizes that what we in the West think of as yoga is only one part of an entire philosophical system of which the ultimate aim is enlightenment – oneness with the Supreme Being or, in more modern terms maybe, achieving and maintaining a state of peace and happiness.

Medically and scientifically proven at the physical and mental level, yoga can be successfully used as therapy by people who suffer from backache, arthritis, or rheumatism – in fact, yoga postures can help just about every physical ailment known to date. As a means of encouraging relaxation, normalizing high blood pressure, helping stave off anxiety, or dealing with stress, yoga is as effective today as it was thousands of years ago.

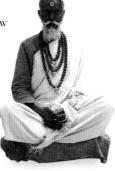

The perfect calm of a yogi in a typical pose.

WHAT CAN YOGA TREAT?

Yoga aims to improve overall health and well-being, and through that, a number of conditions may be resolved. Most of the following will respond to regular practice:

- *stress and stress-related disorders*
- *high blood pressure and circulatory problems*
- *back and neck pain*
- *asthma and other chronic illness*
- *digestive disorders, including irritable bowel syndrome*
- *fatigue and insomnia*
- *arthritis and rheumatism*
- *anxiety and depression.*

CAUTIONS AND CONTRAINDICATIONS

Yoga techniques should not be practiced by anybody who has real difficulty bending the back, especially if this results from spinal injury. Sufferers of high blood pressure, diabetes, hernias, and those with a history of ophthalmic problems should seek medical advice before taking up yoga. Certain postures should be carefully adapted for pregnant women.

clear, relaxed mind

The full lotus position (padmasana), is the classic position for meditation. It lengthens the spine, allowing you to control breathing. The mind is better able to focus and concentrate on problems or empty itself of worry.

controlled breathing

loose hip and knee joints

thumb and first finger closed together to "lock in" energy, allowing it to circulate freely around the body

Forms of Yoga

Traditionally there are many forms of yoga. The best-known traditional forms, such as Hatha, Raja, Ashtanga, Kundalini, and Tantra, have been adapted, and in some cases mixed-and-matched, by such great modern masters (yogis) as Iyengar, Sivananda, and Jois.

HATHA YOGA Now usually understood to be the form that emphasizes physical positions or postures (or asanas) and breath-control techniques (or pranayama).

RAJA YOGA Now regarded as primarily involving meditation, being based on the mental aspects of yoga rather than on the physical asanas.

ASHTANGA YOGA Combines elements of Hatha and Raja. The basis of the practice is the linking of strenuous Hatha positions and

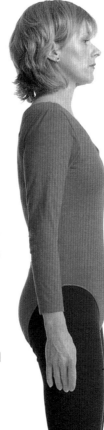

1 This is the cat posture, chakravakasana, which increases spinal flexibility. Kneel up with back straight, arms by your side and look forward.

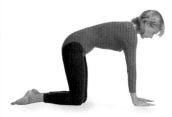

2 Bend forward, placing hands flat on the floor, keeping the spine straight and the body square.

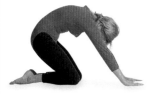

3 Round the spine, moving the legs at an angle by pushing the spine up and the buttocks down.

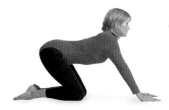

postures into a flowing, almost continuous movement while using the mind to affect breath control, periodically divided by a number of physical "locks."

KUNDALINI YOGA Traditionally referred to as the "coiled serpent" at the base of the spine. Some Kundalini practitioners concentrate on "raising the Kundalini" – a process of awakening this dormant subtle energy so that it moves up the spine to the head, activating major energy centers (chakras) as it does so, and ultimately causing changes in consciousness.

TANTRIC YOGA Based on texts that emphasize the importance of awakening the Kundalini force and that give detailed descriptions of the body's subtle energy centers. One part of Tantric yoga seeks to use sexual pleasure, awakened and sustained through ritualized intercourse, as a means of heightening awareness. But classic Tantra also includes the asanas and pranayama of Hatha yoga.

The different styles of yoga suit different temperaments and physical capabilities. Ashtanga yoga, for example, has a reputation as the most physically demanding. Some yogic teachers recognize this by "prescribing" individual programs of asanas for their students and altering them as the students progress.

round spine as far as is comfortable

use hands for support only, not to push your spine up or down

4 Bring your buttocks up and spine down. Keep legs and hands as position 3.

5 Now push your spine up into the arched position once more.

6 Repeat exercise up to six times, ensuring that the spine is stretched as fully as possible.

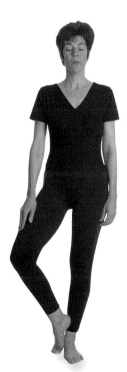

1 This is the tree pose, vrksasana. Start with your arms by your side, bend one leg, and rest the toes of the bent leg on the heel of the straight one.

YOGA AS THERAPY

When yoga is used as therapy, certain positions and postures may be recommended to speed healing or recovery from illness or injury, based not only on traditional wisdom but on the modern medical and scientific research that confirms yoga's benefits. In this way, yoga – like chi kung and t'ai chi – is accessible to all ages and all levels of fitness, and likewise noncompetitive.

The asanas have profound effects on the body and work progressively at many levels. As the muscles are toned up, the spine returns to a natural alignment and the inner organs are revitalized. Breathing and breath control are used as a bridge between body and mind. Positions and postures that at first are just awkward to get into are held longer and longer – a process intended to redirect the flow within blood and lymph vessels, alternately flushing and emptying. This has the effect of giving the internal organs a healthy massage.

The pranayama are yoga's equivalent of chi kung. They promote an ability to focus and control the flow of life energy in the body. And, on a purely physical level, they have beneficial effects on the heart and lungs.

hands in prayer position

other leg as high as possible

balance on one leg

2 Bring the foot of the bent leg farther up the straight leg. Keep arms by your sides, but support the bent leg if necessary.

3 When you feel balanced, bring your hands into a praying position in front of you.

4 This is the ideal position. Bring the foot of the bent leg as far up the straight leg as possible and raise the arms, with the flats of the hands together, above your head.

You can stop this exercise at any stage and practice until you have learned to balance well enough to go on.

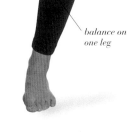

Yoga for the Beginner

Beginners generally start with a set series of postures that can be repeated many times. A famous example is the series of 12 movements known as the Salute to the Sun, in which the final five postures represent the first five in reverse order, so ending once more at the beginning.

From such relatively simple exercises, practitioners may progress to more complicated asanas that involve twists and stronger stretches. Two exercises are shown here. One combines the seated forward bend and the head-knee posture. The other is the half spinal twist.

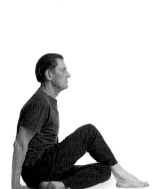

This is an exercise to twist the spine and increase its mobility. It is called ardha matsyendrasana, the half spinal twist. This is a progressive sequence; you can stop at any stage and practice until you feel confident.

1 Keep one leg as straight as possible on the floor and place the other leg over it with the foot flat on the floor as far as is comfortable. Keep the spine straight. Repeat on both sides.

This is a seated forward bend, dandasana, moving into the head-knee posture, janu sirsasana.

1 Start by sitting in a dandasana pose with legs straight, hands by the side of your hips. Keep the back straight.

2 Bring the bent leg underneath you, keeping the other straight. Keep the spine straight. Repeat on the other side.

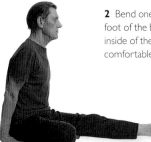

2 Bend one knee so that the foot of the bent leg touches the inside of the straight one at a comfortable position.

3 Use your hand behind you to help balance before you twist. Some people have to work toward this stage.

3 Stretch both arms above the head in this position. This is the start of the janu sirsasana.

flexible spine

4 Twist the torso from hips upward – spine, stomach, shoulders, head – using hands to balance. Reverse the process to work on the other side of the body.

better breathing

mobile joints

4 Bend over into the forward bend position as far as you are able. Repeat the exercise on the other side. The aim is to get your head on to your legs. You may need to bend your knees but aim to keep them straight.

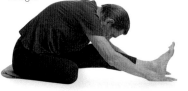

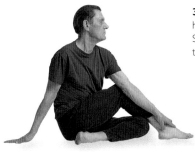

Themes and Variations

There are hundreds of other yoga postures, all of which have a therapeutic effect. Two are shown here. The warrior posture is considered one of the most auspicious asanas; there are several versions of it. It strengthens the legs and hips, firms the muscles of the back and chest, and tones the nervous system. The other posture shown here is the shoulderstand, also known as the complete posture or the candle posture.

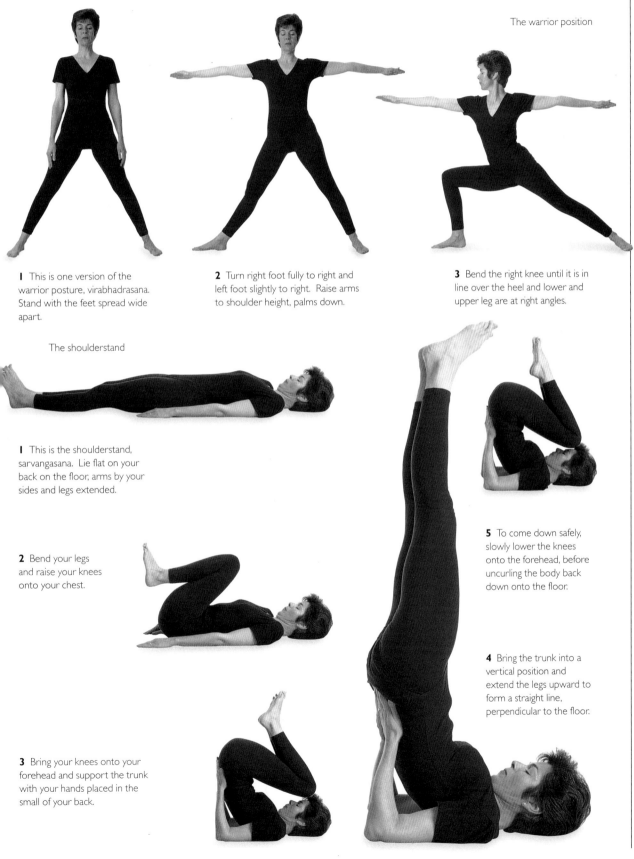

The warrior position

1 This is one version of the warrior posture, virabhadrasana. Stand with the feet spread wide apart.

2 Turn right foot fully to right and left foot slightly to right. Raise arms to shoulder height, palms down.

3 Bend the right knee until it is in line over the heel and lower and upper leg are at right angles.

The shoulderstand

1 This is the shoulderstand, sarvangasana. Lie flat on your back on the floor, arms by your sides and legs extended.

2 Bend your legs and raise your knees onto your chest.

3 Bring your knees onto your forehead and support the trunk with your hands placed in the small of your back.

4 Bring the trunk into a vertical position and extend the legs upward to form a straight line, perpendicular to the floor.

5 To come down safely, slowly lower the knees onto the forehead, before uncurling the body back down onto the floor.

Plant, Food, and Mineral Therapies • Herbalis

Californian poppy
*Eschscholzia
california.*

THERAPIES involving plants, foods, and nutritional elements are some of the oldest and perhaps easiest to understand of all the therapies available to us. Over the last decades, we in the West have been encouraged to believe in "a pill for all ills," and we take comfort in medical treatment that can be taken orally and that appears to be prescribed in a conventional manner.

Almost every culture has a history of herbalism, each depending on the local flora or vegetation to nourish and to heal. Herbalists were, in the past, dealers and collectors of herbs; we refer to them as herbal therapists or medicinal herbalists, to make clear the distinction. Much of modern medicine is based upon early herbal practices; indeed, most conventional drugs contain synthesized extracts and essences of herbs and plants. The active constituents of many ancient natural remedies are the key ingredients of many proprietary drugs. The tradition of herbalism is best established in North America and the Far East, and it was these cultures that encouraged the development of our modern-day herbal medicine.

▲§ **PLANT ESSENCES** Herbalism and aromatherapy and homeopathy use the pure essences of plants to treat illness and disease, and find that this prevents side effects and provides a more effective form of treatment.

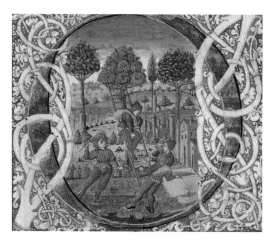

A page from a manuscript by Pliny the Elder (c. A.D. 23–79), the Roman scientist and historian, who wrote a treatise on the nature of plants and was regarded as an authority by medieval herbalists.

Each of these disciplines uses different types of plant in different forms, and, therefore, the technical terminology within herbalism and the plant- and food-based therapies varies widely; for example, homeopathic remedies include a dilution quotient, and herbal remedies and aromatherapy use the Latin taxonomic term for the plant, with or without additional descriptions. Herbalism may sound complicated, but everyone can grow herbs and experience the profound effect they have on the body.

▲§ **FOOD AND NUTRITION** Food and nutrition are fundamental to all life, and the therapies that have evolved around the implementation of diet and the elements of nutrition to address health problems are correspondingly essential to most kinds of treatment – conventional or complementary. Diet has always played an important role, both spiritually (diets for religious purposes) and physiologically (diets for medical purposes), and as an understanding of nutrition has evolved, that role has become more defined. Nutritional therapy focuses on tailoring diet to the person, examining the individual condition and treating accordingly. Through it, diet has become more than the sum of its parts; it has become a tool for living.

Finally, the wide-ranging and holistic disciplines of homeopathy and flower and plant essences have become more popular than ever, promoting good health and well-being by gently encouraging the body's own life force in order that it may heal itself. All flower and tree remedies are based on herbal sources, as are many homeopathic medicines.

The power of plants and their extracts is only just beginning to be understood and recognized; their interaction with the human body provides scope for some of the most exciting developments in modern medicine.

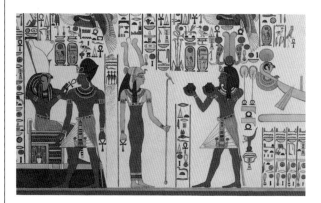

The Egyptians used herbs in medicine, and many friezes depict the manufacture and use of herbal remedies.

Berberry *Berberis vulgaris*, an excellent herbal remedy for a malfunctioning liver.

Herbal Medicine • 1

Herbal medicine is one of the most ancient forms of remedial treatment, evolving with humanity, as we learned through trial and error, and by watching animals. Almost every major culture has at one time used herbs as its main or only source of medicine.

As long ago as 3000 B.C. the ancient Egyptians compiled lists of herbs and their properties. Later, the ancient Greeks followed suit. It was the Romans who brought herbs to northern Europe, and there herbalism was nurtured and molded by other cultural influences, including the Arabs, who invaded the Iberian Peninsula.

In the Middle Ages, herbal lore was often created around superstition, but underlying this was a basic comprehension of the body and the effects that different herbs had upon it. When the reasons why herbs worked on a medical basis were unclear, a philosophy or didactic myth would be woven to explain them. It was believed that people tended to embody one of four dispositions associated with bodily humors, being either cheerful, sluggish, hot tempered, or gloomy, depending on which of the humors predominated. Herbs were thought to possess their own characteristic temperaments, and were therefore prescribed according to their individual characteristics to correct imbalances. There was also a belief that each part of the body was governed by one sign of the zodiac, and each herb by one of the known planets.

Others believed in the Doctrine of Signatures, which held that any herb showing a physical similarity in shape or coloration to the symptoms of a disease could be used

Elderflower *Sambucus nigra* is used to treat colds, flu, hay fever, and sinusitis.

to effect a cure for that disease. When based on this ideology, prescribing became a complex business, but this was later simplified slightly by the advent of the printing industry. Herbals outlining these elaborate theories could be purchased, studied, and exchanged, and the practice of herbalism flourished, coexisting alongside developing orthodox medicine for centuries. However, as modern drug- and surgery-based medicine became more established, the use of herbs became nearly extinct.

Pharmaceutical companies have encouraged the belief that their drugs containing synthesized plant ingredients were somehow more effective than plants themselves. While eagerly examining the enormous potential of medical botany, the pharmaceutical industry actively campaigned against herbalism – going to great lengths to find a toxic element in many herbs that would, in suitable quantities, be entirely harmless.

The growing concern about the side effects of drugs has meant that herbalism has been called upon once more to provide natural medicines. In particular, pregnant women, children, people with chronic conditions that have refused to be shifted by conventional medicine, and those with immunosuppressed conditions have had successful and safe treatment without the use of toxic drugs. As research into the active constituents of herbs continues, increasing numbers of ancient treatments and tonics are becoming recognized once more and brought back into widespread use.

Bladderwrack *Fucus vesiculosus*, or kelp helps problems presented by underactive thyroid glands.

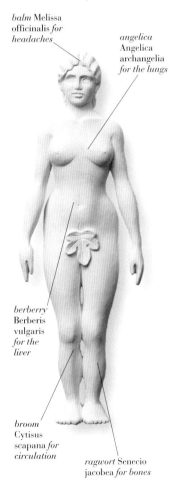

balm Melissa officinalis *for headaches*

angelica Angelica archangelia *for the lungs*

berberry Berberis vulgaris *for the liver*

broom Cytisus scapana *for circulation*

ragwort Senecio jacobea *for bones*

There is almost no part of the body that herbs cannot help to heal.

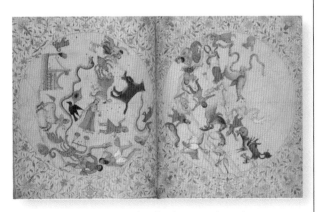

Herbs were once assigned a planetary ruler and were associated with particular signs of the zodiac.

Herbal Medicine • 2

In 19th-century North America, a form of herbalism currently known as physiomedicalism (intended to refer to the study of healing through the use of organic substances) became the basis for therapeutic herbalism, as we know it in the United States today. This had strong elements of traditional Native American plant knowledge and rural settlers' folklore remedies. In Europe, herbalism struggled to become reestablished on scientific grounds and remained more closely linked to plants. This form of herbalism is more correctly called "phytotherapy." In France today all phytotherapists are qualified physicians, although herbal therapists elsewhere in Europe may have no such qualifications.

The Chinese, Japanese, Indian, and Native (North and South) American cultures all have traditional systems of herbal medicine. In China and Japan the use of herbal remedies is officially promoted by a government ministry and included in national health systems. In India, herbalism is part of the ancient but still widely used system of Ayurvedic medicine. Native Americans use herbs in a spiritual sense, placing emphasis on their purifying and cleansing properties, both physically and mentally.

Among the varied approaches to medical herbalism, there is one important governing principle – that of "synergism," which maintains that the strength of the sum of the parts is greater than the strength of individual parts. Therefore, herbalists prefer to use plant parts in their entirety in their remedies, rather than trying to isolate the plant's chemically active constituents (as conventional medicine does). They believe that the combination of each and every element of a plant forms its healing properties, and that each element has specific roles within the body outside the active ingredient itself. The combination of elements also works to prevent harmful side effects.

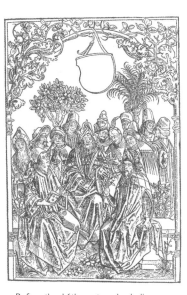

Before the 16th century, herbalism was more or less the only medical system in use. Many herbal manuals were written; this is the frontispiece of one.

Gravel root *Eupatorium purpureum* is a specific herb for kidney stones.

PREPARING AND USING HERBS

Effective herbal remedies can be prepared in the kitchen, but the dangers of self-diagnosis cannot be stressed too highly. Any unusual medical problems should be diagnosed and treated by a qualified medical herbalist, or a conventional medical doctor.

Herbs may be natural, but they are powerful healing tools and can be toxic in excess. To gain maximum benefit from herbs, it is important to prepare them correctly. Some methods are listed below.

INFUSIONS Flowers with their leaves and stalks make the best infusions because they release their active ingredients easily. Measure the required amount of herb into a warmed china teapot. Pour boiling water over, and steep (soak) for 10 to 15 minutes before straining. All infusions should be discarded after a few hours.

DECOCTIONS Woody stems, roots, seeds, and bark are preferred for decoctions. Chop or crush the herb in order to break down the active ingredients. Put the required amount in a nonreactive saucepan and cover with water. Bring to a boil, cover, and simmer for 10 to 15 minutes. Strain, and use while still hot. As with infusions, all decoctions should be discarded after a few hours.

TINCTURES Tinctures are highly concentrated mixtures of alcoholic spirit and herbs. Put the chopped or ground herb into a container with a lid, and cover with vodka. The ratio of herb to liquid by volume is 1:5. Leave in a warm place for two weeks, shaking twice daily. Strain through a cheesecloth, squeezing well. Store in a well-sealed, dark glass bottle.

COMPRESSES A compress enables the skin at the site of an inflammation or wound to absorb the active ingredients of an herbal infusion or decoction. Soak a clean cloth in the heated herbal liquid and apply to the affected area.

POULTICES A poultice is a compress that contains solid (but soft or mushy) constituents. Wrap the herbs from a hot infusion or decoction in gauze and apply to the skin at the site of an inflammation or wound. Place a hot-water bottle over the top in order to maintain the heat within the compress.

Growing Medicinal Herbs

Creating a herb garden can be a fascinating and rewarding experience. Most herbs are easy to grow and require little maintenance, once established. Herbs for the kitchen generally need well-drained soil, plenty of sunlight, and protection from wind. For medicinal herbs a partly shaded site is better because many of them are native to woodland and grow best in moist, rich soil.

Some medicinal herbs can grow spectacularly tall. If space is limited, choose only two or three large ones. Plant them at the back of a border, leaving plenty of space between, and interplant with shade-tolerant creeping herbs.

Blood root *Sanguinaria canadensis* is used in bronchitis and asthma.

A PLANTING PLAN

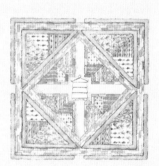

⅌ Tall herbs:

angelica, comfrey, elecampane, fennel, foxglove, lovage, sweet cicely, valerian

⅌ Sun-loving herbs:

camomile, fennel, hyssop, lavender, marjoram, mint, rosemary, sage, St. John's wort, thyme

⅌ Damp-loving herbs:

angelica, comfrey, elecampane, Jacob's ladder, meadowsweet, sweet cicely, valerian

⅌ Shade-loving herbs:

evening primrose, lily of the valley, valerian, woodruff

⅌ Herbs requiring partial shade:

angelica, foxglove, Jacob's ladder, lady's mantle, sweet cicely

COMMON HERBS AND THEIR USES

⅌ HERB	⅌ Therapeutically beneficial for:
⅌ ANGELICA	The common cold, coughs, respiratory infections; flatulence, indigestion, loss of appetite
⅌ ARNICA	Bruises, sprains; (not for internal use)
⅌ BALM OF GILEAD	Eczema, psoriasis; sore throat, laryngitis
⅌ BORAGE	Fever, inflammation; respiratory infections; stress
⅌ CAMOMILE	Anxiety, insomnia; flatulence, indigestion; inflammation, conjunctivitis; healing wounds
⅌ COMFREY	Bruises, burns, ulcers, healing wounds; (use externally only)
⅌ DANDELION	Gall bladder problems, water retention, jaundice; general debility
⅌ FENNEL	Colic, flatulence, indigestion; coughs; conjunctivitis
⅌ GARLIC	The common cold, coughs, adenoid problems, respiratory infections, other bacterial infections; high blood pressure (hypertension); acne
⅌ HYSSOP	The common cold, coughs, sore throat, respiratory infections, loss of appetite; bruises; anxiety
⅌ LAVENDER	Nervous exhaustion, insomnia; headache; rheumatic pain
⅌ LEMON BALM	Flatulence, indigestion; anxiety, depression
⅌ MARIGOLD	Bruises, burns, healing wounds, skin inflammation, conjunctivitis, some fungal infections; adenoid problems
⅌ MEADOWSWEET	Fever, nausea, digestive problems, constipation, urinary infections; rheumatic pain
⅌ NETTLE	Constipation, water retention; bleeding; eczema; allergies
⅌ OREGANO	The common cold, coughs, sore throat, headache; muscular pain; bites and stings, healing wounds
⅌ PEPPERMINT	Flatulence, loss of appetite, nausea, colic; headache, menstrual problems; skin irritation
⅌ ROSEMARY	Headache, muscular pain, neuralgia, general debility; digestive problems; baldness
⅌ SAGE	Laryngitis, inflammation, healing wounds; anxiety, depression; (do not use during pregnancy)
⅌ ST. JOHN'S WORT	Burns, healing wounds, shingles; neuralgia, rheumatic pain; anxiety; tension
⅌ THYME	Coughs, sore throat, laryngitis, respiratory infections; infections in wounds
⅌ VALERIAN	Sedative
⅌ WITCH HAZEL	Astringent
⅌ YARROW	Menstrual problems
⅌ YELLOW DOCK	Skin problems

RED CLOVER
TRIFOLIUM PRATENSE

WHITE COMFREY
SYMPHYTUM OFFICINALE

How a Herbal Therapist Works

Most herbal therapists (sometimes called herbalists – but not all herbalists treat clients medically) believe that the body acts in unison with the psyche (spirit) and emotions to maintain the equilibrium necessary for overall health and well-being. With this holistic approach herbal therapists use their knowledge of plant properties to rebalance a client's life energy levels so that his or her body heals itself.

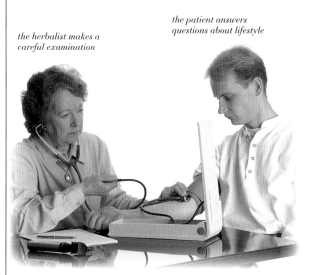

the herbalist makes a careful examination

the patient answers questions about lifestyle

When you consult a herbalist you may find that some of the techniques used are the same as for conventional medicine. Blood pressure and pulse will be measured.

Generally speaking, conventional medicine takes the view that the mind and the body are separate entities. If there is illness or disease in the body, the symptoms and the affected part are treated in isolation. For example, an allergic reaction might be treated with antihistamines by a conventional doctor, while a therapeutic physician would look for the root of the problem, and address that. Every therapeutic herbalist acknowledges that there is a role for surgical procedures and drugs in some situations. The advances of modern medicine can complement medical herbalism, and vice versa.

VISITING A HERBAL THERAPIST

The first session with your herbalist is for gathering information. You can expect to discuss

❋ your current complaint – your symptoms, the length of time you have been suffering, and what medical care you have received

❋ your medical history – every illness or injury that you can remember is important

❋ your lifestyle – every aspect of your lifestyle is also important – how much stress you are under, how you sleep and when, and what you eat and drink; a herbalist will often offer advice on diet and exercise alongside treatment for your illness, so it is important that you tell him or her as much as you can about yourself

❋ your emotional state – some illnesses are exacerbated by emotional trauma or upset, so your emotional health will also be relevant

❋ your work and any occupational or environmental hazards that might be affecting your health.

Any physical examination during the visit is similar to that carried out by your family physician. During the first session, it is likely that most of the following will be done

❋ your blood pressure measured

❋ your eyes and ears examined

❋ your heart or chest listened to by stethoscope

❋ palpation by hand of an area where the tone of the organs or muscles is in question

❋ blood or urine samples may occasionally be required.

An initial consultation lasts about one hour. Once the picture is clear and a diagnosis is made, the therapist prescribes one or a combination of several remedies tailored to suit the client and may advise on which foods to avoid or to favor in order to aid recovery.

The most common forms of remedy include tinctures, capsules or lozenges, ointments, and creams. Many herbal therapists are happy to work together with the client's local physician, especially when the client is already receiving conventional medical treatment.

CAUTIONS AND CONTRAINDICATIONS

Herbal medicines have a much better safety record for everyone from babies to pregnant women and the elderly than that of conventional drugs. But herbs are powerful healing tools, and some herbs are toxic when taken in large doses. Ask your herbalist for guidance, especially if you are taking herbs during pregnancy or giving them to babies. If you want to take herbal medicines in conjunction with conventional medicine, it is best to consult both your physician and a herbalist.

WHAT CAN HERBAL REMEDIES TREAT?

Common complaints that respond well to herbal remedies include

❧ *allergies*	❧ *insomnia*
❧ *arthritis*	❧ *kidney and urinary*
❧ *digestive problems*	*infections*
❧ *headache*	❧ *menopausal problems*
❧ *high or low blood*	❧ *menstrual problems*
pressure	❧ *skin diseases.*

The American Tradition

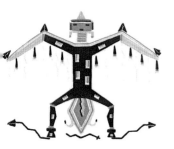

Part of a Navajo sand painting, used to depict the spirit's journey through the diseased state.

The tradition of herbal medicine has always been strong in North America, thanks to the pooling of European and Native American skills during the 18th and 19th centuries. Friendly Native American tribes shared their profound knowledge of healing with the first European settlers and introduced to them countless hitherto unknown medicinal and culinary herbs. Many herbs are particulary useful for women's problems, notably squaw vine and blue cohosh, both uterine tonics.

The settlers in their turn brought with them the seeds and roots of their most valuable herbs, which took hold and flourished in their new environment. The religious sect called the Shakers lived by agriculture and were also the first white Americans to grow and sell herbs in commercial quantities.

The Native Americans of Canada, the United States, and Mexico based their concept of natural medicine on the Great Spirit, and on the Medicine Wheel, within which we are all born and travel on life's journey. The Wheel is made up of the Four Directions, each with its particular qualities and energies. Herbs are thought both to guide and to assist in healing.

The Native Americans of the northeast recognized herbs to cure sore eyes, skin problems, abdominal complaints, and lung disorders, among other ailments. When they gathered the woodland herbs in high summer, the medicine men would begin by offering tobacco to the Four Directions of the Wheel and to the sky and earth. Herbs were gathered after ritual prayers and promises not to take more than was needed.

The Cherokee of the southeast recognized more than 100 types of medicinal herb. Some were used because they resembled the causative agent of the disease or because they looked like the part of the body affected. This compares with the medieval Western Doctrine of Signatures *(see page 67)*, where plants are named for their resemblance to body parts and used in remedies for that part. We know more about Cherokee medicine and herbal repertoire than any other Native American traditions because their great chief Sequoia developed a form of written language that was used to record rituals, prayers, and medicinal remedy recipes. The Cherokee believed that illness was caused by the spirits of dead animals, revenging themselves on human hunters, or by malcontented spirits or ghosts. Diseases were named for their causes not their symptoms. Illnesses were cured by rubbing boiled herbs into the patient's skin or blowing dried herbs over them through a cane pipe. Singing and ritual formulas were also important.

Much of Native American healing centered around purification, not just of the body but also of the spirit. Heat was considered a great purifier, and "hot" herbs were often administered to induce violent vomiting. Sweating out toxins in the "sweat lodge ceremony" was central to curing disease and maintaining health, and also purified the body in preparation for enlightenment. Fresh or dried herbs were burned during the ceremony and the smoke was considered to provide a link with the spirit world. Sage was a particularly important herb, and was believed to be especially sacred.

For modern Native Americans who live on reservations, the use of herbs and other traditional methods of healing remains vitally important and is still preferred to conventional medicine.

A medicine man from the Native American Blackfoot nation in full regalia. His shamanic drum is accompanied by medicine bags hanging from his clothes.

Sage *Salvia officinalis* is a sacred herb for many Native Americans.

Individual Therapies

Herbal Medicine in China and Japan

In China, natural substances have been used medicinally for thousands of years, and their application is encouraged by the present Chinese government. Traditional Chinese Medicine, including herbalism, began to be imported into Japan from about the 5th century A.D., and – with a few modifications – it has to a large extent been incorporated into the system operated by Japanese health insurance authorities.

The use of herbs once belonged partly to the realm of magic, in the healing rites performed by shamans (men and women of "natural wisdom") and also stems from observations of the way in which animals treat themselves to various plants when sick or wounded. But careful study of herbs and their properties over thousands of years has developed Oriental herbal medicine into a highly refined and complex discipline.

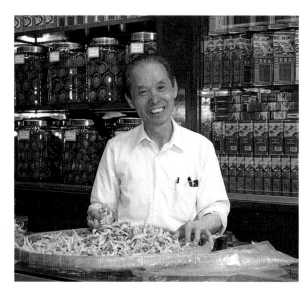

A ginseng shop in Korea. Ginseng is a well-known herbal tonic in Eastern countries and its properties are also recognized in the West.

Medical diagnosis is usually undertaken by practitioners familiar with both Western and Oriental medicine, resulting in a wide-ranging and comprehensive assessment of a patient's symptoms. The yin/yang balance will be appraised, as well as the functioning of the internal organs and systems, the patient's psychological state, diet, and lifestyle. And each of these factors will be considered in relation to the nature of the diseases or disorder involved, and its degree and speed of progression.

Following diagnosis, the therapist selects a combination of natural "herbs," which may include mineral and animal ingredients. Western herbal therapies are often based on using a single herbal remedy at a time; indeed, most rural forms of folk medicine work on this premise. An Oriental herbal therapist will provide an individually tailored cocktail of herbs that will work in conjunction with one another, and with you, and that will probably

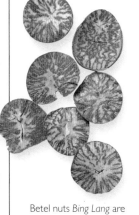

Betel nuts *Bing Lang* are used for intestinal worms and irregular bowel movements.

be readapted several times during the course of treatment as healing proceeds.

Herbs are classified in a number of ways. The nature of each is said to be cold, cool, hot, warm, or neutral. This is the chi or energy value of the herb and is used to balance excess or deficiencies in the "disharmony" that constitutes the illness. The herb's taste and smell are also evaluated, as sour, bitter, sweet, pungent, or salty (and also tasteless or astringent). These characteristics are linked to special affinities with different organs or body systems and the related emotions that can be involved in disease. The herbs are also characterized as having an ascending or descending effect. The herbalist prescribes a mixture of herbs and tells the patient how to prepare and use them. Occasionally ready-prepared remedies such as herbal pills or tinctures may be given.

In Chinese medicine, diet is a matter of great importance in preventing and treating disease, and the Oriental therapist also gives instructions on how to correct the diet and lifestyle. Acupuncture may also be recommended.

Western research now suggests that many of the substances that are used in Oriental medicine may in fact be capable of forming part of the treatment of cancers and other diseases.

Oyster shells are the remedy source for *Mu Li*; it has a sedative effect and calms excess liver yang energy.

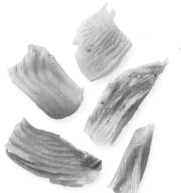

Chicken gizzard *Ji Nei Jin* is used as a remedy for digestive disorders.

SOME ORIENTAL HERBS

Oriental medicine herbs are generally used in combinations. There are approximately 300 herbal ingredients regularly used in prescriptions, and about half of these would be considered to be essential in any Chinese herb store. Some common combinations and essential ingredients are listed below, together with the conditions they can help. Herbs are listed by European, Chinese, and Japanese name. The conditions they can help are grouped together.

ANGELICA *ANGELICA ARCHANGELICA*

ORIENTAL HERBAL COMBINATIONS AND FORMULAS

Constituent	Combination	Formula	Therapeutically beneficial
ANGELICA AND PAEONIA		●	infertility
Dang gui shao yao san		●	endometriosis
Tokishakuyaku-san		●	hysteria
BUPLEURUM AND CINNAMON	●		the common cold, influenza
Chai hu gui zhi tang	●		peptic ulcer
Saikokeishi-to	●		
BUPLEURUM AND PAEONIA		●	menstrual disorders
Jia wei xiao yao san		●	anemia
Kamishoyo-san		●	nervous disorders
CINNAMON AND HOELEN		●	menstrual disorders
Gui shi fu ling wan		●	menopausal problems
Keishibukuryo-gan		●	
GINSENG AND DANG GUI	●		degenerative diseases (such as malignant tumors)
Shi kuan dau tang	●		autoimmune disease, tuberculosis
Juzentaiho-to	●		
HOELEN FIVE		●	edema (swelling)
Wu ling san		●	motion sickness
Gorei-san		●	hangover
MINOR BUPLEURUM	●		chronic hepatitis
Xiao chai hu tang	●		cirrhosis of the liver
Shosaiko-to	●		bronchitis
PUERARIA		●	the common cold
Ge gen tang		●	tonsillitis
Kakkon-to		●	stiffness in the shoulders

AMERICAN REN SHEN

ORIENTAL HERBAL CONSTITUENTS

Constituent	Therapeutic effect
GINGER RHIZOME (fresh ginger) (*Zingiber officinalis*)	Antipyretic (reduces fever), cough suppressant
Sheng jiang	
Shokyo	
GINSENG ROOT (*Panax ginseng*)	mildly stimulant
Ren shen	gastrointestinal soother
Ningin	mildly antidepressant
HARE'S EAR ROOT (*Bupleurum*)	antiallergic
Chai hu	antibiotic
Saiko	mildly anti-inflammatory
LICORICE ROOT (*Glycyrrhiza uralensis*)	sedative
Gan xao	reduces muscular spasm
Kanzo	anti-inflammatory

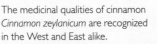

KEY   European Herb   Chinese equivalent   Japanese equivalent

SIBERIAN REN HEN

The medicinal qualities of cinnamon *Cinnamon zeylanicum* are recognized in the West and East alike.

Dietary and Nutritional Therapies

WHAT WE EAT is influenced by many factors, including personal preference, lifestyle, culture, religion, and ethical and moral attitudes. But what we eat can also have a therapeutic effect. The most common reason for a change in diet is to lose weight, but many people also alter their diet to prevent or treat diseases such as cancer, or heart disease, the main cause of diet-related premature death in the West.

Dietary Therapy

Diet as therapy has been practiced for centuries. The father of medicine, Hippocrates, wrote extensively about the therapeutic use of diet, yet until relatively recently modern medicine has largely forgotten the overwhelming role of diet, except as related to problems such as obesity and diabetes.

With the growth of nutritional science in the 20th century, particularly since World War II, specific foods have been recognized as risk factors in disease. For example, too much fat, and saturated animal fat in particular, is now widely recognized as a risk factor of heart disease and some cancers. Equally, too much refined food and too little fiber causes a range of digestive and bowel disorders, from constipation to irritable bowel syndrome – and may even be a cause of some cancers. Too much salt may exacerbate high blood pressure and reactions to food-trigger allergies.

BASIC PRINCIPLES AND DIFFERENT METHODS

Most alternative therapists believe that everybody can benefit from dietary self-help for both prevention and treatment of disease. Many therapies recommend fasting, perhaps drinking only fruit and vegetable juices, or eating salads or single fruits. Fasting is probably the oldest therapy known to humankind. Primitive people, and animals, instinctively stop eating when they are ill, probably because digestion takes up energy and puts extra strain on the body. The aim of fasting and dietary therapy is to rid the body of the toxins that are said to accumulate from the wrong diet, so that it can function at its optimum level.

Self-administered fasts should not exceed two days, and returning to eating should be gradual. Start with raw fruit and salads, followed by wholegrain foods,

> **CAUTIONS AND CONTRAINDICATIONS**
>
> It is essential, during every fast, to maintain your fluid intake. Continue to drink as much as possible, preferably mineral water, throughout.

WHAT CAN DIETARY THERAPY TREAT?

Almost all complementary therapists recommend dietary therapy as part of their treatment, for it works both on a preventive and a therapeutic basis. Specialized diets may be used to treat particular problems, but overall, dietary therapy is aimed at improving general health and well-being. Particular conditions that respond to dietary therapy include

- heart and circulatory disorders
- infections, including fungal infections (i.e. thrush)
- some cancers
- digestive problems
- ME
- Aids and other immune problems
- allergies and catarrh
- arthritis and rheumatism
- sinus problems
- Alzheimer's and Parkinson's diseases.

fish, poultry, or lean meat, and then yogurt and dairy produce. Fatty, sugary, and refined carbohydrate foods, coffee, cola, tea, and other stimulants, alcohol, and tobacco should be avoided completely.

Some of the side effects of fasting – such as headache, bad breath, diarrhea, and vomiting – are unpleasant and if they are intolerable, the alternative is to introduce a very little fruit and/or fresh vegetable juice, into the diet.

cookie   cake
sugar
fudge
hamburger
white rice
french fries
white bread
potato chips

Good food against bad, juxtaposed on a plate to underline the difference.

Special Diets

People on therapeutic diets often experience side effects similar to those from fasting. Symptoms commonly become worse before they improve. Modified diets should only be followed for a limited time to avoid vitamin and mineral deficiencies. Infants and children should never be made to fast, or even put on a restricted diet, except under medical supervision.

✌ **EXCLUSION DIETS** Exclusion, or elimination, diets are used to detect foods suspected of causing food allergies or intolerance, or triggering attacks of illness, such as migraine. Suspected foods are avoided for about two weeks and then reintroduced one at a time.

✌ **VEGETARIAN DIET** Vegetarians eat no meat, fish, or poultry, but most eat eggs and dairy products (this is called lacto-ovo-vegetarianism). A vegetarian diet followed correctly over a long period can reduce risk of heart disease, cancer, and other major illnesses.

✌ **VEGAN DIET** Vegans eat no animal products. They need vitamin B12 from fortified foods or supplements. A vegan diet shares most of the benefits of a vegetarian diet when carried out correctly.

✌ **FOOD COMBINING DIET** Food combining (the "Hay diet") advises against combining starch and sugar with protein and acid fruits *(see page 28)*. At least four hours should separate starch and protein meals. Protein, starch, and fats are eaten in small quantities, and all refined and processed foods are prohibited. This diet is said to improve arthritis and digestive problems.

✌ **ANTI-CANDIDA DIET** Anti-Candida diets for the treatment of thrush avoid yeasts and mold – as in malted cereals, cheeses, fungi – sugar and sugary foods, and peanuts.

fresh fruit

nuts

lentils

oily fish

wholemeal pasta

brown rice

wholemeal bread

vegetables

✌ **LIVER DIET** In a liver diet the following foods are avoided because some alternative therapists believe they are difficult for the liver to process: meat, poultry, eggs, sugars and sugary foods, dairy produce, nuts, coffee, tea, alcohol, chocolate, fried food.

✌ **LOW BLOOD SUGAR DIET** A low blood sugar diet is based on three meals a day, plus small, two-hourly snacks of nuts or seeds, milk, oatcakes, or wholewheat toast. Sugar and sugary foods must be avoided.

MACROBIOTIC DIET

A macrobiotic diet classifies all foods as either yin or yang. The aim is to eat a perfect balance, taking into account the individual's different yin/yang needs. If the equilibrium is upset, ill-health results.

Food is prepared, cut, and cooked in particular ways to preserve yin/yang characteristics. To create balance, people living in a yang environment (hot and dry) need to become more yin (cold and wet), and vice versa.

Yin foods grow in hot dry climates (such as the Middle East), have stronger smells, are hotter, more aromatic, and contain more water, and are therefore softer and juicier. Yang foods grow in cold wet climates (such as Britain) and are drier, shorter, harder (as in stems, and roots, and seeds), and are saltier and more sour.

The diet is similar to that of the traditional Japanese peasant, which consists of:

✌ *50 percent cooked whole cereal grains, pasta, bread, porridge, stir-fried rice, or noodles*

✌ *25 percent local seasonal vegetables, cooked in a variety of ways (for example, raw, pickled, steamed, sautéed, and boiled)*

✌ *10 percent protein, drawn from local fish, beans, and soybean products, such as tofu or tempeh*

✌ *5 percent sea vegetables, used in soups, stews, and condiments*

✌ *5 percent soups, including miso soup, fish soup, bean soup, and vegetable soup, among others*

✌ *5 percent desserts and teas, including simple teas and grain coffees, and desserts using fruits and fermented rice (amaskae), agar agar (sea vegetable), seeds, and nuts.*

Individual Therapies

Nutritional Therapy

Nutrients are the chemical components of diet and are essential to life and health. Nutrients are classed as either macronutrients or micronutrients:

❋ macronutrients are carbohydrates (sugars and starches), fats (including essential fatty acids), proteins (including essential amino acids), and fiber

❋ micronutrients are vitamins, minerals, and trace elements that cannot be manufactured in the body, and so must be eaten daily.

If micronutrients are absent or too low, illness results. Scurvy, for example, is a disease resulting from lack of vitamin C. It used to be the curse of sailors who had to make long trips at sea with no access to fresh fruit or vegetables. Once the connection between scurvy and fresh fruit had been made, and the sailors issued lime juice to drink, scurvy virtually disappeared.

Micronutrients have only been identified extensively and researched since 1913 when an American biochemist, Elmer McCollum, discovered the first vitamin, vitamin A. Their use in treatment has now become a major, and rapidly growing, therapy in its own right throughout the world. Another nutritional therapy is megavitamin therapy *(see page 80)*, established by the Nobel prize winner Dr. Linus Pauling in the United States. He believed that schizophrenia and other mental problems were the consequence of vitamin deficiency and originally called his therapy "orthomolecular psychiatry."

The therapeutic prescription of nutrients is known as nutritional therapy, and practitioners specializing in it are nutritional therapists. Nutrients prescribed in this way are called "dietary" or "food supplements," and they come in the form of tablets, capsules, powders, or liquids. Nutrients may sometimes also be injected for greater effect, but in most countries only conventional medical doctors may do this.

WHAT CAN NUTRITIONAL THERAPY TREAT?

Nutritional therapy aims to find where individual health has become unbalanced, and to put it right using nutrition as a therapy. Most treatment is preventive and restorative, but because it is holistic, many conditions will respond, including

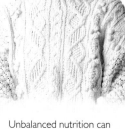

Unbalanced nutrition can lead to low-grade flu symptoms such as mild depression and fatigue.

⋟ *stress and stress-related disorders*

⋟ *pregnancy problems*

⋟ *arthritis*

⋟ *circulatory disorders*

⋟ *eye conditions*

⋟ *women's problems, including PMS, infertility, PNI, and menopause*

⋟ *joint and bone problems*

⋟ *general infections, including coughs, colds, and influenza*

⋟ *cancers*

⋟ *MND, MS, Alzheimer's and Parkinson's diseases*

⋟ *many others.*

SUPPLEMENTS AND THEIR SOURCES

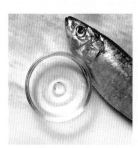

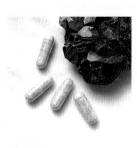

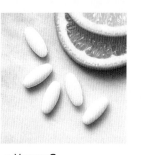

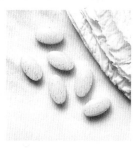

⋟ **FISH OIL**
Fish liver oils are available as supplements in many strengths; you could also step up your intake of oily fish such as herrings or mackerel.

⋟ **IRON**
Iron supplements are usually prescribed for anemia and for pregnant women. If you take supplements choose those that combine iron and vitamin C.

⋟ **VITAMIN C**
Vitamin C needs to be replenished daily. If you don't eat enough fruit and vegetables for your daily requirement, supplements are a good idea.

⋟ **FOLIC ACID**
Folic acid is a B vitamin found in green leafy vegetables such as spinach. It is essential in fetal development and blood formation.

Vitamins and Minerals

While most people eat enough calories they are often from the wrong foods. For example, fatty or sugary foods are low in vitamins and minerals from processing, and this is why many experts believe the typical modern Western diet allows disease to develop, if it does not actively promote it.

Furthermore, even a diet rich in fresh, unprocessed foods can be deficient in micronutrients, for intensive farming methods have largely robbed the soil of nutrients. A mineral-rich vegetable, for instance, cannot be produced from soil that is empty of minerals. Fruits and vegetables are force-grown and ripened; by the time they reach our supermarket shelves, there is little or no nutrition in them.

Other factors can also increase the need for vitamins and minerals. Examples are poor digestion and absorption, smoking, and drinking. Rapid growth in childhood and adolescence, pregnancy, lactation, and old age, all increase the need for nutrients. Requirements are also raised during illness, when we are under stress, taking drugs, or affected by environmental toxins and pollutants. It is in these situations that nutrients such as vitamins, minerals, amino acids, and essential fatty acids may be recommended and prescribed.

➵ **SPECIAL NOTE** Nutrients not listed have not yet been allocated recommended daily levels *(see "Safe intake" on page 79)*. This is because experts either do not consider them essential (they believe most people get enough of what they need in their daily diet) or they disagree on what the levels should be.

VITAMINS AND MINERALS

Recommended daily intakes for vitamins and minerals

➵ EUROPE

➵ VITAMIN	➵ RDA	➵ MINERAL	➵ RDA
Vitamin A	800ug	Calcium	800mg
Vitamin B6	2mg	Iodine	150ug
Vitamin B12	1ug	Iron	14mg
Vitamin C	60mg	Magnesium	300mg
Vitamin D	5ug	Phosphorus	800mg
Vitamin E	10mg	Zinc	15mg
Biotin	0.15mg		
Folacin	200ug		
Niacin	18mg		
Pantothenic acid	6mg		
Riboflavin	1.6mg		
Thiamin	1.4mg		

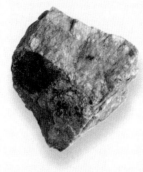

➵ USA

➵ Vitamin	➵ Men (25–50)	➵ Women (25–50)	➵ Pregnancy	➵ Lactation
Vitamin A	1,000ug	800ug	800ug	1,300ug
Vitamin B6	2mg	1.6mg	2.2mg	2.1mg
Vitamin B12	2ug	2ug	2.2mg	2.6ug
Vitamin C	60mg	60mg	70mg	95mg
Vitamin D	5ug	5ug	10ug	10ug
Vitamin E	10mg	8mg	10mg	12mg
Vitamin K	80ug	65ug	65ug	65ug
Folate	200ug	180ug	400ug	280ug
Niacin	19mg	15mg	17mg	20mg
Riboflavin	1.7mg	1.3mg	1.6mg	1.8mg
Thiamin	1.5mg	1.1mg	1.5mg	1.6mg

➵ Minerals

	➵ Men (25–50)	➵ Women (25–50)	➵ Pregnancy	➵ Lactation
Calcium	800mg	800mg	1200mg	1200mg
Iodine	150ug	150ug	200ug	200ug
Iron	10mg	15mg	15mg	15mg
Magnesium	350mg	280mg	355mg	340mg
Phosphorus	800mg	800mg	1200mg	1200mg
Selenium	70ug	55ug	75ug	75ug
Zinc	15mg	12mg	19mg	16mg

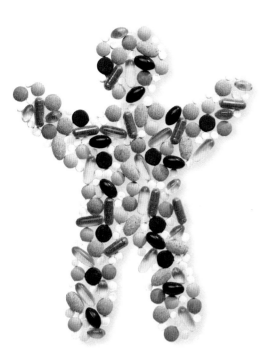

While supplements should not replace a good balanced diet, they can help, if maintaining such a diet is not possible.

Phosphorus, the source of an essential trace element.

Food Supplements

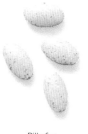

Pills for nourishment.

Food supplements may be prescribed to prevent certain long-term chronic imbalances or to establish a sound constitution, but they also have a role to play in acute common conditions such as indigestion, premenstrual syndrome, sore eyes, coughs and colds, and general infections. Obviously, they cannot relieve pain instantly, but the condition can improve within 24 hours or so.

Initially, self-diagnosis and prescription are to be discouraged, but once you have established your needs in acute situations, you could take the supplements as and when required, remembering always to adhere to the recommended daily intake.

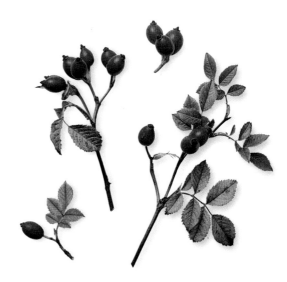

Rosehips *Rosa canina* are one of the richest sources of vitamin C.

SUPPLEMENTS FOR COMMON CONDITIONS

The following table provides general guidelines as to what supplements might be useful in the treatment and prevention of common conditions. For dose levels it is best to see your family doctor or a qualified nutritional adviser, not only for a proper diagnosis of your condition but also, and as important, to ensure that particular supplements will not affect the action of any regular medication you may be taking. A good practitioner should also discuss changes in diet and lifestyle that may be worth trying at the same time as well as, or even instead of, taking supplements.

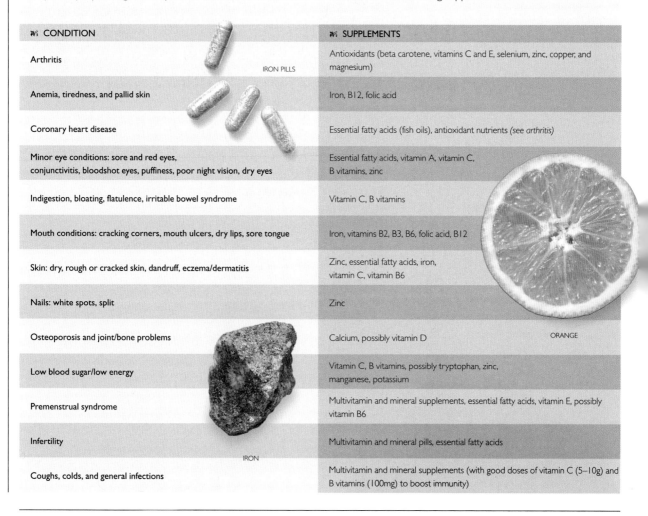

🪶 CONDITION	🪶 SUPPLEMENTS
Arthritis	Antioxidants (beta carotene, vitamins C and E, selenium, zinc, copper, and magnesium)
Anemia, tiredness, and pallid skin	Iron, B12, folic acid
Coronary heart disease	Essential fatty acids (fish oils), antioxidant nutrients (*see arthritis*)
Minor eye conditions: sore and red eyes, conjunctivitis, bloodshot eyes, puffiness, poor night vision, dry eyes	Essential fatty acids, vitamin A, vitamin C, B vitamins, zinc
Indigestion, bloating, flatulence, irritable bowel syndrome	Vitamin C, B vitamins
Mouth conditions: cracking corners, mouth ulcers, dry lips, sore tongue	Iron, vitamins B2, B3, B6, folic acid, B12
Skin: dry, rough or cracked skin, dandruff, eczema/dermatitis	Zinc, essential fatty acids, iron, vitamin C, vitamin B6
Nails: white spots, split	Zinc
Osteoporosis and joint/bone problems	Calcium, possibly vitamin D
Low blood sugar/low energy	Vitamin C, B vitamins, possibly tryptophan, zinc, manganese, potassium
Premenstrual syndrome	Multivitamin and mineral supplements, essential fatty acids, vitamin E, possibly vitamin B6
Infertility	Multivitamin and mineral pills, essential fatty acids
Coughs, colds, and general infections	Multivitamin and mineral supplements (with good doses of vitamin C (5–10g) and B vitamins (100mg) to boost immunity)

IRON PILLS

ORANGE

IRON

How to Use Supplements

Most dietary supplements are designed to provide our daily requirements of vitamins and minerals, expressed on packaging as a percentage of the Reference Nutrient Intake (RNI). This is the amount that is thought to be enough for virtually everyone, including those with particularly high requirements.

Other measurements used are Estimated Average Requirement (EAR), set for average needs but recognizing that some people need more *(see RNI)*, and that others need less, which is expressed as Lower Reference Nutrient Intake (LRNI), the amount needed by those with low needs. However, if you habitually eat (or take) less than LRNI you are likely to find that you are deficient.

Supplements are usually taken in pill or tablet form with water or fruit juice.

When taking food supplements it is important to follow the doses stated on the package in order to prevent any dangers of overdose *(see "Safe intake")* and to avoid imbalances. All nutrients work in conjunction with others, and with substances in the body, so taking too much of one vitamin, mineral, or other food supplement could upset the balance of delicate mechanisms within the body such as enzyme production. Minerals that could be harmful, however, are rarely sold except on prescription.

As a general rule, vitamins and minerals work "synergistically." That means they both need each other to work properly and that neither works as effectively on its own. A classic example is the combined effect of vitamin C and the mineral zinc, which is used in the treatment of the common cold and influenza.

In most cases food supplements should be taken with or just after meals (exceptions are amino acids, which are most effective taken on an empty stomach).

You should avoid taking iron pills with certain antibiotics. Check with your supplier about the suitability of taking supplements with medication you are taking.

CAUTIONS AND CONTRAINDICATIONS

Fat-soluble vitamins, such as vitamins A, D, and E, can be toxic in excess. Doses above 20,000iu of vitamin A can, for example, cause severe intercranial pressure. The maximum intake of vitamin D is 400iu, unless you suffer from hypoparathyroidism. See your nutritionist about the correct dosages before beginning any vitamin therapy.

iu = International Unit

SAFE INTAKE

There are no recommended levels for the following nutrients, which are known to have important functions. Safe intake is judged to be a level or range of intake at which there is no risk of deficiency and below a level of undesirable side effects.

✽ NUTRIENT	✽ SAFE INTAKE
Pantothenic acid	Adult 3–7mg Infants 1.7mg
Biotin	10–200ug
Vitamin E	Men above 4mg (as polyunsaturated fatty acids) Women above 3mg, Infants 0.4mg
Vitamin K	Adults 10ug/kg Infants 0.1ug/kg
Manganese	Adults 16ug Infants and children 1.4mg
Molybdenum	Adults 50–400ug Infants/children/adolescents 0.5–1.5ug/kg
Chromium	Adults 25ug Children and adolescents 0.1–1.0ug/kg
Fluoride	Infants only 0.005mg/kg

KEY g = gram, mg = milligram, ug = microgram, kg = kilogram
(as in an amount of a nutrient per kg body weight per day)
*Source: "Dietary Reference Values for Food Energy and Nutrients,"
UK Department of Health (Coma, 1991).*

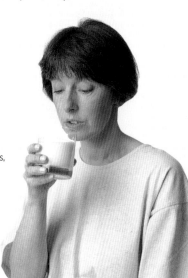

Some supplements, notably vitamin C and fish liver oil, are available in liquid form.

Megavitamin Therapy

Vitamins A, E, and C are usually available in a combination form.

Megavitamin therapy involves taking doses of vitamins far larger than are considered necessary for general health. The megadose approach has been used for conditions as diverse as the common cold and cancer, but there are drawbacks.

POSSIBLE ADVERSE EFFECTS

VITAMIN A (retinol) Large amounts of retinol can cause liver and bone damage. Since retinol is fat soluble, it can build up in the body. Women who are pregnant or planning to be should not take vitamin A supplements because of the risk of birth defects.

THIAMIN (B1) More than 3g a day is toxic to adults causing headache, irritability, insomnia, rapid pulse, weakness, contact dermatitis, pruritis, and even death.

NIACIN (B3) Very high doses of nicotinic acid, 3–6g a day, can damage the liver. Around 200mg a day can cause flushing (although it can be avoided by taking B3 as nicotinamide).

VITAMIN B6 Nerve function can be damaged at doses of between 2–7g a day, and some sensory loss is reported in some people between 50–500mg a day with symptoms disappearing after withdrawal of supplements. High intakes in pregnancy may be risky.

VITAMIN C May cause kidney stones in a small group of people who produce too much oxalate in response to high doses.

VITAMIN D Infants are most at risk at doses over 50ug a day from calcium deposits in the arteries and excessive calcification of bones and internal organs.

MAGNESIUM High doses between 3–5g a day over a prolonged period can be fatal.

PHOSPHORUS Maximum daily intake is 70mg per kg of body weight or about 4.5g for a 65kg man.

POTASSIUM Intakes above 17.6g a day could be toxic.

IRON Poisoning occurs in children above 20mg per kg body weight a day with between 200–300mg per kg body weight being a lethal dose.

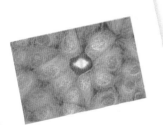

Skin cancer cell; megavitamin therapy may help such preventable cancers.

WHAT CAN MEGAVITAMIN THERAPY TREAT?

Large doses of vitamins/minerals may also benefit the following:

SMOKERS *Large doses of vitamins B, C, and other antioxidant nutrients can combat the damaging effects of smoking (although megadoses do not prevent cancer and other illnesses caused by smoking)*

HEAVY DRINKERS *Alcohol increases demands for vitamin C and the B vitamins*

HIGHLY STRUNG PEOPLE *Anxiety, irritability, and nervousness can be helped by increased intake of the B vitamins.*

People whose diets are high in:

FAT — *particularly saturated fats: fats increase the need for vitamin E and other antioxidants as well as essential fatty acids*

PRESERVATIVES — *these may increase the need for vitamin C, selenium, and bioflavonoids*

CAFFEINE AND DIURETICS — *tea, coffee, colas, and other such drinks may increase the need for potassium.*

ZINC Poisoning can occur at daily intakes of 2g or more. Long-term exposure to 75–80mg a day can lead to anemia. As little as 50mg a day interferes with the metabolism of iron and copper.

COPPER High intakes are toxic but how much is not known.

SELENIUM Serious problems occur at intakes above 750ug a day. In the absence of more details, a safe intake is set at 450ug a day for adult males.

IODINE High intakes can cause goiter and hyperthyroidism. Upper limit on intakes is 17ug per kg body weight a day.

COBALT Doses of 29.5mg a day have produced serious toxic effects.

GERMANIUM Doses of 50–250mg a day for between 4 and 18 months can cause serious harm and even death.

Mineral Salts

The body also needs to maintain certain levels of mineral salts. Biochemic tissue salts, or Schuessler salts, are mineral remedies for everyday ailments. They are prepared in the same way as homeopathic remedies *(see pages 82–5)*, and are used to make up mineral deficiencies believed to underlie many common health problems.

The salts are nontoxic and have no known side effects, although the tablets are made with lactose (milk sugar) so people with lactose intolerance should not take them.

CELLOID MINERALS

Celloids are pharmacological doses of minerals taken to rebalance cell chemistry. They were developed by the Australian naturopath practitioner, Maurice Blackmore.

The name "celloids" comes from colloid, the form in which minerals are found in living plants. It is believed that the human body can assimilate these quickly and completely. In their colloidal form larger doses of minerals do not cause problems of toxicity, so only children under two years take a smaller dose than adults.

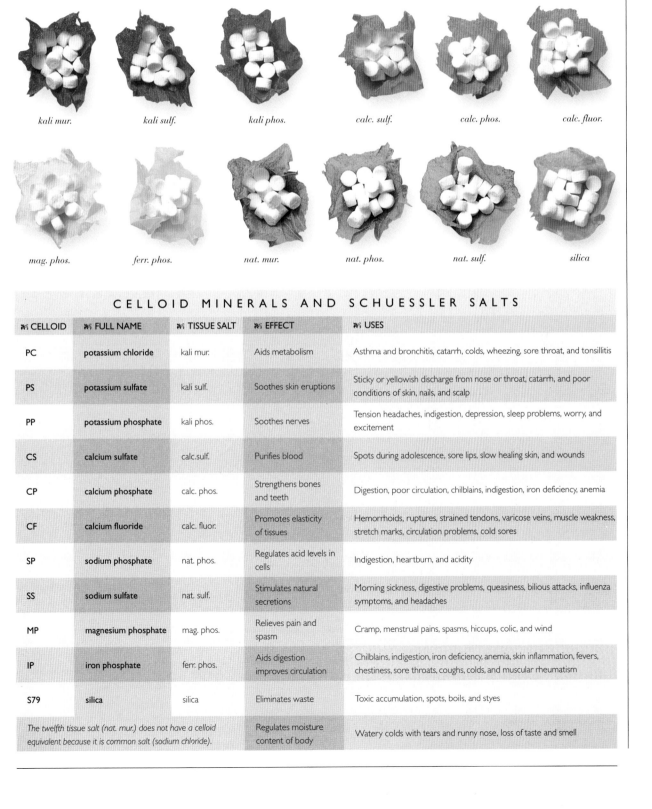

kali mur.   *kali sulf.*   *kali phos.*   *calc. sulf.*   *calc. phos.*   *calc. fluor.*

mag. phos.   *ferr. phos.*   *nat. mur.*   *nat. phos.*   *nat. sulf.*   *silica*

CELLOID MINERALS AND SCHUESSLER SALTS

CELLOID	FULL NAME	TISSUE SALT	EFFECT	USES
PC	potassium chloride	kali mur.	Aids metabolism	Asthma and bronchitis, catarrh, colds, wheezing, sore throat, and tonsillitis
PS	potassium sulfate	kali sulf.	Soothes skin eruptions	Sticky or yellowish discharge from nose or throat, catarrh, and poor conditions of skin, nails, and scalp
PP	potassium phosphate	kali phos.	Soothes nerves	Tension headaches, indigestion, depression, sleep problems, worry, and excitement
CS	calcium sulfate	calc.sulf.	Purifies blood	Spots during adolescence, sore lips, slow healing skin, and wounds
CP	calcium phosphate	calc. phos.	Strengthens bones and teeth	Digestion, poor circulation, chilblains, indigestion, iron deficiency, anemia
CF	calcium fluoride	calc. fluor.	Promotes elasticity of tissues	Hemorrhoids, ruptures, strained tendons, varicose veins, muscle weakness, stretch marks, circulation problems, cold sores
SP	sodium phosphate	nat. phos.	Regulates acid levels in cells	Indigestion, heartburn, and acidity
SS	sodium sulfate	nat. sulf.	Stimulates natural secretions	Morning sickness, digestive problems, queasiness, bilious attacks, influenza symptoms, and headaches
MP	magnesium phosphate	mag. phos.	Relieves pain and spasm	Cramp, menstrual pains, spasms, hiccups, colic, and wind
IP	iron phosphate	ferr. phos.	Aids digestion improves circulation	Chilblains, indigestion, iron deficiency, anemia, skin inflammation, fevers, chestiness, sore throats, coughs, colds, and muscular rheumatism
S79	silica	silica	Eliminates waste	Toxic accumulation, spots, boils, and styes
The twelfth tissue salt (nat. mur.) does not have a celloid equivalent because it is common salt (sodium chloride).			Regulates moisture content of body	Watery colds with tears and runny nose, loss of taste and smell

Homeopathy

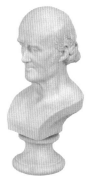

Samuel Hahnemann, (1755–1843), founder of homeopathy.

HOMEOPATHY is a holistic form of medicine that aims to help the body heal itself. It works for both acute (short-term) illnesses and chronic (long-term) ailments, and the prevention of illness is as crucial to its philosophy as the treatment. The name homeopathy comes from the Greek word *homios* meaning "like" and *pathos* meaning "suffering." The word "homeopathy" simply means treating like with like. This means that a substance that causes symptoms of illness in a well person can also be used to cure similar symptoms when they result from illness.

The minute substances used in treatment are called homeopathic remedies. There over 3,000 homeopathic remedies, which are usually referred to by their abbreviated name, for example Arsenicum album becomes Ars. alb. and Mercurius solubilis becomes Merc. sol.

BACKGROUND AND HISTORY

Hippocrates understood the basic precepts of homeopathy, and he had a selection of remedies in his personal medicine chest. But homeopathy as we know it was founded by a German doctor and chemist named Samuel Hahnemann (1755–1843). Disillusioned by the medical practices of his day, and by the rampant spread of disease, he gave up conventional medicine in order to work as a translator.

It was this work that led to his discovery of homeopathy. While translating Dr. William Cullen's *A Treatise on Materia Medica* he noted that quinine was listed as an effective treatment for malaria because of its astringent properties. Hahnemann was puzzled, for although he knew that quinine was antimalarial, he also knew that its astringency had little to do with it. For several days he took low doses of quinine and noted his reactions to it. One by one, he developed the symptoms of malaria even though he did not have the disease. Each time he took another dose of quinine, the symptoms recurred, and when he didn't take it, they went away. He believed it was quinine's ability to cause the symptoms of malaria that made it such an effective treatment for the disease. From here he experimented with other popular medicines, including arsenic and

The wooden box in which Hahnemann stored his repertory of remedies, which were kept in small glass phials.

mercury. From this system of testing he built up a drug picture for each of the hundreds of substances that he tested.

Next, he attempted to build up a "symptoms picture" of each client before he prescribed for them. He discovered that the more information he had about a client, the more accurately he could prescribe a remedy that would work.

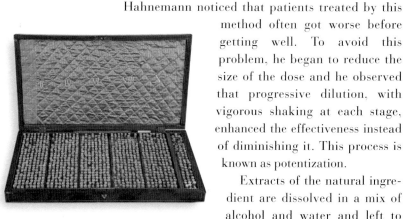

Marigold *Calendula officinalis* is the remedy source for Calendula.

MAKING THE MEDICINES

Hahnemann tested numerous medicinal substances on himself and his followers who, although healthy, took them until they produced symptoms similar to the illnesses for which they were prescribed. These experiments were known as provings, and homeopathic medicines are tested on healthy people to this day.

Hahnemann noticed that patients treated by this method often got worse before getting well. To avoid this problem, he began to reduce the size of the dose and he observed that progressive dilution, with vigorous shaking at each stage, enhanced the effectiveness instead of diminishing it. This process is known as potentization.

Extracts of the natural ingredient are dissolved in a mix of alcohol and water and left to stand for two to four weeks. During this time they are shaken occasionally and then strained. The strained solution is known as the mother tincture. The mother tincture is then diluted to make the different potencies. The various dilutions are then added to tiny lactose tablets, granules, or powder and stored in dark bottles. The higher the dilution number, the more heavily it has been diluted. It is the higher dilutions that prove the strongest.

Medicines produced in this way are safe, nontoxic, and relatively inexpensive, and can be used for young and old, as well as pets and farm animals.

Honey bees are the remedy source for the Apis remedy.

How Homeopathy Works

Homeopaths prescribe remedies for the "whole" person, and the practice of homeopathy is still based on the three principles established by Dr. Hahnemann. This is the "law of similars," the principle of the minimum dose and prescribing for the individual.

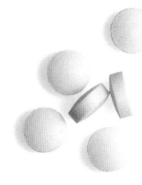

Most homeopathic remedies are administered in the form of lactose pills; tinctures or ointments are also available.

The law of similars states that a substance that can produce symptoms of illness in a well person can, in minute doses, cure similar symptoms of disease. The minimum dose states that by diluting a substance, its curative properties are enhanced and any side effects are eliminated.

Whole-person prescribing is probably the most important part of homeopathy, for the fundamental philosophy behind the practice is that each person is an individual and must be treated as such. A homeopath studies a person's temperament, personality, emotional and physical responses, even the food they like and dislike before prescribing.

Homeopaths believe that treatment works according to a set of rules known as the "Laws of Cure," and these state that:
❋ a remedy begins to work from the top of the body downward
❋ it works from the inside out and from major to minor organs
❋ symptoms clear in reverse order of their appearance.

Homeopaths also believe that a person's constitution is made up of inherited and acquired physical, mental, and emotional characteristics and that these can be matched to a particular remedy that will improve their health, no matter what their illness.

Furthermore, people with similar characteristics and constitutions can be grouped under one of the constitutional remedy types, if they all share specific physical and emotional characteristics. Your constitutional type can change as your physique, health, and attitudes change, and some people can be a combination of constitutional types.

CAUTIONS AND CONTRAINDICATIONS

Homeopathic remedies are completely safe for everyone from children to the elderly, in all states of health. It is essential, however, to take remedies only for as long as you need them, and to advise both your physician and your homeopath if you wish to take remedies alongside conventional medical treatment.

It is not clear exactly how homeopathy works, but studies have proved that it does. Hahnemann believed that remedies worked to balance the body so it was able to heal itself.

THE CONSULTATION

The first consultation will take upward of an hour. Your homeopath will ask you numerous questions about yourself in order to build up a complete picture of you and your mental, physical, and emotional health. You will be asked about your family health, past illnesses, lifestyle, and diet, and then more specific and unusual questions such as how you react to cold, or what sorts of food you like, and how you sleep, feel about darkness, and face responsibility. It is these last, seemingly trivial details, that help your homeopath to pinpoint the remedy most suitable for you.

Remedies are usually prescribed one at a time and may change as your symptoms clear. The remedy will come in the form of small pills, tablets, granules, powder, or liquid, which should be taken a half-hour before or after eating and drinking.

Diet and lifestyle changes may be suggested, and you can expect to have a followup visit in order to check how the remedies are working. Treatment may only take one or two visits, but long-term conditions may take much longer. You should see some change in your condition within a few days.

HOMEOPATHIC ANTIDOTES

A number of substances have the ability to counteract the homeopathic remedies, and these include coffee, alcohol, tobacco, minty flavorings, highly perfumed cosmetics, strongly smelling household cleaners, and aromatherapy oils. Avoid these when taking homeopathic remedies.

WHAT CAN HOMEOPATHY TREAT?

Homeopathy can treat almost any complaint – physical and psychological – although its efficacy appears to be dependent on the individual. Everything from indigestion, catarrh, childhood illnesses, gallstones, depression, burns, sports injuries, allergies, and stress to travel sickness, peptic ulcers, kidney disorders, hyperactivity, cold sores, and bursitis will respond, depending on the other steps that are taken by the sufferer to attain and maintain good health.

Individual Therapies

When to Use Homeopathy

Health problems that come from within the patient respond particularly well to homeopathy. Examples include eczema and other skin problems, asthma, allergies, indigestion, irritable bowel syndrome, and ME. Illnesses of this nature should always be treated by a fully trained and registered practitioner. Homeopathy is safe for everyone, from babies to pregnant women, and the elderly, and can address almost any condition, but it does not always work for everyone who tries it. Take the remedies only for as long as you need to. Homeopathic remedies may safely be taken alongside conventional treatment although some drugs may affect their action.

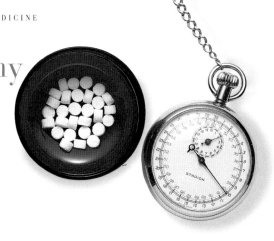

The timing of homeopathic remedies is very significant and part of the prescribing process.

HOME USE

Homeopathy can be safely used in the home for simple, self-limiting ailments, and first aid. The medicines are not expensive and since they all have a wide range of applications, a home kit can be gradually built up. If this is stored correctly it can be kept almost indefinitely. You may have to look for a specialist homeopathic pharmacy if you want to buy some of the more unusual remedies or potencies.

Sulfur is one of the most important homeopathic remedies.

The names of all homeopathic medicines are followed by a number that indicates its potency or "strength." As a general rule, low potencies like 3 or 6 are used for long-standing or chronic conditions. Higher potencies like 30 or 200 are used for acute conditions such as colds or influenza, or following an accident. Higher potencies are also used constitutionally. When the correct remedy is chosen, symptoms should begin to clear immediately. Symptoms may become worse before they get better. In acute conditions, doses should be taken every half-hour to begin with, up to a maximum of about ten doses. As soon as there is some improvement, the interval between doses should be increased to 8 or 12 hours for two to three days at the most. In chronic conditions, 6c remedies are usually taken three times a day for up to 24 days, and 30c remedies every 12 hours for a few days. Because the medicine acts by stimulating the body's ability to heal, once that healing is well-established there is no need to continue the treatment.

Sarsaparilla is prepared from wild licorice *Smilax officinalis*. It is indicated for cystitis.

PROVING A HOMEOPATHIC REMEDY

If a chosen remedy does not have a noticeable effect within a short period of time, then stop taking it. Long-term use or high doses of an incorrect remedy can cause the symptoms of the condition that the remedy is designed to treat to manifest themselves.

RESEARCH

French researcher Professor Jacques Benveniste claimed that diluting in water and succussing (vigorously shaking) a homeopathically prepared ingredient releases its energy into the water and the water "remembers" or retains an imprint of that energy. This confirms Hahnemann's belief that it is the energy or "vibrational pattern" of the remedy, rather than its chemical content, that stimulates healing, by encouraging the body's own healing force.

Spongia is made from natural sea sponge, toasted and crumbled.

Recently, another homeopath, Dr. David Reilly, has published the results of a number of trials in leading medical journals that show that homeopathically prepared allergens are effective in the treatment of asthma, hay fever, and perennial rhinitis. Other trials are taking place all over the world, but shortage of money is an obstacle to more work being done.

Undoubtedly, the growth in homeopathy is consumer-led as patients, aware of the side effects of many modern drugs, seek a gentler return to health. The low cost and safety of homeopathic medicines is leading governments to consider using them in order to reduce their huge drug bills. Medical students in Britain are asking for homeopathy to be included in their training, and yet in the United States it is banned in some states. Homeopathy has always been widely used in France and Germany, and there is growing interest in other European countries.

A HOMEOPATHIC FIRST AID KIT

Arnica 6 and 30c	For symptoms brought on by shock after injury and bruising, cramp, burns, stings, black eye, nose bleed, sprains, strained or torn muscles, eczema, boils, whooping cough, and bedwetting in children
Apis 30c	For insect stings that are hot and swollen, cystitis, hives, edema, arthritis, allergic reactions in eyes, throat, and mouth. (Avoid during pregnancy)
Argentum nit. 6 and 30c	For fear before a big event, such as exams, public speaking, a driving test
Arsenicum alb. 6 and 30c	Used for fear and panic when alone. Also good for food poisoning with severe vomiting or diarrhea, insomnia, mouth ulcers, and shingles
Belladonna 30c	For feverish colds with hot head and red face, sore throat, earache, painful periods, bursting headaches, high, burning fever, and abscesses
Bryonia 30c	Used for swollen painful joints, swollen painful breasts, heat exhaustion, bursting headache, nausea, screaming colicky babies, colds, and influenza
Cantharis 6c and 30c	For burns, scalds, and blisters, cystitis, burning diarrhea, any burning or stinging sensation
Chamomilla 6c and 30	Excellent for teething babies, but also used for extreme pain with irritability in adults, following surgery or dental work. Good for insomnia with restlessness
Euphrasia 6c	Used for eye injuries, conjunctivitis, eye strain or foreign bodies in the eyes, hay fever where the eyes are mainly affected, bursting headaches, constipation, and measles
Gelsemium 6c and 30c	For fear, stagefright, influenza with heaviness of body, aches and pains all over, sneezing, absence of thirst but a need to urinate often, heavy eyelids, hammering headache, and occasionally ME
Glonoin 30c	For heat exhaustion, bursting headache, hot flushes
Hypericum 30c	For wounds with shooting pains, for injuries where the nerves are affected: crushed fingers or toes, head wounds and cut lip, nausea, indigestion, diarrhea, and depression
Ignatia 6c and 30c	A valuable remedy for grief and shock following immediately after bad news, also for hiccups after shock, facial tics, headaches that feel as though a nail has been driven into the skull, and a cough that improves after eating solid food
Ledum 6c	For insect stings and wounds that feel numb and cold and for a painful black eye, prevents infection. Useful for any puncture wounds, including immunization and surgery
Natrum mur. 6c and 30c	One of the most commonly used remedies, for the ill effects of grief, depression in people who bottle things up, migraine, colds with much sneezing in the morning, colorless catarrh, and cold sores
Nux vomica 6c	For travel sickness and nausea with a headache, digestive problems, heavy periods, hangovers, morning sickness, cystitis, insomnia due to mental strain, colic due to overeating, and labor pains
Phosphate 6c	Excellent for nosebleeds caused by severe blows, or injury
Pulsatilla 6c and 30c	Helpful for measles, headaches, and stomach upsets following rich food or ice cream, recurring styes, cold with thick, bland yellow discharge, depression, palpitations, acute sinusitis, nosebleeds, and bedwetting
Rhus tox. 6c	Can be used for red, swollen, itchy blisters, diaper rash, painful stiff muscles, cramp, rheumatic or arthritic pain that is eased by moving. Excellent for herpes infections (such as chicken pox and cold sores), and for sore throats
Ruta grav. 6c	Use this for pain and stiffness in pulled muscles, eye strain, rheumatism, deep aching pain in bones and muscles, headaches, tendon injuries, bruised bones, and sciatica
Sepia 6c	Helps many women with the symptoms of the menopause; also useful for postnatal illness, headaches accompanied by nausea, indigestion, low blood pressure, palpitations, bedwetting, and menstrual upsets
Silica 6c	This can be used for splinters that could cause infection, migraine, recurrent colds, and infections, spots, weak nails, fractures, and glue ear
Sulfur 6c and 30c	Suitable for conjunctivitis, hypoglycemia, chronic diarrhea, anal fissures, headaches, catarrh, sore, burning lips, lower back pain, stiff joints, and muscle cramps
Tabacum 6c	For motion sickness, nausea, vomiting, faintness, dizziness, and anxiety
Urtica 6c	For stinging burns, scalds, and allergic skin, insect stings, cystitis, neuritis, rheumatic pain, and hives
Also:	Mother tinctures of Calendula, Hypericum, and Euphrasia, and ointments of Hypericum, Calendula, Urtica, and Arnica

RUTA GRAVEOLENS

Flower and Tree Remedies

Oak leaves, source of one of Dr. Bach's remedies.

Remedies from flowers and trees are subtle "elixirs" that claim to be able to help to rekindle a feeling of mental and emotional, as well as physical, well-being. Some aim to bring relief from unsettling moods and emotions such as anxiety, fear, guilt, and anger, and others encourage people who use them to recognize and let go of deep-seated behavioral patterns that give rise to such feelings. Above all, they claim to be able to help people feel calm and content in times of stress. Flower and tree remedies are so safe and harmless that they are often used as self-treatment. They are not targeted at particular symptoms but at states of mind accompanying illness.

Though flowers have played a role in healing for centuries – Australian Aborigines and Native Americans were using remedies made from flowers to ease emotional upsets and achieve peace of mind thousands of years ago – the healing power of flowers was only rediscovered in the West in the 1920s when it was revived by Dr. Edward Bach.

Bach (pronounced Batch) was a British Harley Street physician specializing in pathology and bacteriology, with a practical understanding of homeopathy. As a young practitioner he quickly noticed that patients with "physical" complaints often seemed to be suffering from some form of anxiety or "negative" emotional problem. He came to think that the emotional background was the cause of the illness.

Disenchanted with the standard medical approach of relieving the symptoms rather than the cause of illness, he began a quest for a new healing system that could help with the psychological aspect of illness. His search ended with the flowers blossoming in the fields and hedgerows around his cottage.

Bach decided intuitively upon the plants that would give relief. It is said

that he put himself into the frame of mind corresponding to that which he saw as being a cause of illness, before trying out the effects of plants on himself. The first of the plant remedies pinpointed by Bach related to what he saw as 12 key personality types. The next 26 flower remedies brought relief from different kinds of emotional discomfort and distress. The table shown below summarizes the 38 remedies developed by Bach during the 1920s and 1930s.

SUMMARY OF THE BACH FLOWER REMEDIES

❧ REMEDY	❧ FOR
Agrimony	Worry hidden by a carefree mask, apparently jovial but suffering
Aspen	Vague, unknown, haunting apprehension and premonitions
Beech	Intolerant, critical, fussy
Centaury	Kind, quiet, gentle, anxious to serve
Cerato	Distrust of self and intuition, easily led and misguided
Cherry Plum	For the thought of losing control, of doing dreaded things
Chestnut Bud	Failing to learn from life, repeating mistakes, lack of observation
Chicory	Demanding, self-pity, self-love, possessive, hurt and tearful
Clematis	Dreamers, drowsy, absent-minded
Crab Apple	Feeling unclean, self-disgust, small things out of proportion
Elm	Capable people with responsibility who falter, temporarily overwhelmed
Gentian	Discouragement, doubt, despondency
Gorse	No hope, accepting the difficulty, pointless to try
Heather	Longing for company, talkative, overconcern with self
Holly	Jealousy, envy, revenge, anger, suspicion
Honeysuckle	Living in memories
Hornbeam	Feels weary and thinks can't cope
Impatiens	Irritated by constraints, quick, tense, impatient
Larch	Expect failure, lack of confidence and will to succeed
Mimulus	Fright of specific, known things – animals, height, pain, etc.
Mustard	Gloom suddenly clouds us for no apparent reason
Oak	Persevering, despite difficulties, strong, patient, never giving in
Olive	Exhausted, no more strength, need physical and mental renewal
Pine	Self-critical, self-reproach, assuming blame, apologetic
Red Chestnut	Worry for others, anticipating misfortune, projecting worry
Rock Rose	Feeling alarmed, intensely scared, horror, dread
Rock Water	Self-denial, stricture, rigidity, purist
Scleranthus	Cannot resolve two choices, indecision, alternating
Star of Bethlehem	For consolation and comfort in grief, after a fright or sudden alarm
Sweet Chestnut	Unendurable desolation
Vervain	Insistent, wilful, fervent, overstriving, stressed
Vine	Dominating, tyrannical, bullying, demands obedience
Walnut	Protection from outside influences, for change and stages of development
Water Violet	Withdrawn, aloof, proud, self-reliant, quiet grief
White Chestnut	Unresolved, circling thoughts , constant worry
Wild Oat	Lack of direction, unfulfilled, drifting
Wild Rose	Lack of interest, resignation, no love or point in life
Willow	Dissatisfied, bitter, resentful, feeling life is unfair and unjust
Rescue Remedy	For any sudden difficulty or crisis, accidents, and emergencies

CENTAURY
CENTAURIUM ERYTHRAEA

Rescue Remedy is a combination of Cherry Plum, Clematis, Impatiens, Star of Bethlehem, and Rock Rose

Reproduced courtesy of Julian Barnard and the Healing Herbs Company, UK.

Flower Remedies

Flower remedies are made by floating the freshly picked blooms in bowls of spring water and leaving them in sunlight on a cloudless day. In this way, the water is "potentized" by the essence of the flower, which is believed to have entered the liquid. The potentized water is then mixed in fixed proportions with brandy, which acts as a preservative, and stored in a dark glass bottle.

Although there are now many varieties of flower remedies made around the world, most are prepared in this way. Unlike many modern herbal medicines, flower essences do not contain any artificial chemical substances, except for the brandy preservative.

HOW FLOWER REMEDIES WORK

The remedies are normally taken by dropping a few drops of the essence into a small amount of still mineral water. This mixture is then slowly sipped.

Though plant-based, flower remedies are more homeopathic than herbal in the way they are said to work. That is, they work psychologically and psychically at the energy level, rather than chemically. Supporters describe them as "liquid energy" because they believe they encapsulate the flowers' healing energies and present them in a form that can be used therapeutically in the simplest and most effective way.

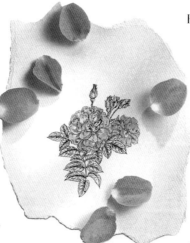

Damask rose *Rosa damascena* is a favorite source for flower remedies.

Flower remedies are said to deal with and overcome negative emotions, and in this way encourage a sense of enhanced personal well-being, which is then extended to physical health through improved powers of self-healing.

There is no accepted research yet to support this idea of a psychic-psychological effect, but flower remedies remain widely popular throughout the world and a large number of people swear by them. The concept behind this therapy is often difficult to grasp, but there are several clinical studies that suggest that the therapy does work on the mental and physical health of clients. Perhaps the most successful and popular example is Bach's Rescue Remedy, which acts as emergency treatment to reduce the effects of trauma and shock after an accident, or in stressful situations, and through that stimulates the healing powers of the body. This remedy has attracted an extraordinary amount of interest from other alternative practitioners and, increasingly, conventional medical doctors.

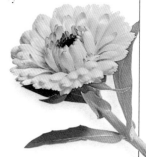

Marigold *Calendula officinalis* is a versatile flower that appears in herbalism, homeopathy, and flower remedy therapies.

CAUTIONS AND CONTRAINDICATIONS

Flower remedies are suitable for people and animals of all ages, and there are no contraindications known.

WHAT CAN FLOWER REMEDIES TREAT?

Treatment with flower remedies is both restorative and gentle, and because they work on the premise that good health is based on emotional balance, most conditions will respond to their use. In particular, the following may benefit from treatment:

- ❧ *nervous disorders*
- ❧ *depression, anxiety, and mood swings*
- ❧ *asthma, eczema, psoriasis, and other deep-seated conditions*
- ❧ *first aid (bruises, bites, burns)*
- ❧ *ME and Aids.*

Spanish broom
Spartium junceum

Choosing and Using Flower Essences

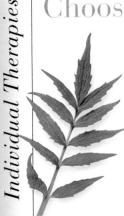

Many naturopaths may prescribe flower essences as part of their treatment, but they are also designed so that they can be safely self-prescribed, or prescribed for others. Simply choose essences whose qualities best describe your particular problem. It could be an emotional upset such as mood swings, a physical weakness such as poor immunity, or a spiritual predicament ("What is the purpose of my life?").

Successful choice is said to depend on being as specific as possible, using just two or three essences at a time. As well as being sipped in a glass of spring water, drops can be taken directly on the tongue or with herb tea. They can also be dropped into a bath.

Valerian Valeriana officinalis *is a well-known sedative.*

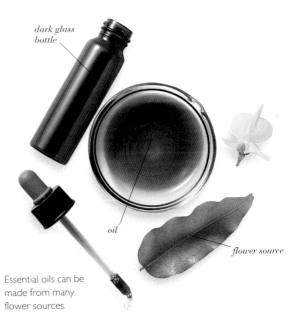

dark glass bottle

oil

flower source

Essential oils can be made from many flower sources.

FLOWER ESSENCES FROM AROUND THE WORLD

Symptom to treat / Essences	Effect
Shock and trauma Star of Bethlehem (Bach) Arnica (FES) Hibiscus (Himalayan Aditi) Fringed violet (Australian Bush)	Soothes after all kinds of unexpected shocks such as receiving bad news, receiving an unexpected tax demand, losing your job, as well as physical shocks such as cutting your finger
Exhaustion Alpine mint bush (Australian Bush) Olive (Bach) Life Force (gorse, elder, sycamore, valerian, grass of Parnassus) (Findhorn)	When emotionally drained, burned out, and apathetic. Restores vitality, enthusiasm, motivation, and joie de vivre
Mood Swings Chamomile (FES) Scleranthus (Bach)	Restores a sense of balance and calm when feeling touchy, tearful, irritable, and restless
Mental Clarity Paw Paw (Australian Bush) Brown Boronia (Australian Living) Madia (Flower Essence Society)	Aids concentration and decision-making when confused, and unable to think clearly, and solve problems because your mind is overwhelmed and befuddled
Stress Black-eyed Susan (Australian) Yellow flag flower (Australian) Impatiens (Bach) Indian Pink (FES)	For when you feel extremely tense, anxious, and unable to cope with the pressure of life. Helps you unwind and relax
Relationship Problems Ixora/Red Hibiscus (Himalayas)	For enhancing compatability between couples, bringing renewed vitality and sexual excitement to relationships
Emotional Pain Violet Butterfly (Australian Living) Bleeding Heart (FES)	Soothes emotional pain and lets you get on with life when shattered by breakups. Good for those going through a separation or divorce
Sadness/Depression Bluebell (Bailey) St. John's wort (FES) Mariposa Lily (FES)	Restores feelings of happiness and optimism in those feeling emotionally low often for no particular reason. Mariposa Lily is especially good for children
Worry White Chestnut (Bach) Filaree (FES)	When everything seems to give cause for concern and distressing thoughts fill your mind, often causing headaches and insomnia
Fear and Panic Rock Rose (Bach) Scottish Primrose/thistle (Findhorn)	Brings courage and inner peace in times when you feel terrified and powerless to control yourself
Confidence Five Corners (Australian Bush) Larch (Bach) Lehua (Hawaii)	Restores faith in yourself at times when you feel inadequate and lack self-esteem. Lehua is especially good for women

ARNICA
ARNICA MONTANA

KEY	Essences	Symptom to treat	Effect

Flower Essences

For many years Bach's flower remedies stood alone, but in the mid-1970s American therapist Richard Katz, looking for ways of dealing with the increasing varieties of stress in people's lives, established the Flower Essence Society in California.

Katz's aim was to research new flower essences and gather together those working with various essences to exchange ideas and information.

The Flower Essence Society now has a database of more than 100 essences from different flowers in more than 50 countries.

The newer flower essences are made from a wide variety of flora, ranging from modest hedgerow and alpine flowers to exotic orchids, antique roses, and the blossoms of fruits such as avocado and banana. Some flowers, especially those native to the Australian "bush," Himalayan mountains, and Hawaii have a long tradition of being used in natural medicine.

The waratah flower from Australia, for example, comes from one of the oldest plant groups in the world, its origins dating back 60 million years to Antarctica. Known by its aboriginal name (meaning beautiful), the waratah is said to be a survival remedy. It is said to embody the Australian bush-dwellers' qualities of adaptation and the ability to cope with all kinds of stress, especially emergencies.

From the foothills of the Blue Ridge Mountains of Virginia comes a family of rose essences that are claimed to help people cope with spiritual issues in their lives. Orchids growing in the Amazon jungle are said to have the same effect.

Tree Remedies

Humans have regarded trees as having healing qualities for centuries, with each species of tree having its own different characteristics. Intuitive people even claim they can sense these energies when walking in woodlands or forests.

Remedies made from the flowers of trees are found in many of the flower essence families. For example, olive, beech, hornbeam, aspen, red chestnut, white chestnut, walnut, pine, elm, larch, and oak, all feature in the Bach flower remedies range. Another range, also from Britain, is the Green Man Essences, also made entirely from tree blossoms.

A slightly different approach was taken in France by healer Patrice Bouchardon. His "energetic tree oils" are created from other parts of the tree as well as the flowers, such as the buds and leaves. He cuts nothing from the tree to make his oils.

Scots pine *Pinus sylvestris* is the source of an important tree remedy.

Instead he dips whatever part of it he wants into a bowl of saline solution to extract the essence, which is then preserved in sesame or sunflower seed oil.

According to Bouchardon, energetic tree oils can be used for bringing out certain positive characteristics within us to promote the process of self-healing. The oils are massaged into specific areas of the body such as the soles of the feet.

FLOWER ESSENCES FROM AROUND THE WORLD

⚘ AFRICA AND THE AMAZON
Andreas Korte Essences

⚘ AUSTRALIA AND NEW ZEALAND
Australian Bush Flower Essences
Living Essences of Australia
New Perception Flower Essences

⚘ BRITAIN
Bach Flower Remedies /Healing
    Herbs Company
Bailey Essences
Findhorn Flower Essences
Green Man Tree Essences
Harebell Remedies

⚘ FRANCE
Deva Flower Elixirs

⚘ INDIA
Himalayan Aditi Flower Essences
Himalayan Flower Enhancers
Himalayan Indian Tree and Flower
    Essences

⚘ USA
Alaskan Flower and Environmental
    Essences
Desert Alchemy Flower Essences
Flower Essence Society
FES and Californian Research
    Essences
Master's Flower Essences
Pegasus Essences
Hawaiian Tropical Flower Essences
Petite Fleur Essences
Perelandra Virginian Rose and
    Garden Essences
Pacific Essences

BOUCHARDON'S NINE ENERGETIC TREE OILS

⚘ TREE	⚘ QUALITY
Birch	Gentleness and reconciliation
Fir	Respiration, fluidity
Hawthorn	Being in the present, finding one's own resources
Beech	Being prepared to go farther
Wild rose	Opening
Pine	Bringing in light, rediscovering one's vitality, and connection with life
Boxwood	Freedom, continuity
Walnut	Responsibility, autonomy
Broom	Renewal

Agrimony
Agrimonia eupatoria

Oriental Therapies ● Acupuncture

ACUPUNCTURE, which originated in China, is a way of adjusting the body's "life energy" (qi or chi) flow. It involves the insertion of fine needles into carefully selected acupuncture points along the meridians (energetic pathways) of the body (*see Acupuncture, page 31*). Points are selected on the basis of pulse and tongue diagnosis, observation, and questioning. The points affect the meridian system. Each meridian has a specific effect on a specific body system or organ of the body. Needles are inserted on the points and then manipulated, either by twirling or by a gentle pumping action. This removes blockages or stimulates energy flow. Stagnant energy can be dispersed and the whole energy flow regulated (too much energy in one area adjusted and too little stimulated). Acupuncture can be used to relieve symptoms as well as to promote general health and well-being.

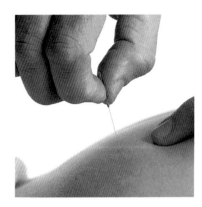

Once in place, the needles are manipulated either by twirling or a gentle pumping action.

RELATED FORMS OF TREATMENT

Moxibustion and cupping are two forms of treatment that are closely related to acupuncture. Both rely on the meridian or channel theory and treat selected points along the meridians. In moxibustion, preparations of the herb moxa (mugwort) are burned close to the skin to have a warming effect. When this is used in conjunction with acupuncture, the moxa is burned on the needles to intensify their effect. Moxa sticks can also be held above the skin and burned. When moxa is burned it becomes extremely hot, and great care is always taken by the practitioner. In cupping, a vacuum is created by burning tapers in purpose-made glass or bamboo cups. The cups are quickly placed on acupuncture points on the body and the vacuum creates suction that draws blood to the surface. Acupuncture is often performed in conjunction with either moxibustion or cupping (*see also pages 30–1*).

Acupuncture needles are made of stainless steel, silver, or gold and are either disposable or rigorously sterilized. The needles vary in diameter and length according to the area of the body where they are to be used. Longer, thicker needles are used in "padded" areas such as the buttocks, and finer, shorter ones where the flesh is thin and close to the bone (as on the forehead). The thinnest are not much thicker than a human hair. The needles are inserted into the skin at varying depths. They are sometimes simply left in place, but usually they are gently manipulated to remove blockages and enhance the flow of chi along the meridians either by lifting the needle, or by rotation, flicking, or stroking.

Acupuncture is one of the most widely practiced and accepted forms of natural medicine in the world today. There are over 500,000 acupuncturists in China, over 50,000 in Japan, over 6,000 in the United States, and around 10,000 in Europe. Acupuncture is used for the relief of common ailments, for the prevention of disease, for health promotion, for anesthesia, for some symptoms of pregnancy, and in childbirth.

WESTERN FORMS

"Scientific acupuncture" is a Western adaptation that rejects the theories underlying Chinese medicine and assumes that in theory acupuncture can be explained in terms of ordinary scientific anatomy and physiology. Tender points have long been known to be associated with pain in relatively distant parts of the body, and massage of these points was known to cure the pain. Acupuncture points are compared to these trigger points.

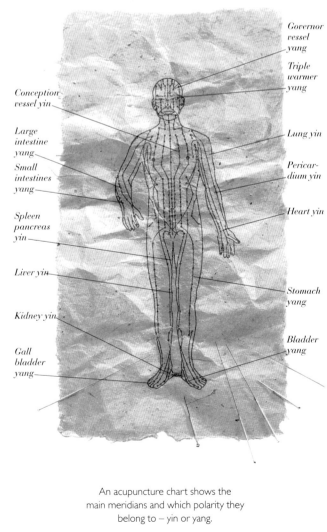

Governor vessel yang

Triple warmer yang

Conception vessel yin

Large intestine yang

Small intestines yang

Spleen pancreas yin

Liver yin

Kidney yin

Gall bladder yang

Lung yin

Pericardium yin

Heart yin

Stomach yang

Bladder yang

An acupuncture chart shows the main meridians and which polarity they belong to – yin or yang.

Acupuncture at Work

All Chinese medicine is a way of keeping people healthy as much as it is a treatment to cure disease. It is often quoted that in Chinese medicine the patient pays the doctor only so long as he or she is well. The doctor would regularly check the patient to spot impending imbalances that, if untreated, could lead to disease. Often only dietary advice or suggestions as to therapeutic forms of exercise would be needed to resolve the problems. If necessary, acupuncture (or herbalism) would be the form of treatment given to adjust energy balance. However, particularly in the West, people often do not seek treatment of any kind until there is something acutely wrong, and often they do not see an acupuncturist until they have been suffering for some time with a chronic problem, which orthodox medicine has been unable to cure. Yet acupuncture is frequently found to alleviate or cure, even in these circumstances. Treatment is thought to improve the functioning of the internal organs and bring the body back into balance.

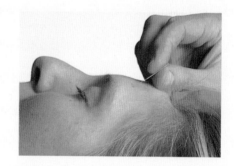

Acupuncture needles rarely draw blood, because their rounded ends let them divide the flesh rather than pierce it.

round-ended needle

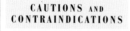

acupuncture point

DIAGNOSIS

Pulse diagnosis is one main form of diagnosis used by the acupuncturist. Visual examination and, especially in the West, "taking the case" are also important. In Traditional Chinese Medicine pulse-taking is a highly refined art, but many Western practitioners take the pulse more simply in much the same way as their orthodox colleagues.

Acupuncture is not necessarily thought to be the most suitable form of treatment in any particular case, although in the West practitioners tend to specialize in either acupuncture or herbalism, so that to some extent the patient chooses the therapy in advance by going to an acupuncturist rather than a herbalist. Some people do not respond well to acupuncture, and in general anyone who is apprehensive about having needles inserted into them is less likely to be suitable for this specific form of treatment.

CAUTIONS AND CONTRAINDICATIONS

Acupuncture can be safely used for most common ailments but should only be practiced by a qualified practitioner. There is no risk of contracting Aids or hepatitis if you consult a registered practitioner who follows correct hygiene and sterilization procedures or uses disposable needles. Care must be taken when treating the chronically sick and the elderly.

WHAT CAN ACUPUNCTURE TREAT?

Acupuncture is rarely used in the treatment of infectious diseases and is never performed on a person who is suffering from a high fever or is under the influence of alcohol or nonmedicinal drugs. Some of the conditions that acupuncture can help are

- *respiratory problems*
- *arthritis and rheumatism*
- *headaches and migraine*
- *insomnia and back pain*
- *urinary infections*
- *menstrual imbalances*
- *sinusitis*
- *tinnitus* (ringing in the ears)
- *eye problems*
- *allergies*
- *digestive disturbance*
- *palpitation and anxiety*
- *mental and emotional problems*
- *morning sickness and labor pains*
- *childhood illnesses.*

Auricular Therapy

Acupuncture points on the external ear can be used to treat disease, relieve pain, and promote anesthesia. The technique is over 1,000 years old but has been further developed in both France and China in recent years.

Points are located in the ear by pressing with a fine, blunt instrument to locate sensitive spots or by using an electrical sensor to find points that have a low resistance to electricity.

The point is then stimulated either electrically or with small conventional needles. The needles are kept in for about 15 minutes and manipulated every now and then. Alternatively, a small ring-needle or seed may be fixed to the point in the ear and retained for several days, providing continuous treatment lasting for a short period of time. These are held in place with small patches of adhesive bandage. The needles work in the same way as traditional acupuncture, but the seed operates more as a mild form of acupressure.

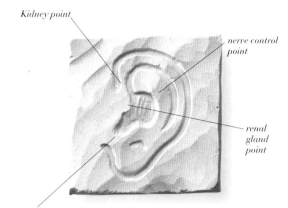

Kidney point

nerve control point

renal gland point

Gall Bladder point

The outer flaps of the ear contain over 120 acupuncture points. Many diseases can be treated by simply applying acupuncture to the ears alone. The spot in the center of the fleshy part of the ear lobe is used to treat eye problems.

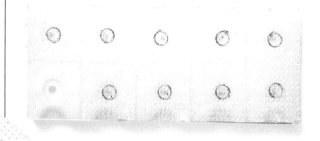

Special press needles are stuck onto the relevant point on the ear with small patches of adhesive bandages so that they stay in place for a week or more.

Since there are over 120 points on each ear, they are very close together and, therefore, it is very important that they are located exactly in order for the treatment to be effective.

During treatment a dull or tingling sensation is generally felt in the ear, and sensation may also be felt in the affected part of the body.

Ear acupuncture is based on the idea that each part of the ear is a mirror of the body as a whole. There are, for example, Kidney meridian points on the ear. As a result almost any ailment can be treated with ear acupuncture. Sometimes it is used together with body acupuncture, but some practitioners use ear acupuncture on its own for diagnosis and treatment.

WHAT CAN AURICULAR THERAPY TREAT?

Traditionally, auricular therapy is used for addictions and for pain control (during labor, or in terminal illness, for example). Today, its use has been expanded to include

- *respiratory disorders*
- *local injuries*
- *musculoskeletal problems*
- *headaches, migraines, and sinus problems*
- *overall imbalances causing long-term illness such as arthritis, gastrointestinal conditions, and skin problems.*

CAUTIONS AND CONTRAINDICATIONS

Because this therapy can be noninvasive and adapted to suit the age and health of the sufferer, it is safe for most people. It is still, however, considered to be unproved in the West, and it is advised that you consult your physician before undergoing treatment.

Auricular acupuncture allows needles to be left in for long periods. These needles are being stimulated electrically.

Modern Acupuncture

Although acupuncture is believed to have been practiced in China for as long as 5,000 years, it is a recent introduction in the West. It was first introduced into Britain at the end of the 18th century, when it was initially taken very seriously by the medical profession. In 1827 there was a fully reported case of a man having been cured of dropsy by the method at the Royal Infirmary of Edinburgh, and in the same year the medical journal the *Lancet* reported the results of a long-term trial in which more than 100 patients with rheumatism had been successfully treated at St. Thomas's Hospital, London. But as scientific medicine rapidly developed, acupuncture soon fell into decline and came to be derided.

TWENTIETH-CENTURY DEVELOPMENTS

In France interest in acupuncture developed at the end of the 19th century, and in 1928 the returning French consul to China, who had translated many treatises on the subject from Chinese into French, fostered a great interest in the subject. Ever since that time it has been a recognized method of treatment in France.

It was not until 1958 that it was discovered, in China, that acupuncture could be effective as an anesthetic and operations began to be performed using this method. East–West relations improved in the 1970s, and President Richard Nixon visited China with three of his physicians, who were able to observe acupuncture in action.

In the last decade or so there has been much research into acupuncture in both East and West. Early studies aimed to verify the existence of the meridians and acupoints and to determine how the therapy works. One theory suggested that acupuncture activates "pain barriers" in the nervous system. Other research has suggested that during acupuncture the brain releases endorphins, chemicals that naturally reduce pain and enhance the feeling of well-being.

The World Health Organization has recognized the value of acupuncture for treating around 100 common ailments, and it is increasingly being incorporated into Western healthcare systems.

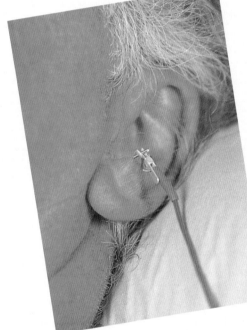

Modern ideas in acupuncture include electrical acupuncture, in which needles are vibrated by a weak electrical current.

WESTERN FORMS OF PRACTICE

Traditionally, acupuncture has always been performed by hand, with the practitioner developing sensitivity in the hands and fingertips for both diagnosis and needle manipulation. In recent years, however, many "hands-off" types of treatment have been developed using electrical or laser stimulation of the acupuncture points.

In the West, especially in Germany, a number of electroacupuncture measuring devices have been developed that claim to measure precisely the amount of electrical energy in each of the meridians and determine appropriate points for treatment. 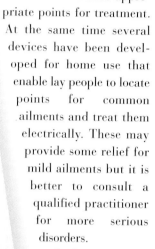 At the same time several devices have been developed for home use that enable lay people to locate points for common ailments and treat them electrically. These may provide some relief for mild ailments but it is better to consult a qualified practitioner for more serious disorders.

In Japan a form of electroacupuncture known as "Ryodoraku" is quite popular and it has already been adopted by some Western acupuncturists. The procedure involves attaching small clips to the needles after they have been inserted and passing a small electrical current through them. A tingling sensation is felt around the point, and the electrical stimulation is said to remove blockages and promote circulation in the tissues. This technique is effective for pain relief.

More recently some acupuncturists have experimented with innovations such as stimulating the acupuncture points with light, sound, and plant essences. Laser therapy is also becoming popular and is applied by means of a laser pen or "gun" that emits a laser beam directly into the acupuncture point. This is thought to promote rapid healing and is popular with some medically trained acupuncturists, but traditional acupuncturists still prefer to use their hands and senses rather than machines.

Acupressure

CUPRESSURE is thought to be one of the oldest healing traditions in the world, pre-dating even acupuncture. The Chinese are credited with having discovered that pressure on specific points of the body could relieve common ailments and discomforts. As far back as 300 B.C. there is mention of acupressure in Chinese medical texts, and it came to be widely adopted as a self-help and first aid technique for lay people, as well as an important part of massage therapy for professional physicians.

Acupressure is based on the same concepts of meridians and acupoints as acupuncture, but fingertip pressure is used rather than needles *(see Acupuncture/Acupressure, page 31).* The aim is also the same, namely to balance the flow of energy within the meridians, thereby creating healthy functioning of the internal organs and preventing or curing disease.

Massage on the acupressure points 1 ½ in/3.5cm either side of the spine in the small of the back will ease pain in the lumbar region.

adjunct to treatment by professionals. In some cases the effects may be immediate, such as acupressure applied to points at the base of the nostrils that can clear a blocked nose almost instantaneously. In other cases, the results may be slower, since acupressure can be used on a daily basis to treat more chronic conditions.

HOW CAN ACUPRESSURE HELP?

Acupressure can be used to relieve common ailments such as headaches, back pain, fatigue, constipation, and so on. It is also useful for prevention of illness and for first aid, for example, in the case of asthma where it has been known to reduce the frequency and decrease the severity of attacks.

To be most effective it has to be repeated little and often and be used on a daily basis.

THE PRACTICE OF ACUPRESSURE

An acupressure practitioner has to learn how to locate the acupoints accurately and to determine the correct ones to use for different ailments. Gentle pressure is applied using the tips of the index or middle fingers, or the thumb, or the edge of the nail. Pressure must be even and is generally applied in the direction of flow of the meridian.

Small rotations may be used to stimulate the flow of energy within the meridian and promote circulation. Alternatively pressure may be applied using small wooden sticks with rounded ends for single acupoints or rollers for covering several points at once, say on the back.

Treatment lasts from half a minute for small babies to several minutes for adults. The acupoints are massaged on both sides of the body, and the procedure is repeated several times during the day. Acupressure is safe and easy to perform and can be used as a self-help therapy as well as an

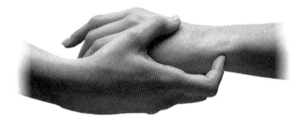

Acupressure can be self-administered. Massaging on this point on the forearm can relieve nausea and motion sickness.

CAUTIONS AND CONTRAINDICATIONS

Some physicians believe that acupressure may mask symptoms of serious disease, such as cancer. Ensure that your acupressurist is aware of any health problems, any medication you are taking, and pregnancy, since treatment will be altered accordingly. Consult your physician before undergoing treatment.

WHAT CAN ACUPRESSURE TREAT?

cupressure can be used to relieve many common ailments or conditions such as:

- headaches
- back pain
- constipation
- asthma
- fatigue.

It is also useful in first aid.

Other Forms of Acupressure

As acupressure has increased in popularity, it has been synthesized with other approaches to create new traditions. Acuyoga combines acupressure with yoga exercises, while Shen Tao, developed in recent years by practitioners at the Middle Piccadilly Healing Centre in Britain, combines acupressure with an understanding of the subtle energetic body.

The ancient Japanese system of Do In, or exercises for physical and spiritual development, is enjoying a revival and incorporates acupressure with breathing exercises, stretches, and meditational exercises for health of body, mind, and spirit. An indication of how a Do In facial massage is performed is given below.

Jin Shen and Jin Shen Do, developed in the United States, use prolonged massage (several minutes) on acupoints together with other therapeutic techniques to obtain good results.

Acupressure has links with Western massage systems such as reflexology *(see pages 52–3)* and is an important part of Japanese shiatsu therapy *(see pages 96–7).*

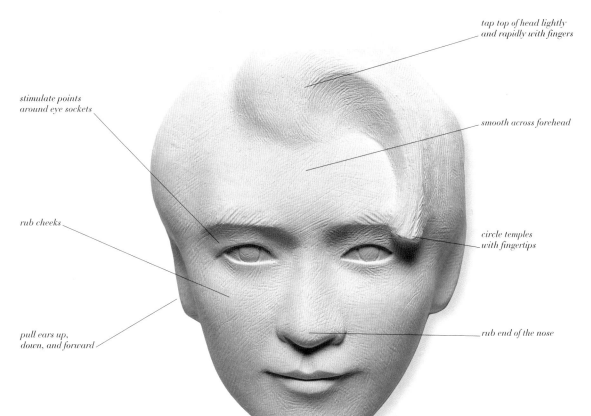

tap top of head lightly and rapidly with fingers

stimulate points around eye sockets

smooth across forehead

rub cheeks

circle temples with fingertips

pull ears up, down, and forward

rub end of the nose

pinch along the lower jaw

A gentle Do In facial massage can help you start the day refreshed and renewed. It stimulates circulation and drains the toxins from the lymph glands.

SHEN TAO

Shen Tao combines the spiritual concepts of Taoism, the philosophy that underlies the soft martial arts, with the techniques of acupressure. Shen means spirit or mind.

DO IN

Do In is a form of self-shiatsu treatment consisting of gentle stretching exercises. A Do In session makes a good start to the day.

TSUBO

Tsubo therapy is concerned with the acupressure points themselves, the Tsubo, and the various methods that there are to stimulate them, either by massage, with needles, or electrically.

SHIATSU

Shiatsu is Japanese for finger massage; it uses the meridians and pressure points of acupressure, but employs different techniques to stimulate or massage them.

Shiatsu

The term "shiatsu" means "finger pressure" and is the name of an ancient and widely practiced form of Oriental massage. It dates back thousands of years to the massage systems developed in ancient China that were brought to Japan, then gradually changed, and developed into separate therapies.

Shiatsu is based on the same principles as acupuncture and aims to restore a balanced flow of energy within the meridians and to enhance vitality and well-being. However, it does not rely solely on acupressure or massage techniques but also incorporates elements from physiotherapy, osteopathy, and from other forms of healing tradition.

HOW IT IS PERFORMED

Shiatsu is usually practiced on a mat on the floor and is performed through clothing so there is no need to undress. Diagnosis is made by pulse-taking, questioning, and palpating the abdomen to determine areas of strength and weakness in the internal organs and the meridian system.

Pressure is applied to individual acupoints and along meridian lines using the fingertips, thumbs, knuckles, elbows, or knees as appropriate. In some forms of shiatsu, the practitioners use their feet. In this way specific points or whole areas of the body may be treated. Some areas of the body may feel sensitive, or even painful, to the touch but this soon eases as the course of treatment progresses.

in shiatsu it is important that the therapist is as comfortable as possible so that they are able to "feel" and treat the patient

client may be treated lying on her front (prone), back (supine) or on her side, a good position for pregnant women or people with neck problems

BASIC SHIATSU TREATMENT

1 Arm rotation is used to relax, open, and stretch joints. This facilitates meridian work and gives the practitioner insight into the patient's overall relaxation picture.

2 The stomach meridian is worked on with the fingertips. This is zen shiatsu; there is no stimulation with rotating thumbs, but sustained stationary pressure.

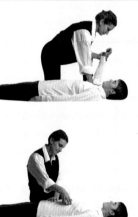

3 One leg is bent so that its toe rests beside the ankle bone of the straight leg. This is the Spleen channel stretch. The Spleen channel is then worked on with the palms.

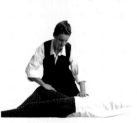

the pressure depends on what the therapist feels, but will probably need to be less when working on the face than on the legs

work may be done with fingers, palms, knuckles, or elbows

CAUTIONS AND CONTRAINDICATIONS

Shiatsu should not be performed directly after eating or on anyone with a high fever or an infectious disease. Techniques are not applied to areas of inflammation, wounds, or scar tissue. Caution is also needed when treating sufferers of cancer or heart disease, the elderly, or frail. In these cases only the gentle, holding techniques may be used, not the more vigorous ones.

Much of the pressure applied in shiatsu is sustained and stationary, rather than vigorous and moving, and it is this unique holding and supportive touch that enables the muscles and soft tissues to relax.

Body stretches are used to release muscular tension and to promote relaxation. In this process, the breathing of both practitioner and recipient is important. Various gentle manipulation techniques may also be used to improve the mobility of the joints.

SHIATSU TREATMENT

Treatment lasts between 60 and 90 minutes and is deeply relaxing. The treatment is holistic in nature, aiming to balance the body as a whole rather than just treat specific symptoms. At the end of a session you feel invigorated and refreshed, as if no part of the body has been left out.

One of the maxims of shiatsu is that "diagnosis is treatment and treatment is diagnosis" since every touch has an effect on the body and also gives information to the practitioner. In this way shiatsu can be used simply for relaxation but can also be effective in treating a wide range of common ailments.

WHAT AILMENTS CAN SHIATSU TREAT?

Shiatsu reduces stress and calms the nervous system. It boosts stamina and improves digestion, menstrual function, concentration, and mental state. It promotes better posture and helps relieve back and neck pain. It enhances body awareness and creates a feeling of well-being.

SHIATSU TODAY

Shiatsu is practiced widely in Japan by both acupuncturists and those trained only in massage and acupressure. In the West it is also enjoying an upsurge in popularity as people come to realize the importance of stress-release and of taking responsibility for promoting and maintaining their own health.

Shiatsu treatment can leave you relaxed, invigorated, and refreshed.

Environmental Therapies • Clinical Ecology

THE BELIEF that our environment can affect our health is not new. Hippocrates, the ancient Greek father of modern medicine (today's physicians still respect the Hippocratic Oath even if they no longer take it), recorded the beneficial and harmful effects of certain foods in the 5th century B.C.

Today our bodies face a daily assault undreamed of by the ancient Greeks: our crops are sprayed with pesticides, our food is packed with preservatives, and the air we breathe is often full of gasoline fumes and pollution.

The overall effect on our bodies is a weakened immune system that makes us even more susceptible to allergies and sensitivities. Air pollution is one of the worst problems, caused by industries, agriculture, power stations, aerosols and other chemicals, coal and other fires. As a result we suffer from headaches, respiratory tract infections and ailments, asthma, bronchitis, emphysema, eye problems, and eventually a profound breakdown in health manifested by

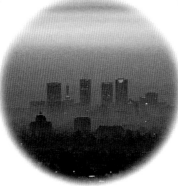

The thick belt of smog that hovers on the Los Angeles skyline demonstrates the power of the car to pollute the atmosphere.

various cancers. Other environmental hazards include lead from gasoline – which causes hyperactivity and birth defects – acid rain, carbon monoxide poisoning, water pollution, and radiation.

Clinical ecologists treat illnesses and disorders that they believe stem from an individual's reaction to these environmental factors. They practice what is known as environmental medicine, and they estimate that between 10 and 30 percent of the population suffer from some form of ecological illness.

Clinical ecologists believe that foods are still the most common environmental factors causing illness. They identify the particular foods or chemicals to which an individual is sensitive and advise on treatment. The simplest treatment is to avoid the foods and chemicals that cause problems. However, people are often sensitive to several different substances. If these are foods, removing them all from the diet could lead to nutritional problems; if the sensitivity is to a very common environmental pollutant, or to a chemical with which an individual works, it may be practically impossible to avoid. In this case treatment concentrates on desensitizing the individual.

Desensitization involves diluting the troublesome foods or chemicals and placing drops of the solution under the tongue. Solutions of varying strengths are used until a tolerance level is established. Then it will usually be possible to withstand limited exposure to the harmful food or chemicals.

CAUTIONS AND CONTRAINDICATIONS

Desensitization is not appropriate for many people; consult your physician before undergoing treatment. Nutritional imbalances and deficiency can result from dietary changes, so it is essential that you seek dietary advice before altering your diet in any way.

The graph plots the rise of carbon dioxide emissions from car exhausts and factories.

RISE IN POLLUTION

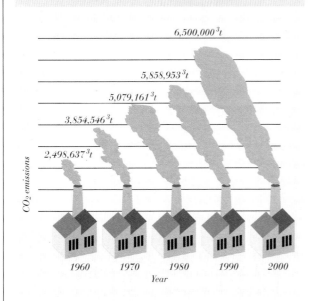

$6,500,000^3t$

$5,858,953^3t$

$5,079,161^3t$

$3,854,546^3t$

$2,498,637^3t$

CO_2 emissions

1960   1970   1980   1990   2000

Year

WHAT CAN ENVIRONMENTAL THERAPIES TREAT?

Environmental stresses manifest themselves in all kinds of ill-health, and therefore, by removing them from our daily lifestyles, many long-term and acute conditions can be resolved. Environmental therapies are, perhaps, most useful in treating

- allergies
- headaches, migraine, general aches and pains
- hyperactivity and sleep problems
- infertility
- asthma, eczema, and psoriasis
- digestive disorders.

ALLERGY TESTING METHODS

ELIMINATION DIET *It is only after troublesome substances in everyday life are eliminated from the diet and then reintroduced that a reaction is seen. First the individual spends at least five days on a diet unlikely to cause adverse reactions and then foods suspected of being harmful are reintroduced one by one.*

CYTOTOXIC TESTING *Here a blood sample is taken and tested by introducing concentrates of suspected substances. Changes in the white blood cells can be seen in people who are sensitive. However, the test often shows people to be sensitive to so many substances that understanding the results can be difficult even for a skilled practitioner.*

INTRADERMAL TESTING *Suspect substances are diluted and tiny amounts injected under the skin. Adverse reaction should occur within three hours.*

HAIR MINERAL ANALYSIS *The hair is tested for toxic metals and other potentially harmful substances.*

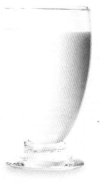

Milk and dairy products are common allergenics.

SUBLINGUAL DROP TESTING *The individual takes only fluids for five days. Then a drop of solution containing a suspected substance is placed under the tongue to test for adverse reaction.*

AURICULAR CARDIAC REFLEX (ACR) *Practitioners check for changes in the client's pulse when food or chemicals suspected of being harmful are placed within the body's electrical field.*

ELECTRICAL TESTING *A weak electrical current is passed into the client's body through an acupuncture point, often at the tip of the toe, and an electrical reading is taken over that point. A glass jar containing a suspected substance is then linked into the electrical circuit. If the individual is sensitive to the contents of the jar, the electrical reading will change.*

KINESIOLOGY (OR APPLIED KINESIOLOGY) *This works on the theory that foods or chemicals to which an individual is sensitive cause muscle weakening as a result of changing the body's electrical field. Practitioners place suspect substances in the hand or under the tongue and then check for muscle weakening.*

Eggs often trigger allergic responses in asthmatics who also have eczema.

dust or pollen enters the nasal passage

mucous membranes become inflamed and irritated

a bout of sneezing as the body tries to get rid of the invader

Sneezing is one way of expelling pollutants from the body. Sneezing can be an allergic response to pollen.

Individual Therapies

Geopathic therapy

The earth's magnetic field generates powerful unseen energy forces that have been recognized for thousands of years. These earth energies were probably easier to detect in the preindustrial age, and it is thought that ancient cultures sited their standing stone circles on sites where the earth's energy could be felt particularly strongly. Not all natural energies are beneficial; for example, granite rock strata emit the noxious gas radon. Other negative energies emanate from the earth and artificial contributions include the local electrical fields generated by power cables.

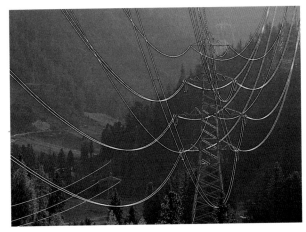

The electromagnetic field generated around pylons has caused headaches, nausea, and general debility in the unfortunate people who live near or underneath them.

Prolonged exposure to these energies – a condition known as geopathic stress – contributes to illness and general debility by weakening the body's defenses against disease and potentially harmful substances in the environment.

WHAT CAN GEOPATHIC MEDICINE TREAT?

Any health condition may be caused by negative energy, and therefore avoiding areas of negative energy may be useful in treating conditions that have suddenly cropped up (acute) or deep-seated problems that seem impossible to shift. In particular, geopathic medicine might be useful for:

- *headaches and migraine*
- *digestive problems*
- *sleep disorders*
- *anxiety and depression.*

In Chinese culture, the effect of earth energies on health and well-being has long been recognized. The discipline known as feng shui aims to modify the flow of energy to produce a balance by making subtle alterations to the landscape. In the West, the importance of earth energies was rediscovered in the 1930s. Even so, the bad effects of negative energies are only just being recognized today.

Geopathic therapy aims to relieve geopathic stress. Practitioners detect these negative energies either by dowsing (using a pendulum or rods), or with kinesiology *(see page 20)*, or by "sensing" or "seeing" them. They then advise on how best to avoid these energies. This may be by moving a bed or a favorite chair away from an affected area, by deflecting the energies with mirrors, or by trapping them in crystals or coils that can then be washed clean.

FENG SHUI

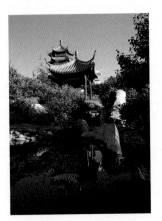

Feng shui in the West; a pagoda in Australia.

Feng shui is the ancient Chinese art of balancing energies by integrating people, buildings, and landscape to create a harmonious whole. Only when balance and harmony are achieved can the chi, the energy or life force of the universe, flow freely, resulting in good health, happiness, and prosperity. In Chinese culture this is taken very seriously and alterations to existing buildings or the construction of new ones are only undertaken after consultations with a feng shui expert. Correcting bad feng shui is considered as much a part of the healing process as prescribing herbs or applying acupuncture or acupressure.

Magnetic or Electromagnetic Therapy

Although the earth forces discussed on page 100 are potentially harmful, magnetic or electromagnetic therapy shows how, in skilled hands, they can be used to help heal the human body. This therapy involves the use of magnetic and electromagnetic force fields to treat a variety of disorders.

In some cases small magnets are attached to various parts of the body, and in others a magnetic field, generated by electricity, is directed onto the individual. The force field makes muscles relax and encourages blood to flow, thereby reducing inflammation and encouraging the healing of tissue and bone.

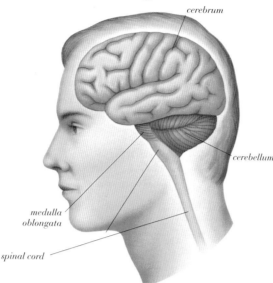

cerebrum

cerebellum

medulla oblongata

spinal cord

The brain (above) is sensitive to electromagnetic fields, such as infrared and ultraviolet waves (below), and may respond to changes in the field outside.

CAUTIONS AND CONTRAINDICATIONS

Magnetic therapy is appropriate for most people, although it is advised that you consult your physician before undertaking any treatment.

METHODS

Two methods are used: the "static" and the "pulsed" techniques. In the static technique, magnets are sewn into a belt or bandage that is worn over the affected area. In the pulsed method, a machine is used to direct an alternating electromagnetic field at the patient.

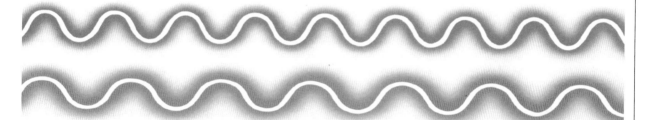

WHAT CAN MAGNETIC OR ELECTRO-MAGNETIC THERAPY TREAT?

Although it is not known which method is the most effective, both have achieved good results in the treatment of back pain, especially where there is muscle spasm. Practitioners also say that magnetic and electromagnetic therapy help prolong the beneficial effects of other natural therapy treatments, such as manipulation and acupuncture.

Magnetic and electromagnetic therapy are reported to be helpful for the following conditions:

- neck and shoulder pain
- sciatica
- lumbago
- joint pain
- torticollis (wryneck)
- rheumatic pain
- whiplash
- fibrositis
- tendonitis
- severe bruising.

TRANSCUTANEOUS NERVE STIMULATION (TENS OR TNS)

This is a method of noninvasive pain relief. Several small pads containing electrodes are taped onto the skin at various points. A low-voltage pulsating electrical current is then passed through them. The technique is believed to work either by blocking the pain pathways to and from the affected nerve endings, or by stimulating the release of endorphins, the body's natural painkilling chemicals.

TENS is considered particularly effective for:

- back pain
- labor pain
- sciatica
- ankle pain
- neuralgia.

Individual Therapies

PSYCHOLOGICAL THERAPIES

JUST LIKE the human body, the human mind is always striving to maintain its health, and the many modern forms of psychological therapy, or "psychotherapies," aim to stimulate and support this process. Traditionally, compassionate personal interaction in soothing surroundings has been used to heal the mind. Alongside this, however, was often harsh treatment for the deranged, who were thought to have been touched by evil, struck down by the gods, or affected by the moon.

A new era dawned in Europe at the beginning of the 20th century with the development of complex and effective therapies reflecting Oriental wisdom.

THE MIND-BODY RELATIONSHIP
The complex relationship between the mind and body has now been acknowledged, and there is strong evidence that many illnesses are caused and exacerbated by psychological factors. All complementary therapies promote the idea of the body as a whole, and promote the idea of treating it "holistically" as a result. Psychological influences, such as stress, worry, depression, and anxiety have an enormous impact on health and are implicated in a number of conditions, including migraine, eczema, asthma, digestive disorders, headaches, and vision problems. Psychological therapies aim to address the parts of the body that some Western medicine has yet to reach successfully – the mind and the sense of well-being necessary to good health.

HEALING THE MIND
What can psychotherapy achieve? By working together, the therapist and the client can transform a problem into a turning point: the beginning of something better. It is done by using any of a variety of methods, usually classified as follows:

BEHAVIORAL Introduced at the beginning of the 20th century and based on learning theories, behavioral psychology aims to predict and control behavior in a scientific way. Cognitive therapy, which developed in the 1960s, is concerned with perception and belief systems: changing the way we view things can change their outcome.

ANALYTICAL Instituted at the end of the 19th century and now comprising many variations (including psychodynamic), analytical theory regards a person's mindset as the outcome of conflict between internal forces and seeks answers from the unconscious. It aims to uncover and analyze the effects of early experience on present difficulties and to look at ways of working to resolve early blocks.

HUMANISTIC This optimistic view emphasizes the essential goodness of human beings and the belief that we all have choices. To realize our full potential we need to get in touch with our inner selves and true feelings, and to be able to express them freely. The attitude of the therapist in achieving and conveying understanding from a position of equality is critical.

INTEGRATIVE Most therapists who work in this way have a humanistic orientation but also use elements of other therapeutic disciplines. Its ruling principle is the integration of "mind, body, and soul" to constitute one whole, aware person.

SPECIAL NOTE Most of the therapies in this section are subtle and complex, and rely on the competence of a trained therapist to be properly effective. This applies particularly to the various psychotherapies and to hypnotherapy.

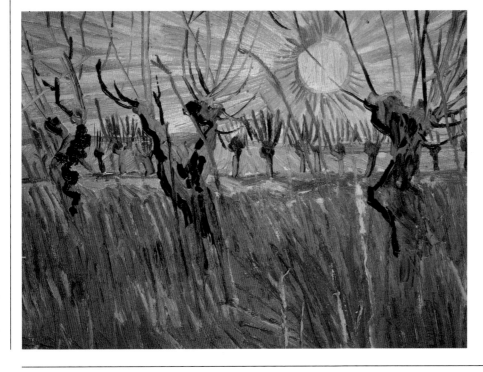

Vincent van Gogh (1853–90), the great Dutch artist, found relief for his tortured feelings in his paintings, many of which can be read as depictions of his inner landscape.

Psychotherapy and Counseling

COUNSELING provides a focused and relatively quick way for clients to review, understand, and sort out their problems.

Talking about problems is an essential part of accepting them, coping with them, and then moving on. In the past, the family unit was larger and tended to stay together; whole networks of relatives across the generations were able to provide a supportive framework. Young mothers were not left on their own, men returning from work had someone to whom they could talk, and the burden of running a household was shared. Priests offered a listening ear to a community, and the local church was a much more social activity. Today, with increased financial pressures and expectations, as well as a smaller family unit, many people find themselves virtually alone. The carefully structured network of friends, family, and fellow parishioners no longer exists to the same extent that it once did. Families have become isolated units, and urban living has resulted in communities where people do not even know their neighbors. Environmental and social factors make modern-day living more stressful than ever, but there are fewer and fewer releases available.

The result is that people are unable to express emotions on a daily level; they bottle up their feelings, causing stress- and anxiety-related symptoms and illnesses. Supportive counseling offers a chance to release the emotions, by talking to someone who will be compassionate and practical, and who will above all listen. Counseling is not a new idea, but it has a new role as the pressures within society increase. Indeed, it has come to be recognized as crucial in the treatment of many conditions, including chronic medical problems, serious abuse, and long-term distress, such as that which is the result of involvement in large-scale disasters and traumas for both victim and observer.

The most immediate effect of good counseling is the gratifying experience for the client of being heard fully, maybe for the first time. This generally leads on to the relieved disclosure of present or long-term difficulties, and possibly also of hitherto unrecognized feelings. The client finds that with increased self-knowledge and understanding, changes in perception and behavior become possible.

In most counseling therapies, patients enjoy a one-to-one session with plenty of time to explore their feelings.

Once the situation has become clear, the work of counselor and client may then involve the setting of specific goals within a plan of action, to be implemented with support from the counselor. Alternatively, it may be directed toward the long-term future – toward achieving greater flexibility, resilience, and strength, along with an improved repertoire of responses in relating to other people or to new situations which may occur.

TYPES OF COUNSELING

PROBLEM-FOCUSED COUNSELING This provides help in overcoming and learning to cope with a specific problem. It is usually a short-term therapy only.

DEVELOPMENTAL COUNSELING This centers on the individual rather than on problems. It aims at altering the client's attitude toward self and toward life, and is often a long-term procedure.

CO-COUNSELING In this type of counseling both client and counselor take turns to act as counselor. By listening and responding to the counselor-as-client for half the session, the client learns about his or her own emotions and mental processes.

PROBLEMS THAT CAN BE HELPED BY COUNSELING

Counseling can be effective in helping people deal with decision-making (particularly professional or career decisions); a crisis or sudden overwhelming change, such as the unexpected breakup of a marriage; post-traumatic stress, where a person is beginning the process of recovery from a deeply shocking experience.

eye contact

relaxed body language to make patient feel nurtured

The Humanistic Movement

The return of shell-shocked and battle-weary troops after World War II prompted the development of humanistic psychotherapy. It was recognized, largely for the first time, that the horrors of war might leave psychological damage that needed help to mend.

Humanistic psychotherapy grew out of a general rejection of old values and authoritarian constraints after World War II. It may be described as optimistic in that it assumes the achievability of transformation in behavior, attitudes, and beliefs. It embodies the view that everyone has an innate tendency to goodness and self-realization. But such a positive tendency may be negated if we become overconcerned with the evaluations and expectations of others, or if our personal and social needs are not met. Humanistic thinking emphasizes the subjectivity of our experiences and our continual freedom to choose how our lives should be; it rebuts the notion that we are controlled by our environment or involuntary internal impulses.

Humanist psychotherapy is aimed at the growth of the individual, and there is more emphasis on personal feelings, well-being, and the response to the immediate environment than on science and sociology. Humanistic psychotherapy has few overall principles and its implementation is very personal. Treatment is undertaken through the development of self-knowledge, and this approach discards the philosophy of the behaviorists who made psychology more scientific and based on more inflexible principles. Each "client" is encouraged to discuss their own characteristics and interpretation of the world around them, and, through this exchange, learns to communicate and feel better about themselves.

Two American psychologists pioneered the idea of the humanist movement – Carl Rogers and Abraham Maslow believed that counseling had to be individual to work and that set ideas and ideologies were irrelevant across the population as a whole. They believed that if clients are encouraged to discuss themselves, they will learn to develop an understanding of situations and how to deal with them. Rogerian therapy grew from this idea, exploring the idea of self-value and teaching people to take charge of their lives. Maslow aimed his theories at self-fulfillment and self-development, based on a list of characteristics that he deemed to be essential to this, which included everything from basic needs like food and water, to love and affection. Today, the humanist therapies are widely used for people with emotional problems.

HOW CAN HUMANISTIC PSYCHOTHERAPY HELP?

Therapists aim to be genuine, to offer unconditional positive regard and focused empathetic understanding. They try in addition to create conditions in which clients can perceive their own motives, assume responsibility for themselves, apprehend the possibilities that exist, and set their own goals.

Existential humanistic psychology believes we create our own worlds, and that what matters is not what we have been but what we are now and what we can become. Existentialists are willing to examine such problematic issues as death, meaninglessness, isolation, and responsibility. They believe it is necessary for us all to question basic assumptions, to face up to our limitations, and to look out for and take advantage of all the possibilities, in order to be fully alive.

Sometimes despair can make us want to hide away from the world. Therapy can help people in despair discover that they can control their lives and solve their own problems.

Jung and Analytical Psychology

Carl Gustav Jung was born in Kesswil, Switzerland in 1875. His concept of "the collective unconscious" may be said to have cast new light on how the world works, and on how the humans in it live and move. Jung was both a friend and follower of Freud, and from 1907 became a devotee of his psychoanalytical theories and a member of a psychoanalytical society created by Freud and his followers. While Freud explained psychological symptoms mainly in terms of repressed infantile sexuality, Jung reached out rather more optimistically, as much forward as backward, into the lives of his clients. Jung eventually rejected Freud's idea that sexual experiences during infancy are the principal cause of neurotic behavior in adults. He believed that Freud overemphasized the role of sexual drive. He developed an alternative theory of the libido, arguing that the will to live was stronger than the sexual drive. Jung also emphasized analysis of current problems, rather than childhood conflicts, in the treatment of adults. In 1912, he resigned from Freud's society and founded his own school of psychology in Zurich.

Jung believed in psychological growth, or "individuation," powered by an innate drive to wholeness. Within this context, neuroses have a positive aim and constructive elements that represent attempts at growth, so it is as vital to elucidate their meaning and lessons as to know their origins.

He considered that at each stage of our lives we progress to deal with different aspects of our development, and that in later years cultural and spiritual needs become paramount.

He classified personalities into two types – introvert and extrovert – and developed a unique theory of the unconscious mind, in which he argued that there were both personal, or individual, and inherited or collected elements.

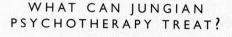

WHAT CAN JUNGIAN PSYCHOTHERAPY TREAT?

Jungian psychotherapy can resolve many psychological conditions, and because the mind-body relationship is so strong, many physical conditions will also respond.

Treatment is most suitable for:

- *anxiety, depression, and other psychological disorders*
- *neurological problems*
- *stress and stress-related disorders.*

CAUTIONS AND CONTRAINDICATIONS

There are no contraindications to Jungian psychotherapy, but it is essential that all treatment is undertaken by a registered, qualified professional.

Carl Gustav Jung, the progenitor of the collective unconscious, drew attention to the significance of our dreams and their meanings.

DREAMWORK

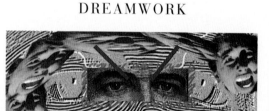

Imagination and dreaming both manifest at the borders of the conscious and unconscious, and provide rich insights into what has happened, what we truly feel, and how we may go forward from where we are now.

The material of fairy stories and myths, primordial images of archetypal figures (such as the Great Mother), and the riches of the collective unconscious – seen as a repository of the whole spiritual heritage of human evolution – may all be used in our dreams to access and process our past and present experiences.

Dreamwork requires accurate dream recall so that, later, in a state of repose, it is possible to "reenter" the dream and continue the experience in "active imagination."

Working with dreams is all part of the search for meaning within ourselves, and for our place in the cosmos. Through dreamwork we can integrate opposing aspects within ourselves, especially any we may seek to deny – male and female, introvert and extrovert, goodness and the dark side of our nature, which it is dangerous to disown.

Bioenergetics

Bioenergetic therapies are based on the concept of the essential involvement of the body in personal development. They stem from the work of Wilhelm Reich during the 1930s and '40s, in Austria and the United States. He was fascinated by the flow of energy through the body and wanted to find out why it became blocked and how to release it.

Reich (and others whose work developed in various ways from his) believed that tensing our muscles is a natural way to defend ourselves against unendurable mental pain, in particular the fear of losing the love of our protectors by displaying unacceptable emotions. Painful experience is split off from the conscious and kept separate by physical "armoring," which also affects our breathing rhythms.

Wilhelm Reich (1897–1957), inspirer of bioenergetics.

HOW IT WORKS

Therapists are trained to read the messages of the body – which, it is said, never lies. Repressed traumas (in primal work such traumas include those that occur at birth) can be brought to awareness, released, and resolved, using a combination of physical and psychological techniques, once the physical location that forms the central focus of the trauma has been determined. Physical exercises, breathing exercises, and various forms of massage may be used, usually in group therapy sessions. This liberating process can also bring back pleasurable memories of past experiences, especially childhood delights.

BIODYNAMIC MASSAGE

Developed by Norwegian therapist Gerda Boyesen out of the integrated form of physical and psychological therapy known as bioenergetics, biodynamic massage combines massage with exercise to release emotional tension. Participants are taught to "connect with" and experience the energy flowing through them in much the same way as they might experience an orgasm. Because it may have a liberating effect on the mind, as well as the body, it is known also as dynamic psychology. *(See also Massage, pages 48–9.)*

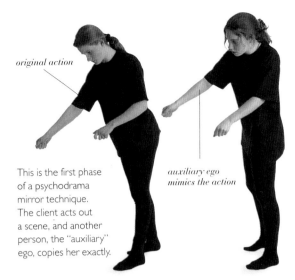

original action

auxiliary ego mimics the action

This is the first phase of a psychodrama mirror technique. The client acts out a scene, and another person, the "auxiliary" ego, copies her exactly.

WHAT CAN BIOENERGETICS TREAT?

Treatment is different for each individual, and some undertake the therapy without expecting to have physical conditions resolved. However, many adherents suggest improvement in some of the following ailments:

- asthma
- migraine and headaches
- irritable bowel syndrome
- ulcers
- sleep disorders
- stress.

In the second phase the auxiliary ego senses the client's unhappiness, and bursts into tears. The client then senses her own situation.

CAUTIONS AND CONTRAINDICATIONS

There are no known contraindications to bioenergetics, although it is recommended that you consult your physician before undergoing treatment.

Gestalt Therapy

This humanistic approach, developed by Fritz Perls, grew rapidly in the United States in the 1960s. Although Perls' methodology became more and more direct, the aim from the first was that clients should learn from their own experience to acknowledge previously denied feelings and aspects of their personalities.

Well-known Gestalt techniques include increasing the awareness of "body language" and of negative internal "messages"; emphasizing the client's self-awareness by making him or her speak continually in the present tense and in the first person; concentrating on a part of a client's personality, perhaps even on just one emotion, and addressing it (or asking the client to address it) as if it were sitting by itself in the client's chair; the creation by the therapist of episodes and diversions that vividly demonstrate a point rather than explaining in words.

Such techniques are widely borrowed by other therapeutic disciplines to support their own practices.

ENCOUNTER GROUPS

Group work can be undertaken in almost any form of therapy but is mostly associated with humanistic and Gestalt approaches, where it focuses on "the here and now." The therapist may work individually with the members of a group, but the purpose is more often to promote interaction among all those who are present.

Members are encouraged to cast off inhibitions and to receive and give feedback. Physical interaction may be significant in open encounter groups.

The success of the group depends on an interplay of energies. The role of the leader in monitoring the dynamics of this interplay is critical to the maintenance of a balance between creating a safe place, avoiding undue pressure, and yet allowing enough challenge to stimulate movement within the group.

CAUTIONS AND CONTRAINDICATIONS

There are no known contraindications for Gestalt therapy or psychodrama, but be prepared for emotional upheavals of any kind once you start work in such a group.

Successful therapy can teach you to lose your inhibitions and live in the now.

PSYCHODRAMA

We all play a role in the drama that is our lives. If that role is painful or frustrating, we may need to express our negative emotions in some way or to create scenarios that make us feel better. Psychodrama, which was developed in the 1920s in Austria and the United States by Jacob Moreno, provides an arena for this.

The openness to self-discovery that is a feature of psychodrama derives from several factors. Once trust has been created, group dynamics encourage disclosure; acting and direction allow for safe exploration of feelings by trial and error; the rare physical freedom of moving at will across an open space promotes expansiveness.

Psychodrama can be used to unlock doors to the past, to explore one person's "dark" side, to empathize with others through role exchange, and to discover and practice fresh ways of relating.

WHAT CAN GESTALT THERAPY TREAT?

The emphasis is on the psychological side of illness, which is most likely to be affected by treatment; however, many physical conditions are improved by the therapy, including

- anxiety, depression, and other psychological disorders
- neurological problems
- stress and stress-related disorders.

Transpersonal Therapies

The spiritual dimension is very significant in transpersonal therapy; the self is seen as integrated into a wider context.

This is a spiritually oriented form of treatment that combines therapy for the individual with a concern for the whole of creation. The transpersonal dimension emerges in the drive of the individual to connect with cosmic forces, and in the impulse to discover an awareness of the soul.

In operation transpersonal therapies involve a wide range of functional techniques. The emphasis is on practical activities rather than verbal interpretations, and so, for example, imagery is used to explore, transform, and expand on ideas.

Transpersonal work shares with other integrative therapies the search for the equal fulfillment of mind, body, and soul. Many people find considerable hope for personal development in such a method that combines a range of diverse elements while looking outward to the world around for meaning.

> ### CAUTIONS AND CONTRAINDICATIONS
>
> There are no known contraindications to transpersonal therapies, but it is essential that all treatment is undertaken by a registered, qualified professional.

PSYCHOSYNTHESIS

Many elements now essential to the transpersonal movement stem from the work of psychoanalyst Roberto Assagioli, whose long career began in Italy in 1926 and encompassed the establishing of important links between Jung's ideas and humanistic thinking. During the 1960s Assagioli's ideas became extremely popular. He saw a need for the synthesis of inner experience and external events, past mystical wisdom, and new scientific knowledge. He believed in the exis-

Half-empty or half-full? What you see indicates your outlook on life.

tence of the soul, and that by achieving our full potential as human beings we actually come to know the vastness of creation. To him, in healing ourselves we heal the world.

Within this broad context, Assagioli placed great importance on exploring practical ways actually to enable people to transform themselves. At various times he used word and free association, free drawing and writing, dance, music, dreamwork, guided imagery, and "becoming the symbol" in visualization.

TRANSACTIONAL ANALYSIS

A humanistic therapy, often drawn on by those working integratively, transactional analysis believes that every social situation produces a "transaction" resulting in a particular presentation of personality and the way we communicate and behave socially.

It was pioneered in the 1950s by Eric Berne in the United States. Some of its concepts have been popularized as the "games people play," the notions of life-stage transition crises, and the awareness of internal voices representing the constantly warring parent-child child-adult aspects of our personalities.

WHAT CAN TRANSPERSONAL THERAPIES TREAT?

Transpersonal therapies are holistic, aimed at balancing and fulfilling the mind, body, and soul. For this reason, a wide range of conditions may respond to therapy, particularly those that are affected by negative feelings or actions. The following conditions may respond to transpersonal therapy treatment:

- headaches and migraine
- anxiety and depression
- arthritis and rheumatism
- asthma, eczema, and psoriasis
- ME.

PSYCHOLOGICAL THERAPIES / PSYCHOTHERAPY AND COUNSELING ● 109

Behavioral Therapy

Since its early 20th-century beginnings, behavioral therapy has prided itself above all on being scientific – and so avoiding such unquantifiables as needs, wants, and motivation, together with excursions into the unconscious and transpersonal.

Instead it has concentrated on observing and analyzing behavioral and cognitive functioning, diagnosing unproductive ways of dealing with life, and instituting systematic changes to improve outcomes. Therapists discuss methods and expectations with clients; the clients' participation is negotiated, and measures to monitor effectiveness are established. Techniques used are practical and direct, including those listed below.

COUNTER CONDITIONING An undesirable response to a stimulus is replaced by one newly elicited.

DESENSITIZATION The client is relaxed deeply, then gradually he or she is exposed to an anxiety-provoking situation.

AVERSION CONDITIONING A stimulus that is attractive to the client, but would lead to undesirable results, is paired with an unpleasant event in order to break the pattern.

ROLE PLAYING The therapist demonstrates more effective behaviors in the session. The client tries these out in real-life situations.

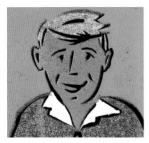

In the pragmatic approach adopted by behavioral therapy, clients are taught to adapt their behavior so that they achieve their goal.

In this instance, the therapist shows that it is more effective to present a happy rather than a gloomy face to the world.

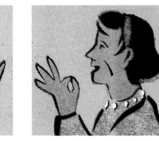

In these two pictures, the client copies the therapist as she "rehearses" a scene that is expected to be difficult so that

the client can learn in advance how to handle the situation and how to be prepared for any eventuality.

BEHAVIOR REHEARSAL The client copies the therapist's staged rehearsal of a forthcoming situation that is expected to be problematic.

COGNITIVE THERAPY

This grew out of behavioral thinking in the 1960s and concentrates on how people's experiences are governed by their perceptions. For example, cognitive theory sees depression as the result of sad thinking, rather than believing conversely that sad thinking is the result of a state of depression.

COGNITIVE RESTRUCTURING Transforming a client's thinking processes so as to influence behavior and emotions.

RATIONAL-EMOTIVE APPROACH Replacing irrational beliefs with rational ones.

ASSUMPTION OF RESPONSIBILITY Getting clients to accept that no one else "makes" them think, feel, or do anything.

QUICK THERAPIES

Using a short series of therapy sessions (between 6 and 25) as a starter to self-help is becoming a popular approach.

Some ways of doing this are listed below.

SOLUTION-FOCUSED *This method looks at the client's existing strong points, seeks possible solutions to the problems, then works out how to get there in the light of both. It provides validation and encouragement within a program that is pared back to just the main current issue: what the client wants and expects from therapy.*

PSYCHODYNAMIC *This focuses on specific problems, with an emphasis on present life and the way it is handled. The method is intense but affords more concrete, manageable goals than longer-term analysis.*

COGNITIVE ANALYTIC *This integrated flexible method allows for a clear focus and framework, and the simultaneous use of a wide range of techniques. It is cognitive in making use of the client's perceptions and thoughts, and analytic in its recognition of the role of the unconscious and of the client-therapist relationship.*

Psychological Therapies

Creative Arts Therapies

Since the early 1900s, as psychology developed and the unconscious began to be explored, the role that the creative process can play in revealing and healing has been studied and clarified. Emotions are experienced – without the filter of words – in the body itself, and emotional memories are encoded and stored there. The psychotherapeutic use of the creative arts enables us to connect with this material directly, and give nonverbal expression to what is driving or crippling us.

Dance, music, art, and other means of imaginative expression can circumvent the blocks between conscious and unconscious in the rational mind. Not only can the meaning and cause of erratic behavior be made explicit, but the clues to its resolution can appear through creative expression and interaction with a therapist trained in both psychotherapy and the arts.

DANCE MOVEMENT THERAPY

Dance movement therapy can enable individuals to integrate their physical, emotional, and cognitive selves. Because "dancing needs the whole living person" (Rudolf von Laban, pioneer of physiotherapeutic choreography in the 1920s), it has the power to affect parts of the mind that direct verbal communication cannot. The system of choreographic notation formulated by Laban (Labanotation) was later developed and used for analyzing movement, and it is on this basis that dance movement therapists analyze and interpret the actions of their clients. Through the therapist's insights, the clients may be led to a greater sense of self-awareness and reach a freer level of self-expression.

In this way it is possible to "read" what the body is already communicating, given that 75 percent of communication is nonverbal. The therapist's interpretation may well reveal new images to the client, possibly representing resolutions of a difficulty or a breakthrough in self-realization. The client may also be pleased that "treatment" seems at least partly physical and is not "all in the head." A group movement session also encourages interactions with others and helps to break down barriers to communication. Solo or in company, however, dance can bring a new and powerful experience of pure enjoyment to the healing process.

WHAT CAN CREATIVE ARTS THERAPIES TREAT?

The arts therapies can benefit people with all types of psychological and emotional problems. They can also benefit people with physical illnesses that are exacerbated by stress. Other conditions that may respond include

- *psychiatric disorders such as schizophrenia or severe depression*
- *eating disorders and addictions*
- *sleep disorders*
- *headaches and migraine*
- *digestive problems.*

ART THERAPY

Art and music therapies have been established now for about 20 years. Because they work on the nonverbal level, they can often help people whose traumas and emotional problems are buried too deep for words, or children who may not have the words to describe their distress. These therapies can be used for people with severe mental problems (although art therapy is not recommended for schizophrenia) but can also help those who find it difficult to express their emotions.

Drawing, painting, craftwork, making models – all such activities may give form to otherwise inexpressible inner feelings and so access truths that have previously gone unrecognized. The goal in therapy is not necessarily to produce skillful finished works, but to follow spontaneous impulses in the use of (for example) line, color, form, and texture. All too often a person's spontaneity has been repressed, and reconnecting with that immediacy and energy of itself provides release. The works created can be interpreted individually or as a series.

Painting and modeling can be more than a chance to express one's creativity. It may be easier for people to represent their inner fears with an image on paper that they can then confront and conquer. Often the actual act of physically painting or sculpting – throwing the clay, making savage paintstrokes – can itself be very therapeutic.

In a session of dance movement therapy, a client turns away from the class, signifying rejection of some kind. The therapist will use this gesture to examine deeper feelings.

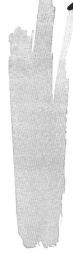

For some people, mind therapy needs to have a physical component. There is great satisfaction handling a paintbrush loaded with paint and capturing your feelings on paper.

It was Freudian analysts who first discovered the significance of paintings made by inmates of mental asylums. Expressing a fantasy in a nonverbal way, according to Freudian doctrine, allows the patient to bypass the ego, which may try to censor the experience for presentation to the world. Painting helps the patient to take part in their own healing process; a series of pictures may chart their progress toward cure.

MUSIC THERAPY

Sessions require both the therapist and the client to play (or beat the rhythm), sing, and listen. The client should create his or her own music while the therapist supports and encourages by responding musically.

Feelings can be conveyed and recognized without words. Through patterns of rhythm, pitch, tempo, and tonality, the client may externalize discordant internal "noise," so effecting release and harmony. Playing in a group creates a social interaction that can develop awareness and the ability to relate in a satisfying way.

Sound therapy *(see page 127)* uses specially filtered recorded music to improve listening skills as a way of energizing and harmonizing the mind. Changing the way people think about what they are hearing can also change the way that they feel and behave.

The most recent development in this rapidly growing area is the use of a "musical bed" – a system of loudspeakers that amplifies vibrations caused by music and transmits them to the client through a specially designed mattress. Some experts consider this to be much more efficacious than sound only.

CAUTIONS AND CONTRAINDICATIONS

There are no contraindications to creative arts therapies, although, like all therapies, it is essential that your therapist is qualified and registered with the appropriate regulatory body.

Hypnosis and Hypnotherapy • Hypnotherapy

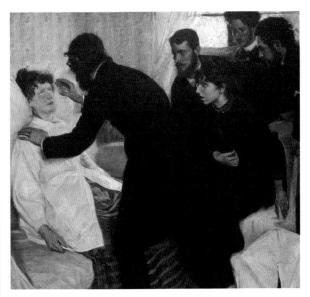

Hypnotherapy was at its most glamorous in the late 19th century, as this genre painting of the hypnotist at work shows.

HEALING a patient who is in a state of trance is one of the oldest therapeutic arts. Ancient cultures all around the world revered individuals deemed to be in contact with supernatural powers and apparently able to use such contacts to cure the sick and distressed while these people were in a state resembling sleep. The supposed connection with the supernatural powers lies behind many of the prejudices and fears about hypnosis that still exist: the vestigial terror, effectively, of possession by some other entity. But the true value of hypnosis – that it is a state that enables inner connections to be made – has at last begun to be universally accepted.

HOW HYPNOTHERAPY BEGAN

The Austrian Anton Mesmer tried in the 18th century to harness mental energy – known at the time as "animal magnetism" – to effect cures. His results were variable, but he developed a ritual around his treatment which genuinely hypnotized those who came to him for help. His "mesmerizing" methods received scientific attention throughout the 1800s. When, in 1841, the Scotsman Dr. James Braid saw a demonstration he began to develop his own theories and techniques. He demonstrated that a trance, for which he coined the term "hypnosis," could be induced very simply, and that hypnotized subjects could not be made to act against their will. The medical profession then

The force behind mesmerism was thought to be animal magnetism.

began to make some use of hypnosis, particularly for anesthesia during surgery.

By 1900 Dr. Pierre Janet in France had come to believe that the effects of hypnosis were partly due to a split in the mind between the conscious and unconscious. He concluded (as Freud did) that neurotic symptoms had a hidden meaning, originating in the unconscious, which could be reached through hypnosis.

Janet's experiments prompted many medical associations, including the British Medical Association (BMA), to investigate further. Freud had translated and studied most of the French works, but he was unskilled at inducing hypnosis himself and dropped it from his psychoanalytical ideology. Most psychoanalysts followed suit, and what was once considered to be a burgeoning and promising field became a therapy for cranks. It wasn't until the 1950s that its use in mainstream medicine and psychotherapy was accepted. In 1958, the American Medical Association approved hypnosis as a useful tool in medicine. Today, in the United States and Britain it has been used to improve physical and mental health at all levels. People suffering from chronic and terminal illnesses can find relief from both the pain and anxiety, as well as other physical symptoms, caused by their condition.

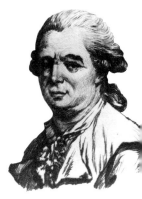

Friedrich Anton Mesmer (1734–1815), the father of mesmerism.

Dentists and dental therapists use hypnotherapy to enable patients to overcome the common phobia of dentists and allow them to experience virtually pain-free treatment.

Many 20th-century scientists have struggled to explain hypnotherapy and how it works. It is one of the few therapies taught in conventional medical schools, and it is widely considered to be a useful method of encouraging healing and altering behavioral states. From the study of hypnosis has come a host of other therapies, including biofeedback, autogenic training, and relaxation and meditation. Many people now use self-hypnosis techniques to manage stress, pain, anxiety, and conditions such as migraine, irritable bowel syndrome, obesity, and addictions.

Hypnotherapy still suffers from a tarnished reputation, due to the continuing tradition of using hypnosis on the stage for its entertainment value (indeed in the wrong hands the therapy can be dangerous), despite the fact that the therapy has been used successfully for generations and is now one of the most scientifically endorsed complementary therapies.

Theory and Practice

There is plenty of clinical evidence that hypnosis can be used to make beneficial changes, even though it cannot be fully explained.

The hypnotic trance is a naturally occurring state of equilibrium somewhere between waking and sleeping. Essentially, it is a state in which inner realities can be contacted and information can be moved around the brain more freely. The conscious mind – the part that uses logic and language – in most people seems to operate principally from the left half of the brain, and the unconscious – concerned with emotions, symbols, and synthesis – from the right.

It would seem that by somehow reaching the right half of the brain through words, hypnosis creates a particular level of activity in both halves and allows a particular type of communication between them.

At a typical hypnotherapy session, the therapist starts by creating a relaxed, calm, and safe atmosphere, and briefly outlines to the client – who is generally sitting or reclining comfortably – what he or she may expect to experience. The room is quiet and has subdued lighting. The therapist then endeavors to relax the client further, using such suggestive terms as "drifting slightly," and "sinking deeper." Sometimes the therapist describes a relaxing scene for the client to visualize. The client's eyes feel heavy, and close.

Under hypnosis, the client is aware of everything that goes on but feels completely detached. Nonetheless, the client is perfectly able to speak if he or she wishes, and to terminate the trance summarily if unhappy. When the client is properly in a state of trance, the therapeutic work can begin. At the end of the session, a simple suggestion brings the client out of hypnosis.

IS IT SAFE?

In the hands of a qualified practitioner, hypnotherapy is completely safe. Modern hypnotherapy does not depend on a deep trance for it to work, and under the guidance of a reputable therapist there is no risk of a woman being taken advantage of, for instance, or a person failing to regain total consciousness. You will always regain total control after a session, and there is absolutely no likelihood of "not coming round." Self-hypnosis is also safe, and most health conditions will benefit.

However, hypnosis is a powerful tool and although there is no danger of anyone forcing you to do something you do not wish to do, the subcon-

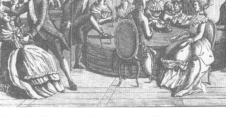

Mesmer's adherents gathered around large circular tubs filled with bathwater and iron filings.

They were endeavoring to feel the power of "animal magnetism" for themselves.

scious will believe anything it is told, so it is possible to reprogram beliefs by the use of suggestion. The therapist must understand clearly what you hope to accomplish, in order to direct you in an appropriate manner. Most modern therapists use very light but efficient trances, which make you suggestible and willing, but do not take you beyond what you subconsciously know is acceptable.

Hypnotism is not effective for people under the influence of drink or drugs, those with psychotic conditions, or children under the age of five.

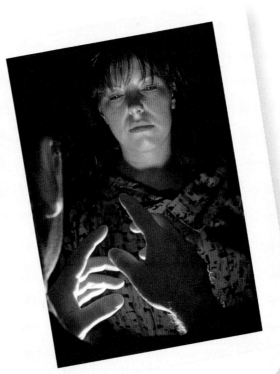

A modern hypnotist at work. The dramatic image shows the "show business" direction that some hypnotists have taken, making it difficult for hypnotherapists to establish a serious discipline.

How Hypnotherapy is Used

In a hypnotic trance it is possible to concentrate totally on the desired goal. A few clients cannot be put into a trance but do come under the hypnotherapist's control, while others enter a deep trance. It is also possible to gain deeper insight into one's own feelings and behavior. Hypnosis is applied in three main ways:

DEEP RELAXATION Letting go of virtually all physical and mental tension is possible under hypnosis.

SUGGESTION THERAPY The aim is to replace negative thought patterns with positive ones.

ANALYTICAL THERAPY Root causes of problems are examined and reviewed from a new perspective.

When your therapist encourages you to relax, she will usually do so through your imagination, talking in a controlled way that ensures that you focus on her voice. Relaxation is normally encouraged through "heavy arms" and "semaphore" techniques.

HEAVY ARMS

You will be asked to relax your arms and concentrate on the fact that your hands are becoming heavier and heavier until they are so heavy that you are unable to lift them.

> ### CAUTIONS AND CONTRAINDICATIONS
>
> The safety of hypnotherapy is a point of considerable concern; however, in the hands of a qualified practitioner, it should be safe for people of all ages. Ensure that you check your practitioner's qualifications before undergoing treatment, and it is advisable that you check with your physician first.

THE SEMAPHORE METHOD Your therapist will ask you to close your eyes and visualize a balloon on your wrist, pulling one arm upward while another is drawn down by a heavy weight. Your therapist will then suggest that the reverse is true.

Therapeutic techniques include those listed below.

DIRECT/AUTO-SUGGESTION THERAPY, in which the therapist offers positive suggestions that your mind will accept. This may be used for addictions, nervous problems, or pain, for instance.

PARTS THERAPY, in which the therapist uses regression to discover why you have certain problems. For instance, your weight may be linked to an overwhelming insecurity, or your aggressiveness may be caused by defensiveness about a problem. This technique addresses factors that may not immediately appear linked but have a common cause.

HYPNOHEALING is aimed at healing pathological disease. Your therapist uses visualization to release the cause of your illness.

AGE REGRESSION, which links illness and other problems to past problems and incidents.

CELL COMMAND THERAPY, which is used to slow down aging and associated degenerative diseases.

HYPNOANESTHESIA, which is used to control pain – for instance in labor, or at the dentist.

apparent sleep

WHAT CAN HYPNOTHERAPY DO?

Hypnotherapy can draw upon all the vast resources of the unconscious mind, which is why it can be so effective in helping a wide range of problems, including

ANXIETY *stammering, phobias, lack of assertiveness, fear of public speaking, panic attacks, difficulties with relationships*

ADDICTIONS *to alcohol, tobacco, drugs, gambling*

MOODS *depression, listlessness, aggression, low self-esteem, lack of concentration*

STRESS *headaches, blushing, dermatitis, impotence, irritable bowel syndrome, obesity.*

Regression

The root cause of a client's recurrent psychological problem may well lie in some incident that at the time inspired extreme fear, disgust, or shame. To recover from the problem, the client – within the peace and security of a hypnotic trance – has to revisit that incident and be able to understand the way in which his or her mind has since dealt with it (the "survival response"). That, after all, is what is currently preventing the client from living life to the full. Equally, hypnosis may reveal that as a child the client had ideas about his or her character, aptitudes, and abilities implanted by adults. Subconsciously he or she feels "useless," "hopeless," or "a failure," for example.

There are various methods by which a therapist may take a client under hypnosis back into earlier years. One is simply to suggest that it is at this very moment a year that is known to be critical in the client's life history, and to ask for a response. Another is "free association," in which an entire series of memories is elicited, each one somehow evoked by the last.

In true regression, the client relives the experience, feeling again all the emotions of the time, with all the perceptions of a younger person or perhaps even of a child or a baby. Releasing these emotions, examining the material recovered (as relayed by the therapist or as recorded), and then reviewing the situation from a present-day perspective are all important parts of regression therapy.

Some healing work – reframing a negative incident in the client's past so that it has a currently positive outcome, for instance – can also be done by looking at the incident under hypnosis.

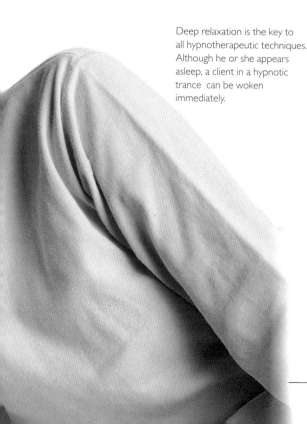

Deep relaxation is the key to all hypnotherapeutic techniques. Although he or she appears asleep, a client in a hypnotic trance can be woken immediately.

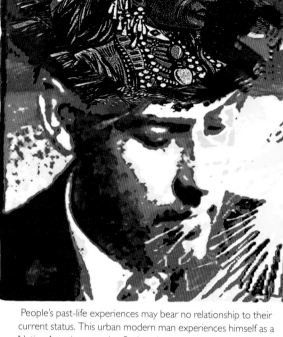

People's past-life experiences may bear no relationship to their current status. This urban modern man experiences himself as a Native American warrior. Such an image may be a metaphor for the way a part of him wants to live or see himself.

PAST-LIFE THERAPY

Since the 1960s, the ability under hypnosis apparently to remember past lives has been the subject of systematic research. Hypnotherapists who work with regression sometimes find that their clients regress not toward their own childhood but into another lifetime altogether, maybe centuries earlier. Moreover, it may appear that in that other lifetime they were of any age, and either male or female, regardless of their age or sex now. They may even speak a different language, or perhaps one that is incomprehensible. Most can also tell how and when that life came to an end.

Some authorities consider this regression to be a genuine memory of an earlier incarnation, while others view it as metaphorical (a mindset referred to another context). In either case, contact with a deeper layer of meaning and associated connotations brings insight into present feelings and behavior.

All therapists have encountered clients who seem "stuck" in their development: who are unable to account for why they feel irrationally wretched about themselves, or who remain stubbornly terrified, even after counseling and/or psychotherapy. Finding the cause of the trauma does not necessarily remove it, but after past-life regression, such clients often say at once, "Now I understand," and start to feel free from the crippling emotion that has dominated them, free from a pattern of behavior that is ultimately destructive.

Individual Therapies

Relaxation Therapies

RELAXATION allows the mind-body complex to get on with its own healing work, restoring internal harmony and creating afresh the conditions for optimal functioning. It is also a very pleasurable experience.

In the therapeutic sense, relaxation is the release of mental and physical tension. Simple as that may seem, not many people can release both mental and physical tension at the same time without help or training. So a wide range of techniques has been developed to promote a profound level of relaxation and enhanced psychological integration. Some go back thousands of years; others are continually being created. All utilize the effect the mind can have on the body.

Choosing a method is a very personal matter, but working with a therapist, individually or in a group, is an excellent way to learn.

WHAT CAN RELAXATION TREAT?

Treatment is gentle and noninvasive, and many conditions will respond, including

- ᴥ *mental and physical problems associated with stress*
- ᴥ *nausea and vomiting (from pregnancy, chemotherapy, etc.)*
- ᴥ *pain*
- ᴥ *anxiety, depression, and panic attacks*
- ᴥ *asthma*
- ᴥ *arthritis*
- ᴥ *high or low blood pressure.*

FLOTATION THERAPY

The beneficial mental effects of weightlessness combined with minimal external stimuli were first researched in the 1950s. Such a combination can be achieved in a flotation tank – a totally enclosed pool about 9ft/2.75m long and 5ft/1.5m wide, holding about 10in/25cm of water at body temperature. The water is highly salted and completely supports a floating human body; the space above the water is air-conditioned. Pressing a switch activates an interior light and, in some tanks, soft music through loudspeakers.

In this comforting environment, with restricted sound and light, or none at all, the mind and body easily enter a state of deep relaxation, the effects of which persist and accumulate as more sessions are undertaken.

Flotation therapy alleviates such physical ailments as arthritis and high blood pressure (hypertension). But it is used more often in psychotherapy to lower stress response levels, thus replacing anxiety with a strong sense of well-being, enhancing creativity and awareness, improving problem-solving, and accelerating learning processes.

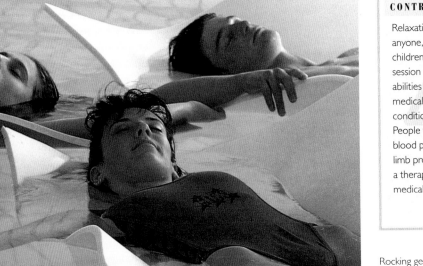

CAUTIONS AND CONTRAINDICATIONS

Relaxation can be safe for anyone, even small children, as long as the session is tailored to their abilities and certain medical and mental conditions are considered. People with very low blood pressure, or joint or limb problems, may need a therapist with a sound medical background.

Rocking gently, securely supported, in a pool of warm water is deeply relaxing, possibly reminiscent of days floating in the womb.

Autogenic Training

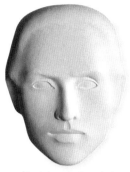

Mental control can help with physical ailments.

Autogenic training (AT) originated in the 1930s as a result of Dr. Johannes Schultz's development of earlier German research into sleep and hypnosis. Physicians noticed that if they emphasized suggestions of environmental heaviness and warmth, their patients tended to enter a mental state in which fatigue and tension disappeared.

AT gives voluntary control over what is normally the involuntary nervous system without the need for being hooked up to any electrical apparatus (of the type that, for instance, biofeedback requires). Changes are achieved through a series of exercises practiced for 10 to 15 minutes two or three times a day. Working in conjunction with a teacher or supervisor is recommended because such exercises may cause occasional muscular strain or dizzy spells as the body spontaneously de-stresses itself.

Autogenic training involves six exercises that are performed sitting or lying comfortably in a quiet place with the eyes closed, and are based on the notion of "talking" silently to each part of the body in turn. The exercises focus on:

✳ heaviness in arms and legs
✳ warmth in arms and legs
✳ calm regular heartbeat
✳ easy natural breathing
✳ abdominal warmth
✳ coolness of the forehead.

WHAT CAN AUTOGENICS TREAT?

Because autogenics is holistic, the whole person is treated rather than specific symptoms. However, many conditions seem to respond to treatment, including

◄§ *irritable bowel syndrome*
◄§ *asthma and eczema*
◄§ *high blood pressure*
◄§ *women's problems, including PMS, PNI, and the menopause*
◄§ *infertility*
◄§ *diabetes and thyroid disorders*
◄§ *headaches and insomnia*
◄§ *stress and stress-related disorders.*

The aim of autogenic training is to teach how to deal with the bodily reactions to stress. In our primitive state we reacted to trouble by running away or putting up a fight, and our bodies prepared us physically for either reaction. Now, physical tension is retained in the body and can manifest itself as high blood pressure, aches and pains, and digestive disorders.

BIOFEEDBACK

Biofeedback is a technologically supported relaxation therapy originally developed in the United States. Clients are taught a series of relaxation exercises similar to those in autogenic training. In biofeedback, however, the client's progress is monitored by machines that assess changes in heart rate, body temperature, muscle tension, skin conductivity, and brainwaves. Once training is complete, clients are able to recognize their body's signals (symptoms of migraines, for example) and to take appropriate steps to deal with them and to reach a state of relaxation. Stress and anxiety-related conditions have been known to benefit from biofeedback.

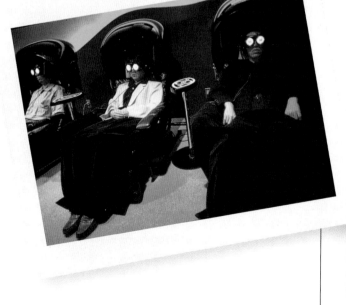

Biofeedback is a high-tech method that uses machines to monitor patients' levels of relaxation.

Meditation

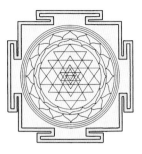

A stylized version of the Shri Yantra, one of the most powerful mandalas.

Meditation is a way of contacting the inner energy that powers the natural processes of healing and self-realization. Many cultures preserve some form of ritualistic technique – in one or two cultures dating from thousands of years ago – that promotes change from the normal levels of perception and that may result in feelings of well-being. This is probably why meditation in one form or another is central to the practice of so many of the world's religions.

Whereas some traditions are strictly mystical, directed toward a unity with all creation and an infusion with sublime joy, others may be described as more pragmatic, striving instead toward what is simply a state of "being" that includes no aspect of movement or sensation. For some people, especially in the Christian faith, prayer is a form of meditation. What is always involved is time out from the world around and a stilling of the mind.

Although it is possible to learn meditation techniques from a book, it is much better to have a teacher. Failing this, a tape can be helpful. It is usual to start by adopting a comfortable posture in a quiet location and closing your eyes. At first it may be difficult to steer the attention gently away from your racing thoughts without forcing the mind to behave in a set way. The vocal repetition of sounds (a mantra), or a visual object of devotional significance to which the attention may be recalled when necessary, is helpful to some people.

CAUTIONS AND CONTRAINDICATIONS

There are no contraindications to meditation, although, obviously, it should not be practiced while driving or operating machinery – heavy or otherwise.

When meditating, staring at a steadily burning candle flame can focus the mind.

WHAT CAN MEDITATION TREAT?

The effects of meditation are wide-ranging, although they may take some time and practice to be fully experienced. Many people feel an improvement in:

- *blood pressure problems*
- *stress and stress-related disorders*
- *circulatory disorders*
- *headaches and migraine*
- *muscular aches and pains*
- *asthma and breathing difficulties*
- *insomnia*
- *chronic pain.*

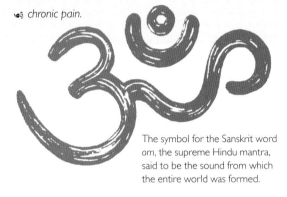

The symbol for the Sanskrit word *om*, the supreme Hindu mantra, said to be the sound from which the entire world was formed.

It has been found that meditating effects changes in heart rate and respiration, helping to reduce stress. As the thoughts slow and the level of tension in the body drops accordingly, feelings of calm, detachment, peace, and sometimes joy begin to fill the mind and spread through the body. Meditation promotes a state of deep relaxation, but also mental alertness and openness. An equilibrium between activity in the rational left side of the brain and the creative right side of the brain is established, and there is an overall increase in the brain's range of operation. Benefits reported include

❋ decreased anxiety, feelings of anger and aggression, depression, nervousness, and physical tension

❋ increased awareness and concentration, mental clarity and resilience, creative intuitive powers, emotional stability and control, and also overall health and well-being.

Transcendental Meditation (TM)

In the late 1950s, an Indian monk named Maharishi Majesh Yogi began teaching a new form of meditation that could be easily practiced by busy, modern people around the world. He called it transcendental meditation and it was based on the concept that a meditation using mantras of short words or phrases, repeated in the mind, could help the user subdue many thought processes and reach a deep level of consciousness. Mantras are selected on the basis of the learner's temperament and occupation. The spirit behind TM is the Vedanta system of philosophy that forms the basis for most modern schools of Hinduism.

The simple technique produces a state of "restful alertness" that, it is considered, transcends thinking to reach the source of thought – the mind's own reservoir of energy and creative intelligence. Through this, people can find great relaxation, inner peace, enhanced vitality, and creativity. TM is ordinarily applied for 15 to 20 minutes twice daily.

Much of the research into the psychological and physiological effects of meditation has been carried out in relation to TM. It shows that the level of rest achieved is deeper than sleep. Another major finding is that meditation produces all the body responses opposite to the flight-or-fight response characteristic of stress. During meditation, breathing slows, the heartbeat becomes shallower, the muscles relax, blood pressure normalizes, and there are compositional changes in blood and skin that indicate a reduction in tension.

Interestingly, Dr. Herbert Benson, the American pioneer of research into the relaxation response, showed in the 1960s that ritualistic techniques employed in various Christian traditions – such as the use of the rosary, prayer-beads, or simple prayers repeated many times over – can be just as effective as TM in achieving the same results.

SIDDHA MEDITATION

This is another practice whose origins are in India. It utilizes both mantra and breath control to still the mind, and thus to allow a spontaneous shift in consciousness. The mantra is recited aloud and serves two purposes. Regarded as pure sound, it causes the body and mind to vibrate at a particular frequency that induces the meditative state: the energy resonates in the unconscious. And its words provide a focus to hold the mind and stop it from randomizing its energy through scattered thoughts and images.

What is known as "breath awareness" is also important: the mind has to become tuned to the way breath enters and leaves the body.

VISUAL MEDITATION

Visual meditation initially involves gazing at a chosen object or symbol that has some personal meaning. The eyes are then closed, and the object is "seen" in the imagination.

⁂ Meaningful objects that may be used for meditation include	
natural items	a flower, a bowl of water, a candle flame
artistic items	icons, spiritual pictures
special words and symbols	the primal sound OM, a crucifix, the yin/yang symbol, the wheel of life

⁂ Religious allegories and illustrations such as:	
mandalas	complex diagrams with a center, contained in a circle, and representing the unity of the personal and transpersonal
yantras	graphic representations of the energy pattern of one aspect of the divine

Smooth regular breathing allows the meditator to focus inward to the almost imperceptible space between breaths and so to the inner self.

Visualization

Visualization is the forming of meaningful images in the mind: it is usually most effective when resting comfortably with the eyes closed. Especially when undertaken in conjunction with hypnosis, this natural ability can achieve therapeutic effects in several ways.

EXTERNAL VISUALIZATION

RELAXATION Imagining a pleasant, relaxing place – a sunny beach, perhaps – releases body tensions.

LIFE CHANGES To visualize yourself competently dealing with your problems, being successful, challenging other people, or playing a musical instrument well, can overcome blocks to being assertive and achieving what you want.

ACCESSING THE PAST Images of childhood may afford access to repressed memories and emotions.

REWRITING THE PAST An event that at the time was traumatic and damaging can be reviewed – this time with a positive outcome.

SPIRITUAL GROWTH Once facility in visualizing is achieved, images may occur spontaneously, increasing insight into your own condition, into the way the world works, and into higher levels of consciousness.

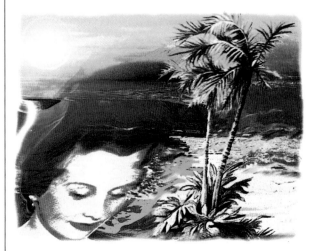

Learning to visualize a pleasant relaxing place and fixing it in your mind makes it easy to recall it when you need "time out" from a tense situation.

WHAT CAN VISUALIZATION TREAT?

Visualization is used to treat most physical and emotional conditions; in particular:

- *asthma and eczema*
- *breathing disorders*
- *heart and circulatory problems*
- *digestive disorders*
- *cancers*
- *anxiety, depression, panic attacks, and phobias*
- *hyperactivity*
- *sleep disorders.*

INTERNAL VISUALIZATION

It is not necessary to be a physician to be able to imagine the workings of your own body.

RELAXATION Just imagining the complete relaxation of specific muscles can help to make it happen.

PHYSICAL STRESS Picturing the heartbeat slowing or the lungs moving evenly and calmly immediately influences these processes.

THE BRAIN Imagining the brain stilling its activity, emptying out unwanted contents, or making better connections between parts of itself can produce changes in mood.

HEALING Forming a clear image of a part of the mind or body that is in need of healing can cause actual improvement to take place.

CAUTIONS AND CONTRAINDICATIONS

Some visualization can trigger physical attacks; for example, visualizing a field of flowers can cause an allergic reaction in hay-fever sufferers. Patients with breathing disorders may experience difficulty and discomfort and it is essential that you consult your physician before undergoing treatment. Patients with spinal disorders may need additional exercises to strengthen the muscles.

ENERGY THERAPIES • Healing

MOST ALTERNATIVE therapies hold that human beings are not only physical, but consist of a "subtle energy" system that relates to the mental, emotional, and spiritual self, all of which may be addressed in diagnosis and treatment. Though not yet scientifically proven, the concept of a sort of invisible "subtle body" appears to have some support in the latest theories in modern subatomic physics.

The idea that we have a "subtle energy body" or "aura" *(see illustration)* is not new. It has been traditionally recognized by Eastern medicine and most religions for centuries, and some psychics claim they can see it. According to these traditions it consists of a series of energy fields around the body, moving out from the "etheric" or electromagnetic field through the emotional and mental bodies, to the spiritual.

Energy flows within the body through channels called "meridians," and seven main energy centers aligned down the spine. These energy centers or chakras (a Sanskrit word for "wheel") absorb and emit life force. Each chakra governs an area of the body together with specific emotional issues. Thus the "root" or "base chakra" connects with the adrenal glands, the hips, and one's security in the world, and the "brow chakra" to the pineal gland, intuition, and will.

Good health depends on the free flow of energy, and ill-health is caused by energy blockages or imbalances resulting from physical causes such as bad nutrition, drugs, or injury, and/or mental and emotional causes such as shock, grief, or negative thinking.

Energy-oriented therapies include acupuncture, biodynamic massage, color and light therapy, craniosacral therapy, crystal healing, homeopathy, kinesiology, polarity therapy, chi kung, shiatsu, sound therapy, spiritual/psychic healing, and zero balancing.

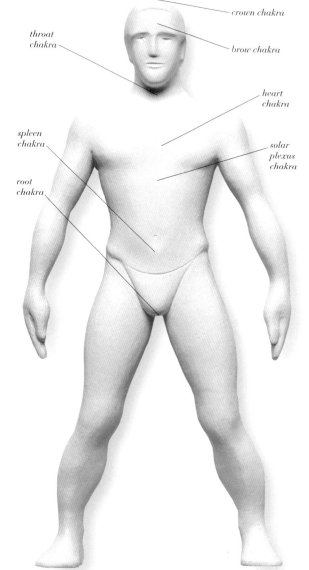

crown chakra

throat chakra

brow chakra

heart chakra

spleen chakra

solar plexus chakra

root chakra

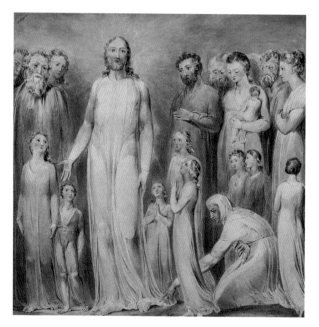

Healers appear in all world religions. According to the Gospels, Jesus Christ (left) healed many sick people during his short ministry.

The subtle energy of the body is thought to flow through the seven chakras, areas in the body that correspond with the endocrine glands.

SUBTLE ENERGY AND ITS LINKS WITH THE BODY

❧ Center (or chakra)	Color	Associated organ
Crown	Violet	Pineal gland
Brow	Indigo	Pituitary gland
Throat	Blue	Thyroid/parathyroid gland
Heart	Green	Heart and thymus gland
Navel/solar plexus	Yellow	Pancreas and adrenal gland
Spleen	Orange	Spleen
Root/sacral	Red	Sacrum/gonads/ovaries

Psychic Healing

Spiritual or psychic healing is believed to transfer healing energy by the laying on of hands. Christians say it works through God or "the Christ energy" and spiritualists claim that the spirits of physicians heal through them. Some healers say they are helped by angels. Many describe themselves as channeling "cosmic" or "universal energy," "light," or "bioenergy." People may experience this energy as a hot or cool current, relieving pain, and promoting well-being and relaxation. Some healers touch their clients, others work only in the energy field. Some combine healing with massage, others use crystals, color, and sound.

Instant "miracle" cures are rare, but most people receive some benefit, from the relief of stress, depression, and pain, to the alleviation of chronic conditions. Treatment may include examining underlying emotional problems. Nowadays healers are encouraged to train in counseling techniques and a few are even qualified psychotherapists. For lasting benefit, regular sessions may be necessary over some weeks or months.

In spite of American researcher Dr. Dan Benor's recent publication of more than 155 controlled studies showing that healing is effective, many physicians and scientists are still skeptical, dismissing any effects as being due to suggestion. Yet babies and animals seem to respond particularly well, and well-conducted experiments have all shown a definite effect on living organisms such as plant and seed growth, blood samples, and cancer cells. Experiments have also shown that distant healing, in the form of prayer or thought sent to people

CAUTIONS AND CONTRAINDICATIONS

By law, healers are not allowed to attend women in childbirth or for ten days afterward and are not to give healing to children under 18 years unless the child's parents or guardian have sought medical help and given their permission for healing to take place. Otherwise, healing is perfectly safe for anyone.

THERAPEUTIC TOUCH

Therapeutic Touch, or TT, is a method of hands-on healing that has been taught to thousands of nurses and healthcare professionals in the United States and 38 other countries. It was developed in the 1970s by an American nursing professor, Dolores Krieger, after seeing the work of Hungarian healer Oscar Estabany, and studying with healer Dora Kuntz. It became popular in the United States as a way around the strict laws against psychic healing imposed in many states.

Tests have shown that nurses trained in TT produce considerable improvements in the physical and emotional states of their patients.

elsewhere, has similarly measurable effects. In many states and also in parts of Germany, it is a prisonable offense to practice healing using "psychic powers," whereas in Britain healing is not only legal but widespread and well organized. Some British physicians even have healers in their clinics, and members of the National Federation of Spiritual Healers in Britain have been allowed to visit patients in 1,500 hospitals since the 1970s. An umbrella organization – the UK Confederation of Healing Organizations – includes 14 member organizations and about 8,000 healers, covering a variety of spiritual beliefs. They run training courses, abide by a code of conduct, and offer healing as a complement to conventional medical healthcare.

When seeking a healer, avoid those who demand a substantial advance financial commitment, or insist that you abandon medication or your religious beliefs.

WHAT CAN HEALING TREAT?

The success of healing often depends upon the relationship between the sufferer and the healer. Healing can help with any problem, mental, physical, or emotional, although it seems to be especially effective for musculoskeletal problems. Chronic and potentially fatal illnesses have been alleviated with healing.

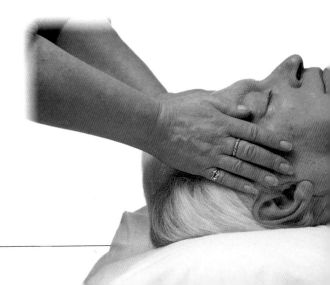

Reiki

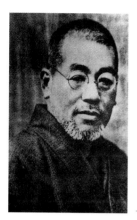

Dr. Mikao Usui,
the rediscoverer of
reiki healing.

EIKI is the Japanese word for "universal life energy" and pronounced "ray-kee." It is a form of healing based on tapping into the unseen flow of energy that permeates all living things.

It is believed that reiki originally evolved as a branch of Tibetan Buddhism and that knowledge of its power and how to use it was transmitted from master to disciple. At some point in the intervening centuries, the secrets of reiki were lost. They were rediscovered in the late 19th century by a Japanese minister, Dr. Mikao Usui. He spent 14 years seeking the ability to heal, which he believed could be discovered through studying Buddhism, learning Chinese and Sanskrit to help his research. It is claimed that he eventually found the knowledge he sought in an Indian sutra, or sacred text. Then, after a three-week meditation on a mountain top, he had a vision of four symbols that could be used to enable healing energy to be passed to others. The ability to channel the healing power was achieved by attunement to each of these symbols. Before he died in the 1930s, Dr. Usui initiated 16 others into the secret of reiki, teaching them the master attunement.

One of these reiki masters was Dr. Chujiro Hayashi, who undertook to preserve reiki and pass it on. He brought scientific training to bear on the method, noting down the results of healing sessions, codifying the sequence of hand movements in a reiki session, and establishing a reiki clinic in Tokyo.

Treatment by a reiki practitioner is intended to promote physical, emotional, and spiritual well-being. Clients lie fully clothed while the practitioner's hands are placed on specific parts of the body, starting with

A healer at work. Healing is based on attuning to the client's energy, finding the area in pain, and channeling his or her healing energy in that direction.

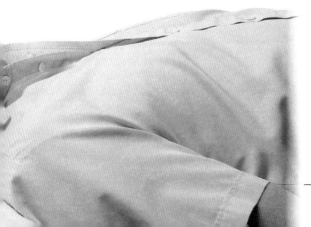

WHAT CAN REIKI TREAT?

eiki is aimed at encouraging the healing energies in the body, and involves transmitting the healer's own energy to the sufferer. Most emotional, physical, and spiritual conditions will respond to treatment, including many that are considered to be untreatable by the conventional medical profession.

the head. Some reiki practitioners do not touch the physical body but transmit healing into the surrounding aura. Reiki can be used to heal the self or someone else, and reiki energy can be projected into the future or directed to a distant place. It can also be used on pets or plants.

Anyone can learn reiki because it is not taught in the strict sense of the word, but transferred from teacher to pupil. This transferral is made though a series of "degrees." The first degree usually takes a weekend and four initiations by a reiki master. It does not involve changing religious beliefs. These initiations impart the ability to transmit healing energy to oneself and others. The second degree deepens participants' experience and enables them to give distant healing. The third degree is taken by those wishing to become reiki masters, able to teach others.

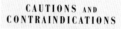

CAUTIONS AND CONTRAINDICATIONS

There are no known contraindications to reiki, although it is suggested that you consult your physician before undergoing treatment.

The results of treatment can be dramatic, or more gradual, showing themselves in general improvements in health and well-being. Reiki healing energies can have lasting results only if the recipient accepts his or her responsibility in the healing process and takes part in it. Daily self-treatment is regarded as preventive, supporting emotional and spiritual growth.

There are more than 200,000 reiki practitioners and centers in North and South America, Europe, and Australasia. The word "reiki" is a generic term in Japanese and is not exclusive to Dr. Usui's healing method; this is more formally known as Usui Shiki Ryoho or the Usui system of natural healing, and is preserved by the international Reiki Alliance, which has agreed professional standards and a code of ethics.

Radionics

R ADIONICS is a means of healing at a distance using special radionic instruments. It originated in the 1920s when an American neurologist, Albert Abrams, invented a "black box" (with no electronic circuitry) that he claimed could pick up a person's vibratory patterns from a "witness" such as a hair clipping, and transmit healing radiations to that person.

Radionics has been the subject of controversy and is banned in the United States. In Britain, by contrast, a committee of medical experts supported Abrams' basic idea as long ago as 1924, and in 1960 a British judge dismissed a case of fraud that had been brought against the therapy.

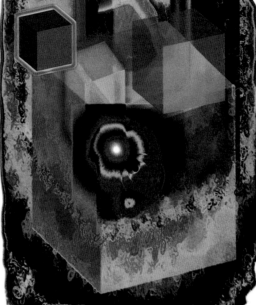

An imaginary vision of the mysterious black box, or radionics, with its secret core radiating energy. How radionics works has not yet been established.

Treatment is holistic, addressing all aspects of the client. After analyzing the condition, the practitioner uses a radionic instrument to direct corrective "energy patterns" to them. Homeopathic or flower remedies, nutritional therapy, lifestyle changes, or conventional medicine if appropriate may also be recommended. Indeed, the British Radionics Association stresses that its work is complementary to conventional medicine, not a substitute for it.

It seems likely that radionics is a form of distant healing (*see page 122*), with the instruments providing a focus for practitioners to create a mental and vibrational link with their patients.

The client may not need to meet the practitioner, although most therapists will wish to meet their client at least once. The diagnosis begins with a questionnaire that will probe the client's medical history. The therapist will also ask for a "witness" of a drop of blood or a lock of hair, which can be used to diagnose or treat the condition. The client is then informed of progress.

The therapy has been shown to be effective in a number of cases ranging from physical pain to emotional problems.

CAUTIONS AND CONTRAINDICATIONS

Radionics is safe for people of all ages, and there are no side effects to the treatment. It is advised, however, that you consult your physician before undergoing treatment.

ACTS

Automatic Computerized Treatment System (ACTS) is a system of computerized radionics developed in Britain by radionics pioneer Major Gordon Smith. This system contains 260,000 treatments, which include homeopathy, acupuncture, herbalism, flower and gem remedies, color, sound, and light therapy, and the energies of vitamins and minerals. The ACTS is connected to you through your witness and delivers the treatment, which it has assessed that you need, at the right time and in the right quantities from its database. From there it may be recommended that you see your physician, or a homeopath or herbalist, according to your needs. ACTS has yet to be independently assessed.

PSIONIC MEDICINE

Psionic medicine was founded in the 1960s by a British doctor, George Laurence, with the aim of treating the basic cause of illness. It is similar to radionics, but practiced only by qualified physicians.

Radionics and psionic medicine are considered to be completely safe, and because it is noninvasive and appropriate for people of all ages, as well as plants and animals, it has grown in popularity.

WHAT CAN RADIONICS TREAT?

R adionics aims to treat the overall health of the sufferer, and in the process, many deep-seated health problems may be resolved; these include

- *asthma and eczema*
- *allergies*
- *chronic pain*
- *arthritis and rheumatism*
- *postsurgical pain and discomfort*
- *headaches and migraines*
- *sleep disorders.*

Crystal and Gem Therapies

HEALERS believe that gems and crystals placed on and around their patients can focus and enhance healing energy.

Placing crystals around your home is said to improve the atmosphere, absorbing negativity, but they should be washed regularly under cold running water and "recharged" in sunlight.

There is no scientific evidence that crystals contain powers or energies but they are often reported by those who use them to have an uplifting effect.

GEM AND MINERAL ESSENCES

More than 200 gem and mineral essences have recently been created in the belief they will assist the healing of specific mental and emotional states. Designed to be taken orally, they are made by immersing the stones in pure water exposed to sunshine, which is said to instill the water with their "healing vibrations." Again, there is no independent scientific evidence for this.

ELECTROCRYSTAL THERAPY

This therapy was developed by the British researcher Harry Oldfield in the 1970s *(see also page 21)*, and is said to promote health by "energy restructuring," rectifying imbalances in the patient's energy flow, so encouraging the body to heal itself.

Crystals are placed in a sealed glass tube in a brine solution, through which an electric current is passed. Tubes are placed on both the client's chakras and their affected meridians. This is said to pass a healing "vibration" into the body without direct contact.

Treatment is painless and has been said to cause improvements in a range of problems from migraine to MS.

SOME POWERFUL CRYSTALS

There are many crystals to choose from, and they have different attributes. Healers believe that uncut stones possess more energy than the polished variety. Crystals should be cleaned in sea salt then rinsed in clear water before you use them for healing purposes.

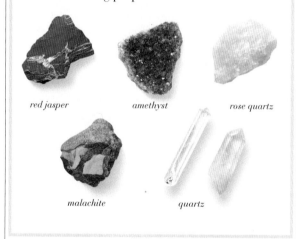

red jasper   *amethyst*   *rose quartz*

malachite   *quartz*

CAUTIONS AND CONTRAINDICATIONS

It is believed that the energy in crystals has as much ability to harm as it does to heal, and therefore your crystal must be dedicated for good. Ensure that your healer is aware of any health problems, so that treatment can be adapted accordingly. There are no real contraindications to crystal healing, although care should be taken with babies, children, and pregnant women.

Crystals are placed around the client to soak up negative energy or replenish low levels of positive energy.

WHAT CAN CRYSTAL THERAPY TREAT?

Crystal therapy is said to work on many levels to encourage healing and to reduce mental and physical problems; in particular, it is used for:

- *healing (for instance of injuries or wounds following surgery)*
- *stress and stress-related disorders*
- *chronic or fatal conditions*
- *arthritis*
- *pain.*

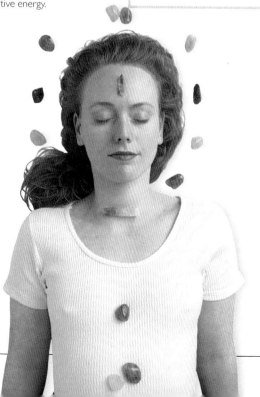

Light and Sound Therapies • Light Therapy

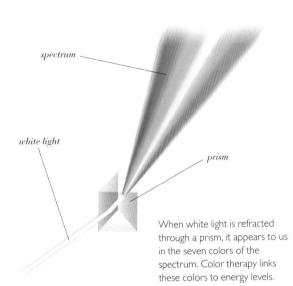

spectrum

white light

prism

When white light is refracted through a prism, it appears to us in the seven colors of the spectrum. Color therapy links these colors to energy levels.

LIGHT AND sound therapies are "sensory" because they act on the human senses through waves of both sound and light. Sitting in the sun or listening to a favorite piece of music can definitely affect your mood. But because not all sound and light waves can be seen or heard, many therapists consider that they work on the energy or "vibrational" planes as well as at the psychological level.

LIGHT THERAPIES

Insufficient natural light can lead to depression, tiredness, or overeating. In the winter, especially in colder countries, the level of indoor light produces only about a tenth of the illumination of a full day of natural light. A form of "winter blues" that can result from this is known as Seasonal Affective Disorder (SAD). It affects around 1 percent of the population (more women than men) but can be successfully treated with special "full spectrum" light units fitted into the home or into the office *(see page 229).*

COLOR THERAPY

Normal daylight (that is, light from the sun) is filtered through the eye to produce the visible colors of the spectrum – red, yellow, orange, green, blue, indigo, and violet. Other colors invisible to the human eye are ultraviolet and infrared, which affect us even though we can't see them, because our skin is receptive to changes in light.

Color therapists work with colors to rebalance the body on both the physical and "psychic" levels. Therapists who work on the physical level believe that as light is received and absorbed through the skin, it works on the nervous system to change the body's chemical balance. By adjusting the amount of specific color input they believe they can affect physical well-being as well as mood. Pink, for instance, is considered to have a calming effect, red speeds up the circulation and raises blood pressure, while blue lowers it.

On the psychic, or subtle energy level, therapists work to influence the seven energy centers, or chakras, each of which is said to correspond to one of the seven colors of the light spectrum, starting with red for the "base" chakra and ending with violet at the "crown" center. So, for example, green is said to influence the "heart" chakra and yellow the "solar plexus."

COLORS AND AURA

Many therapists work with your "aura" and "chakras" *(see page 121).* An aura is an energy field, which is personal to each individual. Some therapists claim to be able to see an aura, which manifests itself in the form of a shimmer or haze of colored light around the body. Every aura has its own colors, and they are affected by your health, well-being, and spirit. If your energy is compromised in any way, that will be reflected in the color of your aura.

Color therapists claim that every subtle change in color affects us on every level of our being. Recent scientific studies have confirmed that every cell of our body is made up of contracted light – and because light responds to color, the as yet unproved theories behind color therapy are believed to make sense.

Color therapy is aimed at restoring cells to an even level of balance, thus stimulating any necessary healing processes and improving overall spiritual and mental health. Your therapist will choose a color that he or she sees as vibrating at a frequency needed to restore the cells; he or she must take care to choose the correct color and offer it in the right "dosage" to ensure that the balance is maintained. Every color has both negative and positive attributes.

Many therapists treat with colored light because this is believed to be the most effective way of using color.

Sound Therapy

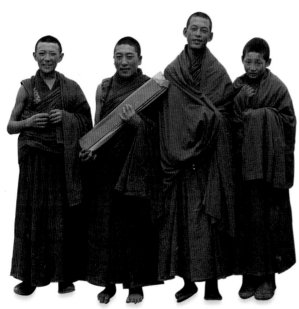

Tibetan monks use chants as part of the healing process.

SOUND THERAPY is a very ancient method of healing. Tibetan monks, for example, have used a method of "overtone chanting" for thousands of years for treating illness. The theory is that since everything in the universe is in a constant state of vibration, including the human body, even the smallest change in frequency can affect the internal organs.

Modern sound therapists consider there is a natural resonance or "note" that is "right" for each part of the human body, and for each individual, so by directing specific sound waves to specific areas they can affect the frequency at which that part is vibrating and thereby restore it to balance and therefore health.

Sound therapy may utilize special machines that transmit "healing vibrations" (the British pioneer Peter Guy Manners has developed a system known as Cymatics that claims to do this). But more usually it involves direct application of the voice, music, or a variety of tonal sounds and sometimes a combination of all three.

The work of voice teachers such as Chris James in Australia and Jill Purce in Britain has been influential in showing many people how to discover and use their natural voice through the use of sound tones. In the United States,

musician Jonathan Goldman has developed the therapeutic use of music through instruments such as the drum, didjeridoo, and flute.

Specifically directed sounds can be used in the treatment of a variety of disorders and have been particularly effective with mentally and physically handicapped children and adults.

CYMATICS

Cymatics grew out of the early research by British doctor and osteopath Dr. Peter Manners into electromagnetic energy. Dr. Manners believes that every condition, illness, or psychological state can be treated or improved by the technique because it releases tension in the system and allows the mind and body to return to a state of equilibrium. Because it is based on scientific evidence and knowledge, it is used and appreciated by the medical profession. Cymatics is painless and has been adopted in many countries.

WHAT CAN SOUND THERAPY TREAT?

Sound therapy and Cymatics are used to reduce pain and inflammation, thereby increasing mobility.

They are particularly useful for conditions such as arthritis, rheumatism, back pain, sports injuries, fractures, and soft-tissue damage. Many practitioners believe these therapies will help all types of illness because they release tension and produce a balance within the body.

CAUTIONS AND CONTRAINDICATIONS

SOUND THERAPY
Sound is a powerful force and must be used with care. Very loud or penetrating sounds should not be aimed directly at the head, and never close to the ears since they can burst the eardrums and cause deafness, and even death.

CAUTIONS AND CONTRAINDICATIONS

LIGHT THERAPY
There are no known contraindications to light therapy, although it is advised that you consult your physician before undertaking any complementary therapy.

The flute is an instrument that can be used in a therapeutic way.

INFECTIONS

SKIN

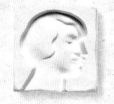

HEAD AND THROAT

DIGESTIVE AND URINARY

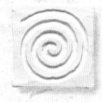

RESPIRATORY SYSTEM

MENTAL AND EMOTIONAL

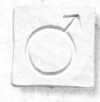

HEART AND BLOOD

MEN'S PROBLEMS

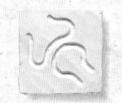

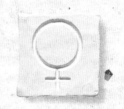

MUSCLES, BONES, JOINTS

WOMEN'S PROBLEMS

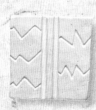

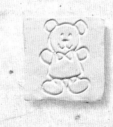

NERVOUS SYSTEM

CHILDREN'S AILMENTS

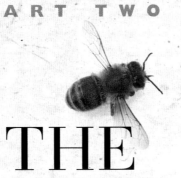

PART TWO

THE AILMENTS

INFECTION AND IMMUNITY • Infections

INFECTION leading to disease is caused by three main groups or types of organism: fungi, bacteria, and viruses. Unlike bacterial and fungal infections, which remain largely local, viral infections can affect a number of body systems at once. Alternative treatments for leading viral infections are described on pages 134–41. Treatments for fungal and bacterial infections are covered under the part of the body affected.

FUNGI

Fungal infections occur mainly on the skin and other warm, damp surfaces such as the mouth, groin, or vagina. Common fungal infections include athlete's foot and ringworm *(see Skin Problems, page 199)*, and candida/thrush *(see Women's Problems, page 240)*. Fungal infections are an unpleasant, sometimes painful, nuisance and inconvenience rather than a threat to life (although they can be life-threatening to people suffering from immunodeficiency disorders). All forms can be successfully treated by various alternative therapies.

BACTERIA

A multitude of bacteria can be responsible for serious illness, but not all bacteria are harmful. Many fulfill a useful purpose by balancing and eliminating other organisms in the body. A good example is the bacterium acidophilus, which is essential for keeping the bowels healthy. The overuse of antibiotics throughout the Western world in recent years has meant that many forms of harmful bacteria have become resistant to conventional treatment, so have become a major, and growing, problem. The bacteria that cause tuberculosis, bacterial pneumonia, and the skin condition impetigo, for example, are now on the increase after decades of being under control.

Alternative medicine can play an important part in effectively treating most bacterial infections.

VIRUSES

Viruses are minute organisms that reproduce only within their host. Viral diseases range from the common cold and influenza to more serious illnesses such as mononucleosis, hepatitis, and Aids. Viral infection is also on the increase among the population. It is widely believed that this is due to a growth in the number of different viruses, coupled with lowered defense systems in many people.

Here again, alternative medicine can be highly effective in treating most viral infections.

HOW BLOOD FIGHTS INFECTION

1 Once a microbe enters the tissues, neutrophils are alerted to surround and immobilize it. Complement and interferon are produced to attract further neutrophils and to prevent the spread of infection.
2 Macrophages collect the microbes and dead neutrophils and return them to the T-cells, while also ensuring more neutrophils are being produced.
3 "Killer" T-cells destroy the foreign organism while "helpers" stimulate the formation of antibodies, in association with the B-cells. "Suppressors" stop antibody production and control the killer T-cells once the infection is over, to prevent them attacking healthy cells.
4 Antibodies travel to the site of infection and activate complement to coat the microbes and attract more macrophages to the area.
5 "Memory" cells record the microbes' details so that the next time one of the same type enters the system, specific antibodies can be produced at once to deal with the infection.

lymph nodes in neck

thoracic duct

lymph nodes in groin

BACTERIAL INFECTIONS *see page 200* • IMMUNE SYSTEM *see page 131*
INFECTIONS *see page 199* • VIRAL INFECTIONS *see page 132*

The Immune System

THE BODY has an impressive array of defenses to block, trap, and kill outside organisms it considers a threat, with a memory to prevent them attacking again. Without this defense system (known as the immune system) most people would constantly fall ill from the wide range of threats to the body. Like an army on constant full alert, the immune system is active night and day to guard against attack and to repel or destroy invaders.

The immune system consists of the blood supply, the lymph system, and small sets of organs known as the tonsils, thymus gland, and the spleen. Defense against disease is essentially a function of white cells in the blood (leukocytes), and it is one of the jobs of this group of organs to produce these cells.

White blood cells produce substances that defend the body against attack from anything harmful such as a bacterium or virus. If an invader (antigen) gets past the barrier of skin, hairs, and body fluid, the defending substances – neutrophils, basophils, eosinophils, and, finally, macrophages – close in and finish off the organism. Some white cells travel in the bloodstream to fight infection while others remain in the lymph "nodes" (glands), situated mainly in the neck, armpit, and groin, where they destroy organisms brought to them by the lymph fluid. It is this battle between white cells and invading organisms that causes lymph nodes to become inflamed and swell; they can often be felt through the skin.

Body cells that become infected produce a wide range of chemical "messengers" to help in the fight against invaders. These chemicals (cytokines) – the main examples of which are interleukins and interferon – send messages to other cells telling them to protect themselves and thus prevent the spread of the infection. Complement, which also travels in the blood when an immune response is activated, coats the invading microbe to attract macrophages to destroy it.

Next in line of defense are T-cells and B-cells, both based in lymph tissue such as the spleen and lymph nodes.

T-cells are divided into "killers" (which destroy microbes), "helpers" (which stimulate the formation of antibodies), "suppressors" (which keep this production in check), and "memory" cells (which ensure a swift response should invaders of the same type return). B-cells produce antibodies, each of which is a response to a specific antigen. These not only protect the body but they also remember the antigen should another return in the future and try to get past the same defenses.

The lymph system consists of vessels, ducts and nodes. The nodes form barriers to prevent infection seeping into the blood-stream.

lymph nodes in armpit

A false color image of the malaria parasite, plasmodium spp, the cause of the parasitical infection that is transferred through the bite of the anopheles mosquito.

A healthy human blood cell. White blood cells are the defenders of the immune system.

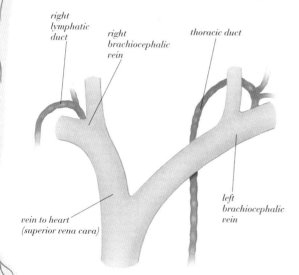

right lymphatic duct

right brachiocephalic vein

thoracic duct

left brachiocephalic vein

vein to heart (superior vena cava)

BACTERIA *see page 130* ❧ BLOOD *see page 164* ❧ VIRUSES *see page 130*

The Ailments

Common Viral Infections • Colds and Influenza

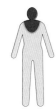

OVER 200 viruses have been identified as being responsible for the many varieties of cold and influenza (or flu) that are now widespread throughout the world. The most common, accounting for about a third of all infections, is the rhinovirus. Conventional medicine has no cure.

The main aim of most natural therapies is to speed up the process or alleviate the symptoms and, in the longer term, to help boost the immune system to fight off infection.

Cold symptoms may include a runny or blocked nose, sore throat, headache, watery eyes, and a cough. Influenza sufferers may also run a fever and have general aches and pains in muscles and joints.

SELF-HELP

Drink plenty of fluids, especially water and fruit juice, to replace fluid loss, and eat extra citrus fruit for vitamin C, or take a vitamin C and zinc supplement. Hot honey and lemon or cider vinegar drinks are also excellent.

❧ TREATMENT

AROMATHERAPY Steam inhalations are effective for alleviating breathing problems. Put a few drops of menthol, eucalyptus, or peppermint oil in a basin of very hot water, cover your head with a towel and inhale. Essential oils *(see box, and Aromatherapy, page 50 for preparation)* may be put in the bath, on a sponge, or vaporized in the room.

HERBAL MEDICINE Catmint is good for congestion, elderflower for catarrh, and camomile for bringing down a fever. There are also specific mixtures that are available in most health stores.

CAUTIONS AND CONTRAINDICATIONS

See your physician if the symptoms of your cold last longer than ten days.

Consult a qualified practitioner/therapist for:

ACUPUNCTURE AND ACUPRESSURE Both of these therapies can be used to strengthen the life force (chi) to fight off a cold and scatter phlegm.

TRADITIONAL CHINESE MEDICINE Massage of the back, chest and arms can alleviate symptoms.

HOMEOPATHY Remedies include Natrum mur., Nux vomica, Allium, and Hepar sulf. (coughs and colds), Gelsemium (for influenza, aches, and shivering).

COLD SORES

Seen as blisters or sores, especially around the mouth, cold sores are caused by the herpes simplex virus, and are triggered by changes in temperature and exposure to direct sunlight.

❧ TREATMENT

HOMEOPATHY Remedies that may help the condition include Hepar sulf. and Rhus tox.

HERBAL MEDICINE Licorice is said to inactivate the virus.

AROMATHERAPY Rub on the spot gently with lavender, geranium, thyme, or tea tree oil.

SELF-HELP

Keep the area clean and dry. Do not share toothbrushes, facecloths, or towels. Avoid nuts and chocolates, and eat plenty of wholegrain cereals, vegetables, fruit, lean meat, and fish. Boost the immune system by taking the antioxidant supplements *(see pages 78-9.)*

Eucalyptus *Eucalyptus globulus var. globulus* used as an inhalant or in a soothing bath is a traditional cure for colds.

ESSENTIAL OILS FOR COLDS AND INFLUENZA

❧ eucalyptus   ❧ lemon

❧ peppermint   ❧ lavender

❧ tea tree   ❧ sandalwood

ACUPRESSURE *see page 94* ❧ ACUPUNCTURE *see page 90* ❧ AROMATHERAPY *see page 50* ❧
HERBAL MEDICINE *see page 67* ❧ HOMEOPATHY *see page 83* ❧ TRADITIONAL CHINESE MEDICINE *see page 30*

Mononucleosis, Herpes, and Shingles

Infectious mononucleosis (glandular fever) is caused by a type of herpes virus known as the Epstein-Barr virus. It is most commonly seen in young people (hence its nickname: "student flu"). The disease is seriously debilitating and can take several months to clear up.

Extreme fatigue, fever, muscular aches and pains, sore throat, and swollen lymph glands, especially in the neck, are the symptoms of this illness.

TREATMENT

AROMATHERAPY Massage with essential oils; lavender has antiviral properties and is particularly effective. (Do not massage with oils while patient still has a fever; dilute oils with tepid water and sponge down instead.)

Consult a qualified practitioner/therapist for:
HOMEOPATHY Homeopathic remedies can help with specific symptoms, particularly exhaustion, sweating, aches and pains, and depression.

TRADITIONAL CHINESE MEDICINE AND ACUPUNCTURE Some sufferers benefit from these therapies.

DIET AND NUTRITION Eat foods rich in antioxidant nutrients (vitamins C, E, beta carotene, B-complex, and minerals copper, iron, zinc, and selenium). Garlic and ginger can be helpful. Sufferers from mononucleosis appear to have lower than normal levels of essential fatty acids (EFAs). A qualified nutritionist might recommend a combination of evening primrose oil and fish oils to help raise these levels and to alleviate the

symptoms of fatigue and malaise. Large doses of vitamin C (up to 100g) given by intravenous injection with the pharmaceutical drug amantadine hydrochloride may remove symptoms and promote recovery. It is the "alternative" treatment of choice in the United States, but must be given by a medical physician.

COUNSELING, RELAXATION TECHNIQUES, AND MEDITATION All of these therapies are helpful for relieving stress and depression.

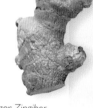

Ginger *Zingiber officinale* promotes perspiration and therefore is a useful cooling remedy in fevered conditions.

THE HERPES VIRUSES

There are over 70 viruses in the herpes family, the main ones being

- **HERPES SIMPLEX:** *causes cold sores around the mouth and sores on the genitals and eyes; after initial infection the virus becomes dormant and recurs after minor infections, trauma, stress, and sun exposure*
- **HERPES ZOSTER:** *causes chicken pox and shingles*
- **EPSTEIN-BARR:** *a variety of herpes zoster that causes mononucleosis.*

SHINGLES

The herpes zoster virus is the cause of shingles, which occurs when the immune system is weakened and the dormant virus is activated. Symptoms include acute skin sensitivity and a classic rash running around one half of the midriff. The face, neck, and (rarely) eyes may also be affected.

TREATMENT
Consult a qualified practitioner/therapist for:
AROMATHERAPY, HOMEOPATHY, AND ACUPUNCTURE All of these therapies are known to be beneficial in cases of shingles. Accupuncture can be effective in the treatment of postherpetic syndrome after infection.

CAUTIONS AND CONTRAINDICATIONS

MONONUCLEOSIS
Because of the risk of liver inflammation, avoid drinking alcohol while suffering from this condition.

SELF-HELP

MONONUCLEOSIS
Take plenty of rest: trying to get back to normal activities too soon is likely to slow down recovery. Boost your immune system by following the tips on page 135.

SELF-HELP

SHINGLES
Eat a balanced diet containing vitamins B complex, C, and E to help revitalize the damaged immune system.

ACUPUNCTURE *see page 90* ❧ AROMATHERAPY *see page 50* ❧ COUNSELING *see page 103* ❧
DIETARY THERAPY *see page 74* ❧ HOMEOPATHY *see page 83* ❧ MEDITATION *see page 118* ❧
RELAXATION *see page 116* ❧ TRADITIONAL CHINESE MEDICINE *see page 30*

Chronic Fatigue Syndrome ● ME

CHRONIC Fatigue Syndrome (CFS), also known as ME (myalgic encephalomyelitis), Post Viral Fatigue Syndrome (PVFS), and Post Viral Syndrome (PVS), appears to be on the increase and still poses a problem to many physicians. Some people believe ME is due to a chronic infection from Epstein-Barr virus (which also causes infectious mononucleosis fever, *see page 133*), but the triggers that spark off the disease are varied. In many cases it follows a viral infection, but vaccination or other hormonal and genetic influences may play a part.

Its wide range of symptoms makes ME difficult to diagnose except by the elimination of other possible diseases. The most common symptoms are chronic fatigue, recurrent sore throat and muscle aches, lymph node swelling, weakness, intestinal discomfort and digestive difficulties, headaches, loss of concentration, visual disturbances, and depression. Symptoms may go on for months or even years.

☙ TREATMENT

Treatment inevitably depends on the individual symptoms, but a combination of physical and emotional treatments may be helpful in this condition where conventional medicine has little to offer.

AROMATHERAPY
Essential oils, used both for massage and in the bath, are relaxing and help relieve stress and depression. Lavender (antiviral), grapefruit (for depression), rosemary and juniper (for muscular aches), and marjoram (for anxiety) are particularly effective. Many others would be appropriate for different symptoms.

HERBAL MEDICINE Golden seal and echinacea may be helpful remedies.

Consult a qualified practitioner/therapist for:
DIET AND NUTRITION Follow a healthy diet, avoiding processed foods, sugars, caffeine, and alcohol. Eat plenty of slow-release carbohydrates, such as pasta, to keep sugar levels constant, and high-energy snacks such as bananas. Evening primrose oil may be helpful – use a product from a recognized manufacturer and take the required daily dose. It may take several months to show any effect.

ME sufferers appear to be significantly low in the mineral magnesium, the amino acid l-taurine, and the hormone dehydroepiandrosterone (DHEA). American alternative physicians claim to have had good results within days with DHEA and intravenous vitamin C. A combination of evening primrose oil and fish oils to raise the levels of essential fatty acids also appears to have had good results. In moderation, B complex vitamins, zinc, and the antioxidants vitamin C and beta carotene may also be of use.

There is hot debate as to whether food allergy plays a part in ME (some sufferers have a milk intolerance). If an allergy is suspected, try excluding one item at a time *(see pages 28, 75, and 99)*. It is unwise to cut out too many foods at once. Chocolate and citrus fruits are common culprits for the irritable bowel symptoms experienced by some patients. In the past some ME patients have harmed themselves by eating an unbalanced diet and overdosing on too many vitamins and minerals. *(For advice on correct dosage and recommended daily intake of vitamins and minerals see pages 77–80.)* The involvement of the candida infection in ME is also contentious *(see Thrush, page 240)*. Some nutritionists believe that the balance of the organisms in the intestinal tract is disturbed in ME, causing an overgrowth of candida and intestinal problems.

SELF-HELP

Take some form of light exercise, but pace yourself – overstretching can bring on relapse. Get plenty of rest and sleep – at least six to eight hours a night – and accept the limitations that ME places on activities.

CAUTIONS AND CONTRAINDICATIONS

Do not take germanium supplements, which are said to encourage the activity of the immune system; studies have shown that they cause severe kidney damage. Avoid alcohol and any foods that exacerbate the condition.

Life in the modern world puts a great deal of strain on the immune system, and ME can strike anyone regardless of age or sex.

ALLERGIES *see page 158* ☙ AROMATHERAPY *see page 50* ☙
DIETARY THERAPY *see page 74* ☙ HERBAL MEDICINE *see page 67*

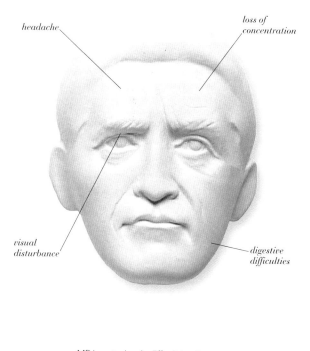

headache

loss of concentration

visual disturbance

digestive difficulties

ME is notoriously difficult to diagnose since its characteristic symptoms could point to many other kinds of ailment.

TEN WAYS TO BOOST THE IMMUNE SYSTEM

Follow the tips below to help fight off many of the more common infections.

◈ *Avoid all junk food and processed products such as margarine, white flour, and sugar; cut down on coffee, tea, salt, red meat, and battery-farmed poultry and eggs.*

◈ *Do not take drugs, especially antibiotics or steroids, unless essential. Overuse of antibiotics, especially, has been shown to damage the immune system, and many organisms are now themselves immune to them.*

◈ *Do not smoke at all or drink too much alcohol regularly (all smoking, even cannabis, is said to lower the immune system, as does too much drinking).*

◈ *Exercise frequently and regularly, ideally in sunshine and natural daylight: walking, cycling, swimming, and other forms of light exercise stimulate blood flow and increase production of killer T-cells (do not overdo it at first if your health is poor).*

◈ *Eat plenty of fresh (preferably organically grown) fruit and vegetables, wholemeal bread, pulses; drink herb or fruit teas and fresh fruit juices.*

◈ *Drink only filtered or bottled water.*

◈ *Reduce your stress levels, get plenty of sleep and take time for relaxation and to nurture yourself: treat yourself to a massage or another stress-reducing therapy you enjoy.*

◈ *Always think positive: there is a great deal of evidence – particularly from Aids and cancer sufferers – to suggest that maintaining a positive attitude to life and health can keep symptoms at bay, and in some cases even reverse the progress of disease.*

◈ *Take supplements regularly to boost your nutrient intake: antioxidants such as vitamins A (or beta carotene), C, and E, and the minerals selenium, zinc, iron, calcium, magnesium, and manganese help protect the body against damage caused to tissues by unstable molecules (free radicals).*

◈ *Make regular use of immunity-enhancing herbs such as echinacea (antiviral, antifungal, and antibacterial), ginseng (particularly useful during the recovery process), and astragalus (a general immunity booster).*

HOMEOPATHY This has been shown to have good effects on some ME sufferers; the results of the first major trial of homeopathic treatment of ME are currently being analyzed. It is essential to note that ME is a complex disease requiring professional homeopathic treatment.

REFLEXOLOGY This therapy is valuable in treating aches and pains, especially when the joint itself is too painful to be touched.

TRADITIONAL CHINESE MEDICINE This treatment approaches ME from a different direction, focusing on integrating the physical and mental areas. It involves the use of herbs such as astragalus, as well as massage and chi kung (self-healing therapy).

ACUPUNCTURE This may also be helpful.

COUNSELING AND HYPNOTHERAPY Emotional support and relaxation are essential in coping with this very stressful and depressing condition.

MEDITATION, YOGA, AND RELAXATION TECHNIQUES Any of these may help a patient come to terms with this chronic illness. They can help sufferers to remain fit yet as relaxed as possible.

ACUPUNCTURE *see page 90* ◈ COUNSELING *see page 103* ◈ HOMEOPATHY *see page 83* ◈
HYPNOTHERAPY *see page 112* ◈ MEDITATION *see page 118* ◈ REFLEXOLOGY *see page 52* ◈
RELAXATION *see page 116* ◈ TRADITIONAL CHINESE MEDICINE *see page 30*

Aids

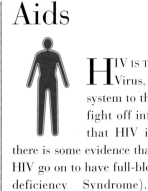

HIV IS THE Human Immunodeficiency Virus, which damages the immune system to the extent that it can no longer fight off infection. Most experts believe that HIV is responsible for Aids, but there is some evidence that not all people who contract HIV go on to have full-blown Aids (Acquired Immunodeficiency Syndrome). Infection by the HIV is followed two to six weeks later by the development of antibodies to the virus. This process may be accompanied by one or more systemic illnesses. Symptoms include

* heavy night sweats and fevers
* lethargy, fatigue, and exhaustion
* weight loss
* diarrhea, thrush, and herpes infections
* mouth ulcers and bleeding gums.

Complete recovery is the norm immediately after this illness, but thereafter the person will test positive for antibodies to HIV (they will be HIV positive) but otherwise appear healthy. Several years typically elapse between the acquisition of the virus and development of full-blown Aids.

Aids is generally believed to be caused by HIV. It is suggested that Aids may be an autoimmune disease (where the immune system turns against itself), but it is now clear that the immune system itself is attacked, especially the "helper" T-cells, so that the body cannot fight infection.

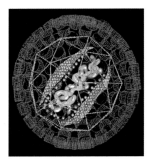

A computer-generated image showing the structure of the HIV virus.

SELF-HELP

DIET AND NUTRITION
Follow a diet (vegetarian, and preferably organic) high in vitamins C, E, and beta carotene, zinc (an antiviral), bioflavonoids (in green leafy vegetables and the pith and skin of oranges and citrus fruits). Eat pleny of sprouted foods for high nutrient content, and cut down on junk and processed foods, dairy foods, gluten grains, and alcohol. Supplements of gammalinolenic acid (GLA) from evening primrose oil can help combat fatigue and boost natural resistance.

LIFESTYLE
Cut down on smoking and drugs. Aim to reduce stress and anxiety levels. Take moderate exercise but do not exhaust yourself.

There is, at present, no known cure for the disease, which, once it develops, is usually fatal. However, a wide range of "natural" therapies have been shown to be effective in treating symptoms of the disease, successfully slowing its progress in many cases, and sometimes even reversing it.

Aids can appear in many forms, but around half of sufferers experience pneumonia (pneumocystis carinii) and a third Kaposi sarcoma, a form of skin cancer. Others suffer from a range of secondary infections as a result of their weakened immune system. Most suffer from fatigue and malaise, as well as stress and anxiety.

◆§ TREATMENT

The alternative treatment for Aids depends on individual symptoms, but is based on four main aims:

* to inhibit the virus
* to prevent and treat secondary infections
* to boost the immune system
* to treat the patient holistically.

Many patients benefit from a combination of several of the following approaches, with or without conventional medicine. Emotional support is essential since Aids is a disease in which physical and mental integration is particularly necessary for good results in treatment.

Consult a qualified practitioner/therapist for:

COUNSELING AND HYPNOTHERAPY These are valuable for helping to deal with stress and depression. The power of the mind over the body is particularly evident in Aids sufferers. Considerable research has shown that a positive state of mind toward the disease and survival has actually helped to raise the T-cell count in some patients and reduced their symptoms.

VISUALIZATION AND MEDITATION These can be used to encourage the body to heal itself.

TRADITIONAL CHINESE MEDICINE
A variety of Chinese treatments has been found extremely effective, including chi kung and the use of Chinese herbs, particularly astragalus, which inhibits the

Du zhong *Eucommia ulmoides* (top) and dang shen *Codonopsis tangshen* are both effective Chinese herbal tonics.

COUNSELING *see page 103* ◆§ HYPNOTHERAPY *see page 112* ◆§
MEDITATION *see page 118* ◆§ TRADITIONAL CHINESE MEDICINE *see page 30* ◆§
VISUALIZATION *see page 120*

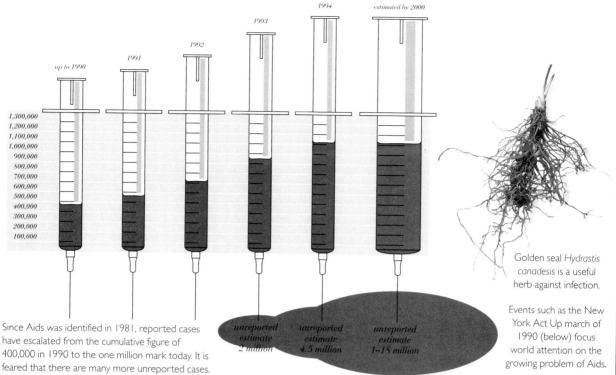

up to 1990   *1991*   *1992*   *1993*   *1994*   *estimated by 2000*

1,300,000
1,200,000
1,100,000
1,000,000
900,000
800,000
700,000
600,000
500,000
400,000
300,000
200,000
100,000

unreported estimate 2 million   *unreported estimate 4.5 million*   *unreported estimate 1–18 million*

Since Aids was identified in 1981, reported cases have escalated from the cumulative figure of 400,000 in 1990 to the one million mark today. It is feared that there are many more unreported cases.

Golden seal *Hydrastis canadesis* is a useful herb against infection.

Events such as the New York Act Up march of 1990 (below) focus world attention on the growing problem of Aids.

spread of the virus. Chinese dietary therapy is based on the idea that foods are hot or cold, dry or lubricating (by nature, not literally). Those with skin problems are advised to avoid "hot" and spicy foods, while those with diarrhea, for example, should not eat cucumbers or dairy products, which are "cold."

ACUPUNCTURE This has been found to be beneficial.

AROMATHERAPY Oils to use for massage and in baths include tea tree (which is antiviral, antifungal, and antibacterial), eucalyptus, lavender, juniper, myrrh, fennel, and sage. Oils can be taken by mouth, but only under the supervision of a therapist qualified in clinical or medical aromatherapy.

CAUTIONS AND CONTRAINDICATIONS

Complementary medicine does not offer miracle cures, and it is essential to ensure that your therapist is qualified before undergoing treatment. Since the Aids epidemic arose relatively recently, many charlatans have entered the arena, claiming to cure this condition.

HERBAL MEDICINE Remedies believed to be of value include golden seal and garlic. Golden seal contains berberine, another antibacterial, antiviral, and antifungal agent. It is particularly effective against diarrhea. Garlic increases "killer" T-cells.

HOMEOPATHY Some patients may find homeopathy beneficial.

MASSAGE AND REFLEXOLOGY These can provide stress relief and relaxation. Lymphatic drainage massage – which stimulates the flow of the lymph carrying waste products away from the blood – may also help.

YOGA, T'AI CHI, AND CHI KUNG These movement therapies are said to be beneficial.

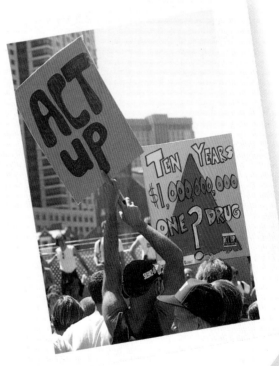

ACUPUNCTURE *see page 90* ❧ AROMATHERAPY *see page 50* ❧ CHI KUNG *see page 59* ❧
HERBAL MEDICINE *see page 67* ❧ MASSAGE *see page 48* ❧ REFLEXOLOGY *see page 52* ❧
T'AI CHI *see page 60* ❧ YOGA *see page 61*

Serious Viral Infections • Polio and Rubella

Polio (or poliomyelitis) is the result of invasion of the intestinal tract by the polio virus. Since the introduction of an effective vaccine in the late 1950s, the disease has been almost eradicated in the Western world, although occasional cases still occur.

Symptoms may vary from very slight to extremely severe, and include headache, gastrointestinal disturbance, and stiff neck and back. The most serious cases can progress to meningitis and paralysis.

❧ TREATMENT
In the acute stage of the illness, hospitalization and conventional medical treatment are the only solution. After the infection has subsided, a number of alternative therapies can help to alleviate the after effects of the disease.

Consult a qualified practitioner/therapist for:
MASSAGE, AROMATHERAPY, AND MANIPULATION These can all help to improve circulation and relax paralyzed limbs.

DIET AND NUTRITION Recent research in the United States has suggested that supplementation with the hormone dehydroepiandrosterone (DHEA) is effective.

COUNSELING AND HYPNOTHERAPY Both these therapies can help alleviate anxiety and depression.

Note In later life, some polio victims experience a kind of "post polio syndrome" – a worsening of their handicap with symptoms similar to those of multiple sclerosis. In such cases, alternative therapy treatment is similar to that for MS *(see page 193)*.

SELF-HELP
Supervised swimming or gentle exercise in a warm pool may help encourage the circulation in the lower limbs.

CAUTIONS AND CONTRAINDICATIONS
Polio is a notifiable disease and any suspected cases must be seen by a conventional medical physician immediately.

RUBELLA SYMPTOMS AND CAUSES

Rubella (German measles) is an acute viral disease that appears to come in epidemics. It is very infectious and, although the symptoms are fairly mild, if caught in pregnancy it can seriously damage or kill the unborn baby. Most young girls in the West are now immunized against rubella, and women planning to become pregnant should ensure they are tested for rubella antibodies.

Symptoms include a slight fever, rash and inflamed glands, lasting just a few days. For treatment *see German measles, page 252.*

Unless there are strong contraindications, babies should be immunized against polio, since it is a disease that could easily regain its hold. Side effects can be treated by a homeopath.

Foot massage (below), with or without essential oils, and gentle manipulation can help improve the blood flow in paralyzed limbs as well as making the sufferer feel relaxed.

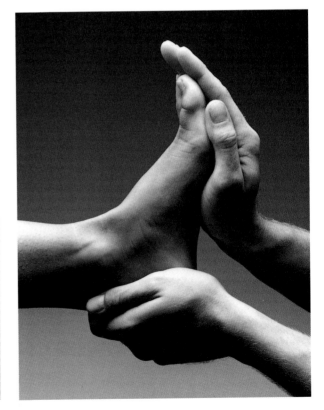

AROMATHERAPY *see page 50* • COUNSELING *see page 103* • DIETARY THERAPY *see page 74* • HYPNOTHERAPY *see page 112* • MANIPULATION *see page 38* • MASSAGE *see page 48*

Hepatitis

Hepatitis is a viral liver infection, caused by a number of related viruses, commonly hepatitis A, B, or C. Symptoms include jaundice, nausea, vomiting, fever, fatigue, and muscle pain.

◢ TREATMENT
In the acute stages of hepatitis, hospitalization and medical treatment are needed since the disease can cause irreversible liver damage and death. But there is a role for complementary therapies during convalescence and to prevent recurrence.

Boost your immune system *(see page 135)*.

Consult a qualified practitioner/therapist for:
HERBAL MEDICINE Catechin is believed to be effective in several types of liver disease, and has antioxidant properties. Dandelion, too, is a well-recognized liver remedy, being high in vitamins, minerals, and particularly carotenoids. Milk thistle, artichoke, and licorice are all established liver treatments.

DIET AND NUTRITION Avoid alcohol, which damages the liver. Eat a diet low in fat and sugars, and high in fiber. Some alternative physicians use 50–100g of intravenous vitamin C with the drug amantadine hydrochloride.

HOMEOPATHY Bryonia 30c, Mercurius 30c, Phosphorus 30c, and Hydrastis 30c may be recommended as constitutional treatments.

TRADITIONAL CHINESE MEDICINE Chi kung and Chinese herbs can be beneficial.

ACUPUNCTURE This may be of use in the convalescent stage.

Meningitis

Both bacteria and viruses may cause meningitis, an acute life-threatening disease that occurs in epidemics and has killed large numbers of children.

A blinding headache, nausea, severe neck stiffness (especially on bending the neck forward), and sensitivity to light (photophobia), coming on very suddenly, can all be symptoms of meningitis. There may also be an angry red skin rash, and in babies the fontanelle (soft spot on the top of the head) may become raised and taut.

◢ TREATMENT
Bacterial meningitis needs prompt conventional medical attention and will be treated with large doses of antibiotics. These will wipe out both the good and bad bacteria that occur naturally in our bodies, and this, in turn, can lead to the growth of fungal infections that those bacteria normally keep in check. During convalescence, alternative therapies can be helpful.

Viral meningitis usually needs no treatment, but complementary therapies, used after the condition has settled, will have a restorative effect and encourage quicker rehabilitation.

Consult a qualified practitioner/therapist for:
HERBAL MEDICINE, HOMEOPATHY, TRADITIONAL CHINESE MEDICINE, AND ACUPUNCTURE All these therapies can help to rebuild strength and immunity.

AROMATHERAPY, YOGA, AND MASSAGE All of these therapies can help strengthen body and mind.

Dandelion *Taraxacum officinale* is a herbal specific in cases of jaundice or liver related problems.

Infection and Immunity

CAUTIONS AND CONTRAINDICATIONS	SELF-HELP	SELF-HELP	CAUTIONS AND CONTRAINDICATIONS
Hepatitis B is infectious for months, so hygiene is essential during this period. Bathtub, toilet, and washbasin should be disinfected after use, as should crockery and cutlery.	Bedrest is advised for as long as the patient feels it is necessary. Drink plenty of fluids to cleanse the system, and take extra vitamin C. Avoid fatty foods and abstain from alcohol to encourage the liver to heal.	Boost your immune system (see *page 135*). Pace yourself when getting back to normal. It can take months to recover fully.	Meningitis is a medical emergency. Speed of treatment is crucial: suspected cases must receive immediate conventional medical help.

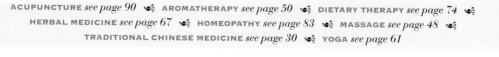

ACUPUNCTURE *see page 90* ◢ AROMATHERAPY *see page 50* ◢ DIETARY THERAPY *see page 74* ◢
HERBAL MEDICINE *see page 67* ◢ HOMEOPATHY *see page 83* ◢ MASSAGE *see page 48* ◢
TRADITIONAL CHINESE MEDICINE *see page 30* ◢ YOGA *see page 61*

The Ailments

Cancer

ANCER is a disease in which certain body cells go out of control and start multiplying rapidly of their own accord. This uncontrolled growth becomes a tumor and eventually, if unchecked, will interfere with the working of a vital organ or organs and cause death.

It is not an infection (although in a few cases it can be caused by a viral infection) but the result, in all probability, of some inherited weakness in the genetic makeup, coupled with poor living habits and surroundings. Unhealthy diet, smoking, prolonged stress, and industrial pollution, for example, are either known to be, or are strongly suspected of being, main contributory or risk factors in cancer.

The human body contains more than 200 different types of cell, which means there are more than 200 different types of cancer. An abnormal growth may be called a tumor or a neoplasm (neo simply means "new" and plasm means "form"). A resulting illness is known as a neoplastic disorder.

If the tumor or growth is purely local and not invasive it will be described as benign. A benign growth does not spread, so is less damaging. Examples are warts, cysts, and polyps. A growth that cannot be contained and continues to spread unchecked is known as a malignant growth. This is cancer.

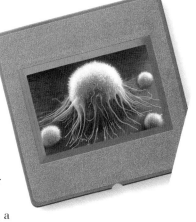

A computer-generated image of the structure of a generic cancer cell (left) compared to the color-enhanced image of a real lung cancer cell (below).

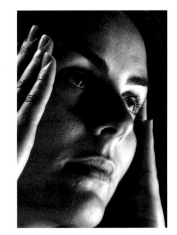

Evidence indicates that positive mental attitude can help when confronting cancer.

Medical terms given to the different sorts of cancer relate to where they are growing in the body:

❊ Carcinoma is cancer of the skin covering the outside of the body and the mucous membrane lining the cavities within (epithelial tissue). This is by far the most common type of cancer and includes cancers of the breast, lung, colon, prostate, and skin. The most serious form of skin cancer is melanoma.

❊ Sarcoma is cancer of the bones, tendons, and muscles.

❊ Lymphoma is cancer of the glands (or nodes) or other parts of the lymphatic system *(see page 131)*

❊ Leukemia is cancer of the blood.

Cancer differs from country to country and from region to region. Some types of cancer are more common in Western countries, such as North America and Europe, than in Eastern countries, such as Japan, or so-called developing countries such as Africa. In Japan, for example, there are many more cases of stomach cancer than there are in the West, and in Africa liver cancer is much more widespread than elsewhere. Overall, the ten most common cancers found worldwide are of the lung, stomach, breast, lower bowel, cervix, mouth, lymphatic system, liver, throat, and prostate gland. None of the therapies described offers a cure for cancer but they can alleviate symptoms and support the immune system.

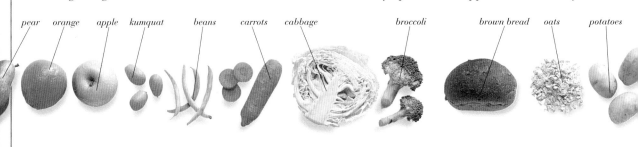

pear   *orange*   *apple*   *kumquat*   *beans*   *carrots*   *cabbage*   *broccoli*   *brown bread*   *oats*   *potatoes*

CERVICAL CANCER *see page 241* ❧ MASSAGE *see page 48*

Early Warning Signs of Cancer

Early detection of all types of cancer is extremely important. It means being continually on the lookout for unusual changes in the body that might signal the start of a cancer. The following are the common early warning signs of cancer:

❋ a lump or thickened tissue in the breast, testicles, or any other part of the body
❋ a sore or ulcer that will not heal
❋ persistent hoarseness or a nagging cough that has blood in it
❋ persistent pain or large lumps in the abdomen or difficulty in swallowing
❋ changes in bowel or bladder function
❋ obvious changes in a wart or mole
❋ unusual bleeding or discharge
❋ unexpected weight loss or loss of appetite
❋ undue fatigue, lassitude, or malaise
❋ persistent pain (though cancer is not always painful)
❋ painless, swollen glands that stay enlarged.

Note These could all be symptoms of a "benign" condition that can be quickly and easily cleared up with the right treatment, but you should always consult a physician right away.

✒ TREATMENT

An estimated 85–95 percent of all cancers are preventable, according to some experts. Prevention, then, is the key in cancer, as it is in heart disease. This means maintaining a healthy lifestyle, and mental and emotional state. And even when it is too late for prevention, the same things that can help prevent cancer are also recommended in its treatment (outside the standard medical treatments of surgery, radiotherapy, chemotherapy, or drug therapy).

DIET AND NUTRITION Eat less fat (trim all the fat off meat, and try fish or chicken instead). Buy only skim or semiskim milk, low-fat yogurt and cheese. Cut down on fried food (bake, broil, or steam instead). Eat butter (in moderation) instead of margarine; give up cream. Eat more fiber (or roughage): at least five portions of fresh fruit and vegetables every day (leave the skin on fruit but wash it thoroughly first); dried fruit, especially prunes (without sugar); plenty of dark green and yellow vegetables (spinach, broccoli, carrots); baked potatoes with the skins left on; plenty of wholegrain cereals (such as brown rice); granola, bran flakes, or porridge for breakfast; wholewheat flour and wholewheat bread only; wholewheat pasta.

Eat less sugar, less salt, and eat organically-grown food as far as possible.

✒ SPECIAL TREATMENT

Nutritional or dietary treatments have a good record for helping some people with cancer. Some are listed below.

THE GERSON THERAPY (OR GERSON DIET) This was created by the late Max Gerson, a German doctor who immigrated to the United States. It involves counseling as well as a strict diet, and requires determination and commitment on the part of the client.

MACROBIOTICS This is an Oriental form of food combining *(see page 75)*.

MEGAVITAMIN THERAPY Supplementation for cancer should only be prescribed by a qualified practitioner.

✒ ALTERNATIVE TREATMENT

Those alternative therapies shown to be most effective for cancer are
❋ psychological therapies: including art, music, and drama therapy; counseling; healing/faith-healing; hypnotherapy; meditation/relaxation; psychotherapy; visualization
❋ physical therapies: aromatherapy; Ayurvedic medicine; homeopathy; herbalism; massage; naturopathy/hydrotherapy; nutritional therapy; reflexology; yoga and t'ai chi.

Healthy eating can help your system. Eat organic food wherever possible, and aim for variety: lean meat and oily fish, at least five portions of fresh fruit or vegetables a day, wholewheat bread and pasta, and fiber-rich foods such as beans and lentils.

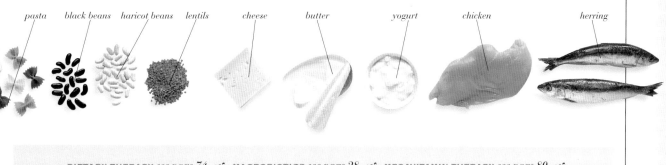

pasta *black beans* *haricot beans* *lentils* *cheese* *butter* *yogurt* *chicken* *herring*

DIETARY THERAPY *see page 74* ✒ MACROBIOTICS *see page 28* ✒ MEGAVITAMIN THERAPY *see page 80* ✒
PHYSICAL THERAPIES *see page 38* ✒ PSYCHOLOGICAL THERAPIES *see page 102*

BODY SYSTEMS • Problems of the Head

THE HEAD contains the brain, the sensory organs, and the throat – the gateway to the lungs and digestive system. Together these organs allow us to think, see, hear, breathe, take in nutrients, and generally make sense of our environment. The bones of the skull surround and protect the brain, the most complex organ of the body. It controls life as we know it, as well as our more spiritual thoughts. Located around the head are the chief sensory organs: the eyes, ears, nose, and mouth. The face is a reflection of our inner health, the way we look, and the condition of our skin and hair, and the brightness of our eyes can all indicate dis-ease, or ill-health.

The nose and throat act as "air-conditioners" or filters to remove harmful particles from the environment around us. The nose warms and humidifies air as we breathe it in, before it passes into the lungs. The throat is a multipurpose tube leading from the back of the nose and mouth to the trachea (windpipe) and esophagus (gullet) and is susceptible to infection that can spread upward or downward. The appearance of the lining of the mouth and throat, gums and teeth can all indicate our state of health. The ears are highly complex organs, made up of three separate compartments – the outer, inner, and middle ears.

The flaps of skin we refer to as "ears" are the least important – unlike some other animals, humans cannot turn them to pick up sounds.

The eyes are delicate and sensitive, yet they contain sets of muscles that can be strengthened with exercise – and can weaken with lack of attention. The eyeball is intricate, made up of layers of tissue. The retina, the inner surface at the back of the eyeball onto which images are focused, contains a layer of light-sensitive nerve cells. Information about light, color, and detail are transmitted from these cells along the optic nerve to the brain.

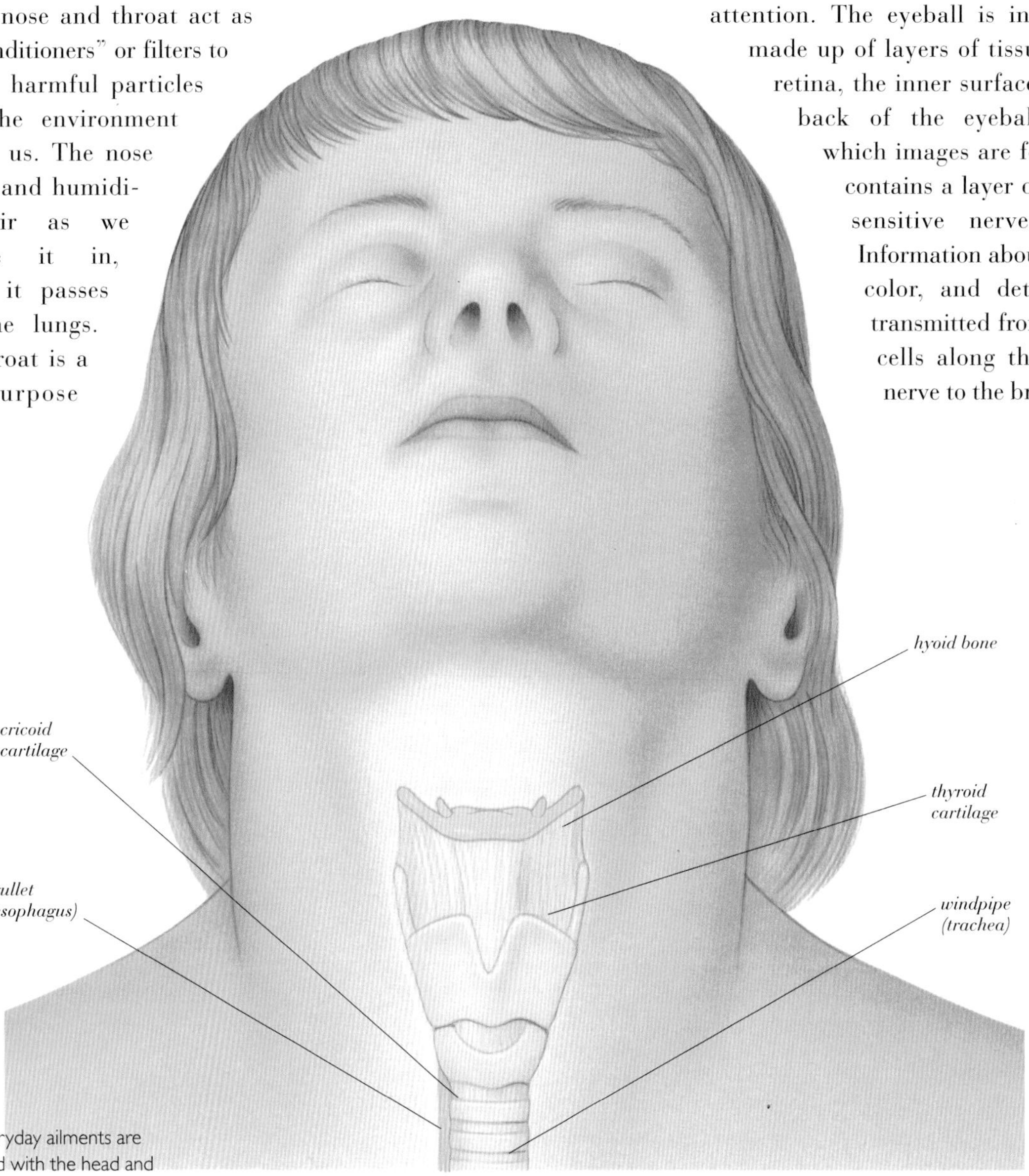

cricoid cartilage

gullet (esophagus)

hyoid bone

thyroid cartilage

windpipe (trachea)

Many everyday ailments are connected with the head and throat, and they can all be treated effectively by natural medicine.

BRAIN *see page 188* ❧ EARS *see page 148* ❧ EYES *see page 146* ❧ MOUTH *see page 150* ❧
NOSE *see page 149* ❧ THROAT *see page 150*

Thyroid Disorders

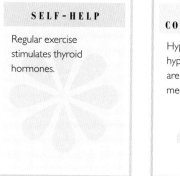

The H-shaped thyroid gland in the lower part of the neck produces the hormone thyroxine, which in turn controls a person's metabolic rate. An essential part of this hormone is the chemical iodine, and therefore an iodine-rich diet (containing seafood, shellfish, organic vegetables, and iodized salt) is a vital self-help measure for thyroid problems caused by iodine deficiency. Hyperthyroidism is overactivity in the thyroid; hypothyroidism signifies a sluggish thyroid.

HYPERTHYROIDISM

Weight loss, increased appetite, and bulging eyes are caused by overactivity of the thyroid gland. There may also be a rapid heartbeat (tachycardia) and tremors. Toxic goiter is another name for this condition, which is usually a result of overstimulation of the thyroid by an abnormal hormone rather than a fault in the gland itself. The conventional treatment for this is surgery.

✧ TREATMENT

HERBAL MEDICINE Infusions of the herb bugleweed three times a day help slow the action of the gland.

HOMEOPATHY A homeopath may prescribe Iodum 30c twice a day for two weeks.

HYPOTHYROIDISM

Lack of energy, muscle weakness, weight gain, and persistent infections are symptoms of this condition. They are a result of underactivity of the thyroid gland. Sufferers may feel cold and have a hoarse voice, coarse skin, and constipation.

✧ TREATMENT

HERBAL MEDICINE Infusions of the herb bladderwrack will help regulate thyroid function.

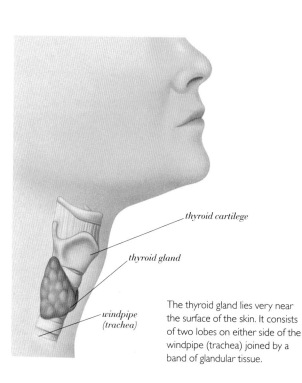

thyroid cartilege

thyroid gland

windpipe (trachea)

The thyroid gland lies very near the surface of the skin. It consists of two lobes on either side of the windpipe (trachea) joined by a band of glandular tissue.

Consult a qualified practitioner/therapist for:
HOMEOPATHY Specific remedies might include Arsenicum alb., but overall, treatment should be constitutional, prescribed by a homeopath.

GOITER

Goiter is an enlargement of the thyroid gland. Symptoms of the condition are palpitations, bulging eyes, irritability, and a high fever. It is not the same as hyperthyroidism *(see above)*. Goiter is often caused by a deficiency of iodine in the diet and can be relieved by taking iodine supplement *(see pages 79–80)*.

✧ TREATMENT

REFLEXOLOGY A reflexologist massages areas that relate to the thyroid, which are found in the big toe and the arch of the foot.

Consult a qualified practitioner/therapist for:
ACUPUNCTURE An acupuncturist may treat the condition with fine needles inserted into positions on the "energy pathways" of the body to clear obstructions of blood circulation and energy, and an accumulation of phlegm, which in Chinese medicine are related to problems with the thyroid gland.

HOMEOPATHY Treatment would be constitutional, but specific remedies include Iodum 30c, Spongia 30c, Calcarea 30c, and Fluoric ac. 30c.

SELF-HELP	CAUTIONS AND CONTRAINDICATIONS
Regular exercise stimulates thyroid hormones.	Hyperthyroidism, hypothyroidism and goiter are likely to need specialist medical advice.

ACUPUNCTURE *see page 90* ✧ HERBAL MEDICINE *see page 67* ✧
HOMEOPATHY *see page 83* ✧ REFLEXOLOGY *see page 52*

Migraine

THIS IS a persistent ache in the head, usually a response to stress or tension, or to toxins circulating in the blood as a result of infection.

Typical migraine symptoms include visual disturbances or hallucinatory "aura"; throbbing headache (classically on one side, known medically as hemicrania); nausea and vomiting; sensitivity to light, movement, and touch; and mood swings. Attacks last between two hours and two days. Migraines are often confused with headaches but are a quite separate disorder of the nervous system, although treatments for the two conditions overlap.

✎ TREATMENT

DIET AND NUTRITION Elimination diets pinpoint trigger foods, but avoid missing meals altogether because low blood sugar levels can bring on both headaches and migraines.

AROMATHERAPY A combination of aromatic oils and massage is an excellent way to soothe head pain. An aromatherapist will prescribe your own personal combination of oils, or you can massage your own head and temples with lavender, basil, or camomile oils. An inhalation, or hot water bath, containing the essential oil of true melissa, rosemary, or sweet marjoram can provide soothing relief.

HERBAL MEDICINE The herb feverfew is one of the most effective natural medicines for migraine. Dried feverfew is sold in capsules by health food stores, and the recommended daily dose is 125mg , or one fresh leaf in a sandwich daily. Valerian is a natural herbal sedative that helps reduce stress and is useful for headaches: pour a cup of boiling water onto two teaspoons of the root and infuse. Willow bark and meadowsweet are natural herbal painkillers. Lavender can also help.

HOMEOPATHY

Treatment should be constitutional but remedies for acute attacks include Natrum Mur., Lycopodium, Silica, and Spigelia.

Feverfew *Tanacetum parthenium* is a traditional herbal remedy for migraine headaches, especially those relieved by applying warmth to the head.

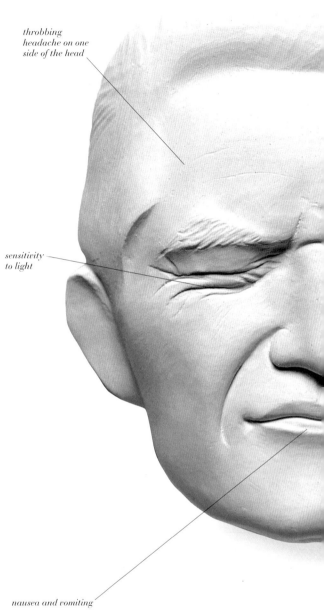

throbbing headache on one side of the head

sensitivity to light

nausea and vomiting

Migraine is not synonymous with the term headache. People suffering a severe headache often believe they have migraine, but the two are completely different.

Migraine pain commonly (but not always) affects only one side of the head and onset is often indicated by a sense of flickering before the eyes.

AROMATHERAPY *see page 50* ✎ DIETARY THERAPY *see page 74* ✎
HERBAL MEDICINE *see page 67* ✎ HOMEOPATHY *see page 83*

mood swings

SELF-HELP

Apply a cold compress over the headache. Massage the temples and back of the head, using deep thumb pressure or knuckles. Alternatively, massage the feet, hands, neck, and shoulders, to relax tense muscles and divert energy from the head.

Another self-help technique is temperature biofeedback, in which the client learns to warm the fingers to 96°F (35.6°C) by using the power of the mind (mental concentration; in other words you will yourself warmer). With 85 percent of clients, the method gives lasting improvement, with a marked reduction in both the frequency and severity of migraine headaches.

CAUTIONS AND CONTRAINDICATIONS

Feverfew can cause sore throats and mouth ulcers and should not be used in pregnancy. Persistent headaches without apparent cause require medical investigation.

SHIATSU

The aim of shiatsu is to disperse stagnant chi, or blocked energy. Gentle massage on the Gall Bladder meridian on the head and neck is an initial treatment to relieve symptoms of migraine, and fingertip pressure on the space between the eyebrows (the Yin Tan point) can relieve a headache. The shiatsu view is that stomach and digestive imbalance provokes headaches.

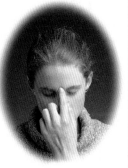

Self-applied shiatsu or acupressure on the point shown can often relieve a headache.

RELAXATION EXERCISES AND MEDITATION These can help to relieve the cycle of tension, stress, and headache.

YOGA Fifteen to twenty minutes a day of specific yoga asanas, or postures, such as neck-rolling or pranayama, can break an established pattern.

ALEXANDER TECHNIQUE Migraine and head pain may be triggered by tensed muscles, and exercises of the Alexander Technique help maintain and develop a stress-free posture and allow the mind to focus on the structure of the body.

ACUPUNCTURE Migraine sufferers respond to treatment on the Liver and Gall Bladder meridians, some of which are on the head.

PREVENTION
❋ Take vitamins B3 and C.
❋ Exercise regularly. Learn to recognize and anticipate stressful situations that are likely to trigger an attack.

Many ordinary foods can induce migraine attacks, and sufferers must learn to pinpoint their particular trigger. Cheese and chocolate are common migraine triggers.

ACUPUNCTURE *see page 90* ❧ ALEXANDER TECHNIQUE *see page 57* ❧ MEDITATION *see page 118* ❧
RELAXATION *see page 116* ❧ SHIATSU *see page 96* ❧ TEMPERATURE BIOFEEDBACK *see page 170* ❧ YOGA *see page 61*

Eye Problems

Severe problems with eyes should always be referred to a specialist, but alternative therapies can support orthodox treatment and may be very useful in conditions that affect the eyelids and tear glands. When treating infections and inflammations of the eyes, wash your hands between treating each eye, and use fresh materials so that you do not transfer infection from eye to eye.

CONJUNCTIVITIS

Conjunctivitis symptoms are red, itchy eyes; a yellow discharge; and inflammation around the eye or eyelid. It is normally caused by infection or allergy and is not serious except in newborn babies.

✎ TREATMENT

HERBAL MEDICINE Herbal eye baths made from infusions of eyebright (euphrasia), chickweed, elderflower, or camomile flowers are a soothing, effective treatment.

Consult a qualified practitioner/therapist for:
HOMEOPATHY A homeopath may prescribe Argentum nit. 6c for "gritty eyes" or Pulsatilla 6c for itchy eyes with a discharge.

EYESIGHT PROBLEMS

Hazy vision, difficulty in reading, tired eyes, headaches are all types of eyesight problems. They may be the result of vision problems, high blood pressure, and eyestrain, among other factors.

✎ TREATMENT

YOGA Candle gazing is a beneficial yoga exercise for eyestrain. Sit comfortably and gaze at a candle about 3ft/1m away, without blinking, for ten seconds. Palm for 30

seconds (p.147), then resume gazing with one eye only, then the other, then together, turning the head. Gradually increase the time (20 then 30 seconds) over several weeks.

Consult a qualified practitioner/therapist for:
HOMEOPATHY Specific remedies to be taken for eyestrain include: Arnica, when the muscles are tired; Natrum mur., when eyes ache upon looking up, down or around; Ruta grav., when the eyes burn or feel strained after close work or reading; Phosphorus, when tired eyes are associated with great nervousness and apprehension.

THE BATES METHOD *(see page 147)* This is designed to strengthen the eye muscles and rectify vision problems, as a natural alternative to wearing glasses.

CATARACTS

Cataracts cause cloudy, distorted vision resulting from changes in the protein makeup of the lens. They are most common in old age, but may be caused by iritis, diabetes, eye injury, and the use of steroid drugs. Some babies are born with cataracts.

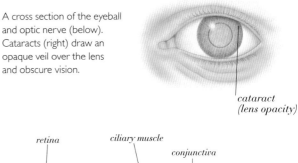

A cross section of the eyeball and optic nerve (below). Cataracts (right) draw an opaque veil over the lens and obscure vision.

cataract (lens opacity)

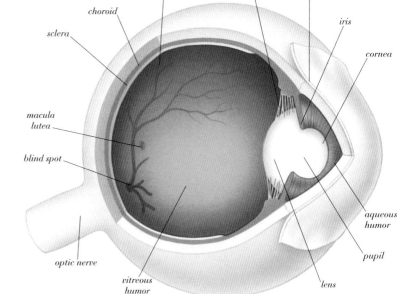

retina
ciliary muscle
conjunctiva
choroid
iris
sclera
cornea
macula lutea
blind spot
aqueous humor
optic nerve
vitreous humor
lens
pupil

CAUTIONS AND CONTRAINDICATIONS

Consult an eye specialist if your eyesight deteriorates.

⚠

BATES METHOD *see page 147* ✎ HERBAL MEDICINE *see page 67* ✎ HOMEOPATHY *see page 83* ✎ YOGA *see page 61*

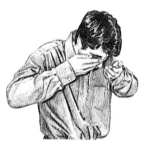

Start by splashing closed eyes 20 times with warm water then 20 times with cold water.

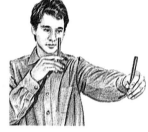

Hold two pencils as shown. Focus on one, blink, then focus on the other. Repeat 12 times.

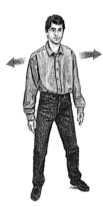

Focus on an object in front of you, and sway, blinking at left and right. Repeat 100 times.

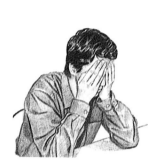

Close eyes and cover but do not touch them with your palms. Focus on pleasant thoughts .

✍ TREATMENT

DIET AND NUTRITION Research suggests that vitamins B2 and C can help improve the condition in which sight deteriorates as the lens becomes opaque. Supplementing with vitamin E and the antioxidant mineral selenium *(see pages 79–80)* can help rectify dietary deficiencies that can exacerbate the condition.

HOMEOPATHY Specific remedies include Phosphorus, when there is a sensation of mist being pulled across the eyes; Calcarea, for the early stages, with circular lines visible in the lens; Silica, for the later stages, when cataract begins to interfere with sight.

GLAUCOMA

Gradual loss of vision, aching pain in and above the eyes, seeing "rings" around lights are the symptoms of glaucoma. The disease is caused by a buildup of fluid in the front chamber of the eye. Glaucoma may be asymptomatic and vision may be lost before the sufferer is aware of the disease. If there is a family history of glaucoma, ensure regular screening by an optician.

✍ TREATMENT

HYDROTHERAPY Home hydrotherapy treatment offers immediate relief – place alternate hot and cold face towels over the eyes.

THE BATES METHOD These exercises can also be used to treat this condition.

HOMEOPATHY Take Belladonna 30c every 15 minutes for up to ten doses when symptoms start.

SQUINT

Squint is the inward or outward turning of the eye or eyes. In adults, squint is normally caused by damage to the eye muscles or the motor nerves that control the eye

THE BATES METHOD

This is a combination of relaxation and exercises to strengthen naturally the muscles that control each eye. It was devised by William H. Bates

Basic Bates exercises (see above)
❋ Splash the eyes alternately with warm and cold water twice a day.
❋ Avoid staring, and shift your sight constantly.
❋ Blink every ten seconds to lubricate the eye.
❋ Practice focusing on objects far and near.
❋ Stand and swing your body gently, letting the eyes move with the body.
❋ Remember particular objects. Bates believed that seeing objects in the mind's eye helped the eyes to see the object in reality.

muscles, usually the result of diabetes, high blood pressure, brain tumor, or brain injury. In children, squint should be treated before the affected eye becomes lazy and ineffective.

✍ TREATMENT

THE BATES METHOD Minor squints can be successfully treated with the Bates Method *(see above)*.

YOGA Palming relaxes the eye muscles and improves squints. Rest with your arms on a table and rub your hands together. Cup hands over closed eyes, shutting out all light, and relax for 20 seconds while being aware of visual sensations. Repeat at least twice a day.

HOMEOPATHY Specific remedies include Gelsemium 6c and Alumina 6c.

The Ailments

Ear Problems

As with eyes, serious infections of the inner ear should be referred to a specialist. Alternative therapies can be very helpful for problems caused by infection of the outer ear and excessive catarrh. Glue ear, a condition that commonly affects children, is discussed on page 250.

EARACHE
Earache is a sharp pain and fever caused by an infection of the outer or middle ear.

SELF-HELP

Hold a hot-water bottle against the offending ear. If earache is due to dental problems, see your dentist as soon as possible.

TREATMENT
HERBAL MEDICINE For immediate relief, carefully apply in the ear two drops of essential oil of St. John's wort, almond, garlic, or mullein and hold a warm hot-water bottle wrapped in a towel to the ear.

Consult a qualified practitioner/therapist for:
HOMEOPATHY Belladonna might be prescribed for acute throbbing.

TINNITUS
Tinnitus is a continuous ringing sound in the ears, usually the result of foreign bodies in the ear, pressure damage, some drugs, wax, and aging.

TREATMENT
YOGA Increase the blood circulation to the head with gentle head and neck exercises.

Consult a qualified practitioner/therapist for:
HERBAL MEDICINE Hopi ear candle therapy is a traditional Native American remedy and a safe and natural way of removing wax from the ear, one of the causes of this condition. A trained practitioner places a specially made cylinder or candle in the ear and lights it, drawing out old wax from the ear and introducing healing herbal vapors.

CAUTIONS AND CONTRAINDICATIONS

Consult a hearing specialist if deafness is sudden or prolonged.

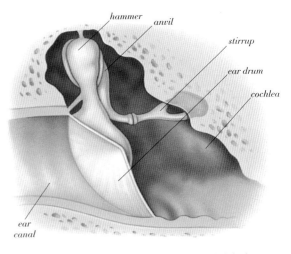

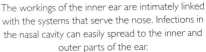

The workings of the inner ear are intimately linked with the systems that serve the nose. Infections in the nasal cavity can easily spread to the inner and outer parts of the ear.

HOMEOPATHY Specific remedies include Salicyclic ac. 6c; Carbon sulf. 6c; China sulf. 6c; and Kali iod. 6c.

DEAFNESS
This is complete or partial loss of hearing. Deafness may be due to infection, Eustachian tube blockage, excessive amounts of ear wax, or otosclerosis. It may also be caused by Menière's disease, drugs, poor nutrition, aging, and congenital conditions.

TREATMENT
NATUROPATHY A naturopathic diet rich in vitamin A promotes repair of damaged tissues in the ear and helps stimulate the auditory nerve. A grapefruit seed extract called Citricidal breaks up hardened wax – a common cause of partial deafness.

Consult a qualified practitioner/therapist for:
HOMEOPATHY Treatment would be constitutional, but specific remedies may include Phosphorus, Graphites, Aconite, China, Arnica, Gelsemium, and Chenopodium, all 6c.

ACUPUNCTURE
Therapists relate the ear with the working of the kidney and bladder, and may use fine needles to unblock these energy pathways and stimulate the nerves of the ears.

CAUTIONS AND CONTRAINDICATIONS

In cases of high fever or severe pain, consult a physician. Antibiotics may be necessary to prevent mastoid infections and more serious complications.

ACUPUNCTURE *see page 90* • HERBAL MEDICINE *see page 67* • HOMEOPATHY *see page 83* • NATUROPATHY *see page 24* • YOGA *see page 61*

The Nose

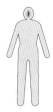

The nose produces extra mucus when there is infection in order to expel it from the body; the runny nose in a cold is a sign that your body's defense system is in good working order.

SNEEZING

Sneezes are a noisy expulsion of air and irritants from the nose, often a result of viral infection or allergy.

✑ TREATMENT

YOGA There are various yoga exercises, including rapid abdominal breathing, and breathing and stretching, that can alleviate nasal allergy. Cleaning the nose in the yogic tradition will help: fill a long-spouted pot with lightly salted warm water and, tilting the head, insert the spout into one nostril and pour water slowly until it comes out of the other nostril. Repeat on the other side.

CATARRH

A cough, blocked or runny nose, "chestiness" caused by a discharge of thick mucus from the lining of the throat, are all symptoms of catarrh.

✑ TREATMENT

HERBAL MEDICINE Use a gargle made from a teaspoonful of salt dissolved in warm water, or a drop of cedarwood oil in half a cup of water.

> **SELF-HELP**
>
> Temporarily exclude mucus-producing foods such as dairy products, eggs, animal fats, white flour, and sugar, and add garlic to the diet.

Consult a qualified practitioner/therapist for:
HOMEOPATHY Treatment would be constitutional, but specifics may include Arsenicum iod. 6c, Graphites, 6c; Hydrastis 6c; Kali bich. 6c; Natrum mur., 6c; Sanguinaria 6c; Calcarea 6c; Sulfur 6c, and Pulsatilla 6c.

SINUSITIS

Sinusitis involves a headache; painful, stuffy nose; and thick nasal discharge. It is caused by inflammation of one or more of the seven bony cavities (sinuses) at the front of the skull.

✑ TREATMENT

DIET AND NUTRITION Persistent attacks may be caused by a food allergy. Supplements of vitamin C and B complex, zinc, and iron are recommended.

HERBAL MEDICINE Use a steam inhalation made from aromatic oils such as eucalyptus or pine, and gently massage the bridge of the nose.

Consult a qualified practitioner/therapist for:
HOMEOPATHY Specific remedies may include Kali bich. 6, Silica 6c, Hepar sulf. 6c, Pulsatilla 6c, Belladonna 30c.

ACUPUNCTURE

This treatment assigns the condition to a deficiency of chi (the flow of energy) in the Lung.

> **SELF-HELP**
>
> Vitamin C and zinc will boost the immune system and reduce colds and sneezing.

> **CAUTIONS AND CONTRAINDICATIONS**
>
> Chronic catarrh and sinusitis may be caused by infection; if your symptoms are not relieved after a day or so of complementary treatment, seek conventional medical advice.

> **SELF-HELP**
>
> Humidify rooms and prepare steam inhalations. Increase your intake of vitamin C and B complex, iron, and zinc.

nasal cavity

organ of smell (olfactory bulb)

nasal bone

nasal conchae

nasal cartilage

hard palate

tongue

soft palate

The inside of the nose is lined with membranes that produce a constant stream of protective mucus to immobilize and remove irritants that come into the nose when we breathe.

ACUPUNCTURE *see page 90* ✑ DIETARY THERAPY *see page 74* ✑
HERBAL MEDICINE *see page 67* ✑ HOMEOPATHY *see page 83* ✑ YOGA *see page 61*

The Ailments

Mouth and Throat Problems

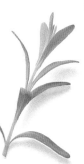

Like the nose, the mouth and throat are open to infection from airborne sources; they are also affected by problems in the lungs, sinuses, and stomach. Throat problems may be the result of constitutional weakness and respond well to the holistic approach offered by alternative therapies.

SNORING

The condition is caused when the soft palate of the mouth vibrates and makes a noise while the person is asleep. Snoring can usually be stopped by waking the sleeper or changing his or her position. However, it is sometimes a result of "sleep apnea," in which the snorer stops breathing for a minute or more during sleep. The body is stimulated by a rush of epinephrine (adrenaline) to make a sudden snoring noise. Sleep apnea, characterized by excessive daytime sleepiness, is a serious condition for which medical advice should always be sought.

◥ TREATMENT
YOGA Relaxing yoga exercises before you go to bed improve breathing techniques. Lie on the floor with your arms and legs apart and breathe deeply and slowly, to a relaxed rhythm. Breathe out for a longer period than you breathe in.

Oil of lavender *Lavandula angustifolia* mixed in warm water makes a soothing gargle.

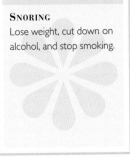

Oil of peppermint can be used to make a soothing ointment for the chest.

SORE THROAT
The main symptom of a sore throat is harsh raw pain on swallowing; this

may be accompanied by fever. Sore throat and pharyngitis *(see page 151)* are essentially the same thing. Most cases (70 percent) are caused by viral infections, the rest by the streptococcus. Viral infections are often accompanied by other symptoms such as a runny nose and a cough, while streptoccocal infection tends to be more severe in form.

◥ TREATMENT
HOMEOPATHY A homeopath may prescribe Hepar sulf. 30c for a very painful sore throat.

HERBAL MEDICINE The following may be gargled or sipped: 2 drops essential oil of lemon and sandalwood in a glass of warm water, or powdered root of licorice dissolved in warm water (it has a mildly anesthetic effect). Or try 30g of the herb red sage (or ordinary sage will do) mixed in warm water. An infusion of the herb golden seal is soothing. Make an ointment using eucalyptus and peppermint oils in a lotion base and apply it to the neck and chest.

LARYNGITIS
Laryngitis manifests as hoarseness, throat pain, cough, and excessive mucus, caused by inflammation of the mucous membranes of the larynx (voice box).

◥ TREATMENT
HERBAL MEDICINE An infusion of sage and thyme gargled – and small amounts drunk – every eight hours eases hoarseness. An infusion of marshmallow leaf drunk several times a day will alleviate the inflammation of the membranes.

HOMEOPATHY A homeopath may prescribe Belladonna for a sore throat, hoarseness, and pain, or Causticum for a raw feeling in the chest and throat, with Spongia for a dry cough (all 30c).

HERBAL MEDICINE *see page 67* ◥ **HOMEOPATHY** *see page 83* ◥ **YOGA** *see page 61*

Lavender
*Lavandula
angustifolia*

PHARYNGITIS

This is a sore throat caused by inflammation of the pharynx, which connects the back of the nose to the back of the throat. The inflammation is normally caused by acute or chronic infection, or is the result of smoking, alcohol, or overuse of the voice.

❧ TREATMENT

HERBAL MEDICINE Gargle with cider vinegar and honey, or warm water with a few drops of sandalwood and lavender oil, four times a day to alleviate the pain and soothe the throat. Use a steam inhalation with olbas oil, apply a cold compress to the throat to alleviate pain, and drink a herbal tea to soothe the throat.

HOMEOPATHY A homeopath may prescribe Lachesis to relieve a feeling of tightness around the throat, and Apis for an inflamed throat and stinging pain.

> ### SELF-HELP
>
> **PHARYNGITIS**
> Avoid cigarette smoke, alcohol, and use of the voice while the condition exists. Drink plenty of fluids and take extra vitamin C, B complex, zinc, and iron.

> ### CAUTIONS AND CONTRAINDICATIONS
>
> Herbs contain drugs so should be used with great care. Consult a physician if a sore throat persists.

The honey bee, whose body is the source of the homeopathic remedy Apis, which is indicated for sore throats accompanied by stinging pain.

TONSILLITIS

Sore throat, pain on swallowing, fever, and sometimes a blocked nose are caused by an inflammation of the tonsils. The disorder is most common in childhood. Tonsillitis is normally the result of an acute infection, although susceptible individuals can have attacks when they become rundown or stressed. Recurrent bouts of tonsillitis may be related to food allergy.

❧ TREATMENT

HERBAL MEDICINE Herbal treatments are among the oldest natural forms of remedy for tonsillitis, and they help cool swollen membranes. Marshmallow, plantain, elderflower, and catnip (catmint) may be used either as tinctures or gargles.

Consult a qualified practitioner/therapist for:
BACH FLOWER REMEDIES Holly, Beech, Agrimony, and Chicory Bach flower remedies are all beneficial for this condition. These concentrated remedies are bought in small amounts and a few drops added to mineral water. The remedy is prescribed not only for the illness but also for the emotional state of mind. An initial visit to a qualified practitioner is advisable.

HOMEOPATHY Treatment would be constitutional if the problem is chronic, but specific remedies are suitable for attacks; they include Belladonna 30c, Hepar sulf. 6c, Mercurius 6c, Lycopodium 5c, Lachesis 6c, and Phytolacca 6c. The remedy chosen depends on the nature of the pain experienced in the throat and the nature of attendant symptoms.

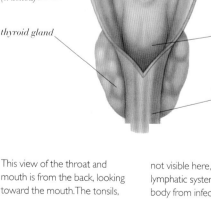

- nasal cavity
- *uvula*
- *tongue*
- *entrance to windpipe (trachea)*
- *thyroid gland*
- epiglottis
- throat
- *gullet (esophagus)*

This view of the throat and mouth is from the back, looking toward the mouth. The tonsils, not visible here, are part of the lymphatic system that defends the body from infection.

> ### SELF-HELP
>
> **TONSILLITIS**
> Bedrest and plenty of fluids will encourage healing and recovery. Chronic conditions will benefit from extra Vitamin C, B complex, zinc, and iron.

BACH FLOWER REMEDIES *see page 86* ❧ HERBAL MEDICINE *see page 67* ❧ HOMEOPATHY *see page 83*

The Ailments

Problems of the Teeth and Jaw

Problems with teeth and gums should not be ignored, as they may be symptoms of underlying disease. Bleeding gums can indicate vitamin deficiency. Ulcers or infections in the mouth, if left untreated, can lead to problems in the digestive system.

HALITOSIS

Halitosis is bad breath, possibly caused by tooth decay, inflamed gums (gingivitis), or digestive disorders.

❧ TREATMENT
HERBAL MEDICINE Chewing parsley and drinking peppermint tea sweeten the breath and neutralize odors.

HOMEOPATHY There are a large number of specific remedies to deal with bad breath, including Nux vomica, when the breath smells sour, especially after a stomach upset; Mercurius, when the breath and sweat are offensive, and the tongue is yellow and furry; Pulsatilla, after eating fatty food.

> **SELF-HELP**
>
> Adopt a vegetarian diet or lower-fat diet, and include leafy green foods.

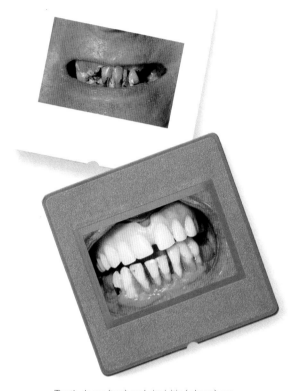

Tooth decay (top) and gingivitis (above) are conditions that can easily be avoided by sensible diet and adequate oral hygiene.

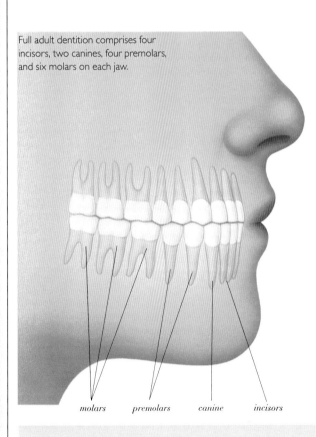

Full adult dentition comprises four incisors, two canines, four premolars, and six molars on each jaw.

molars   premolars   canine   incisors

GINGIVITIS

This is a bacterial infection of the gums caused by a buildup of plaque. Symptoms include sore, bleeding gums. Occasionally gingivitis is caused by vitamin deficiency, drugs, or blood disorders. Avoid the condition by cleaning your teeth regularly and using dental floss.

❧ TREATMENT
HOMEOPATHY Remedies include Mercurius, when the gums are found to be spongy and the breath is bad; Kreosotum, when the gums are red, inflamed, and swollen, and are bleeding easily with the roots of the teeth exposed; and Natrum mur., when the gums are swollen, bleeding, and there are mouth ulcers and also a taste of pus in the mouth.

> **SELF-HELP**
>
> Regular brushing and flossing of the teeth is essential. An effective, natural toothpaste can be made with two parts sodium bicarbonate and one part table salt. Chewing cardamom seeds also helps.

ORAL THRUSH

Oral thrush is small white patches inside the mouth, lips, tongue, and gums caused by a fungal infection, candida. It is most common in the young and elderly, and in the immunosuppressed. Oral steroids, long illnesses and antibiotics may also encourage infestation.

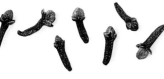

Cloves *Syzygium aromaticum*, chewed raw or as oil, are a well-known folk remedy for the relief of toothache.

> **CAUTIONS AND CONTRAINDICATIONS**
>
> **MOUTH ULCERS AND THRUSH**
> Consult a physician for further advice if an ulcer fails to heal or if the symptoms of thrush persist for longer than a few days.

> **SELF-HELP**
>
> **MOUTH ULCERS**
> Supplement the diet with wheat germ or brewer's yeast in case of vitamin B3 deficiency.

❧ TREATMENT

DIET AND NUTRITION Starve this fungal infection by temporarily excluding sugars and refined carbohydrates from the diet. Adding garlic, olive oil, and live yogurt containing acidophilus to the diet will help kill the infection.

HERBAL MEDICINE For immediate relief, use natural mouthwashes containing aloe vera, myrrh, or marigold.

HOMEOPATHY Constitutional treatment is advisable but specific remedies may include Borax, to be used at the beginning of an attack; Capsicum, when the patches are hot and sore; Natrum mur., when there are cold sores on the lips; and Arsenicum alb., when there are mouth ulcers.

MOUTH ULCERS

These are painful yellowish, round or oval spots inside the mouth. They are often a sign of being run down or under stress but can be caused by injury to the tongue and mouth, or by hot or acidic foods. In some cases they are caused by food allergy.

❧ TREATMENT

HERBAL MEDICINE Mouthwashes containing marigold, myrrh, and thyme are healing, or rub aloe vera gel over the ulcer.

HOMEOPATHY Constitutional treatment is suggested if ulcers are chronic, but specific remedies include Borax, Arsenicum alb., Mercurius, and Nitric ac.

TOOTHACHE

Tooth and gum pain, which may extend into the head, is usually the result of an abscess, dental decay, sensitivity, gingivitis, and sinusitis.

❧ TREATMENT

HERBAL MEDICINE Rub in essential oil of cloves.

HOMEOPATHY Specific remedies which can be given every five minutes for up to ten doses include: Plantago, Coffea, Chamomilla, Mercurius, Pulsatilla, Staphisagria, Belladonna, Bryonia, Apis, and Calcarea.

TEMPOROMANDIBULAR JOINT (TMJ) SYNDROME

TMJ syndrome involves pain in the head, jaws, and face, often caused by teeth grinding (bruxism).

❧ TREATMENT

HYDROTHERAPY Using alternate hot towels and an ice pack on the painful area offers immediate relief.

AUTOGENIC TRAINING This therapy involves special exercises that can successfully relieve muscle tension in the jaw.

HOMEOPATHY There are specific remedies for teeth grinding, including Cina, Santoninum, Phytolacca, Zinc, and Arsenicum alb.

> **SELF-HELP**
>
> **TOOTHACHE AND TMJ**
> Rub oil of cloves into the affected tooth and use a hot-water bottle to ease pain until dental treatment is available. TMJ will benefit from an ice pack on the afflicted area.

> **CAUTIONS AND CONTRAINDICATIONS**
>
> **TOOTHACHE AND TMJ**
> Persistent pain and sensitivity should be seen by a dentist within 48 hours.

AUTOGENIC TRAINING *see page 117* ❧ DIETARY THERAPY *see page 74* ❧
HERBAL MEDICINE *see page 67* ❧ HOMEOPATHY *see page 83* ❧ HYDROTHERAPY *see page 26*

Problems of the Respiratory System

THE BODY'S breathing system is known as the respiratory system and is, with the heart and blood supply, probably the most important system in the body. When working properly it provides us with the oxygen we need to survive and removes carbon dioxide we do not need. The human body can go without food for weeks, without water for days – but without oxygen from the air we breathe we cannot last more than a few minutes.

Of all the muscles in the body, the muscles we use to breathe are the only ones over which we have dual control; that is, they can work both automatically and voluntarily. In healthy people, breathing in and out happens automatically but, when necessary, we can also control it. We do this, for example, to avoid inhaling smoke and fumes, when singing, or when swimming under water.

HOW WE BREATHE

The respiratory system is made up of the ribcage and intercostal muscles, the diaphragm – a sheet of muscle between the chest and stomach – and the respiratory tract, which comprises the airways and lungs.

When we breathe, the muscles in the thorax that link the ribs contract, pulling the ribs up and out. The diaphragm pulls the chest cavity down, and together these two processes cause the lungs to expand. Cold air is drawn in through the nose where it is warmed and then taken down into the lungs. When enough air has been inhaled successfully (which is called inspiration), the muscles and diaphragm relax and the air is exhaled as the lungs compress (called expiration). Then the diaphragm contracts once more and the cycle begins again.

When the air passes through the nose it enters the trachea (the windpipe) and the bronchi, which are small airways that run through each lung. These bronchi become smaller and smaller, eventually taking the form of bronchioles, which end as tiny air sacs called alveoli. The alveoli are linked to blood capillaries, which exchange oxygen and carbon dioxide at a very quick rate.

On average we take about 12 breaths per minute, and that rate is controlled by the body according to its needs at a particular point in time. If there is too much carbon dioxide and too little oxygen, the rate of respiration will increase and the body will gulp or gasp for air. This may, for example, occur during strenuous exercise, an asthma attack, or in fright. When the levels of oxygen and carbon dioxide return to normal, breathing returns to its normal rate of respiration.

When we are stressed, we may breathe at an accelerated rate. Rapid breathing is a general response to stress, and it leads to overall tension of the muscles and

WARNING SIGNS

Consult a physician if you notice or experience any of the following:

- *blood in spit*
- *chest pain and/or shortness of breath*
- *persistent fever*
- *a cough that lasts or worsens over two to three weeks*
- *if you have inhaled a foreign body.*

Aerobic exercise such as swimming helps expand the lung capacity.

DIAPHRAGMATIC BREATHING *see page 25* • **STRESS** *see page 223*

When we breathe, air is drawn in through the nose and passes down the windpipe (trachea), which divides into two tubes called the bronchi. These lead directly into each lung, where they subdivide into small bronchioles.

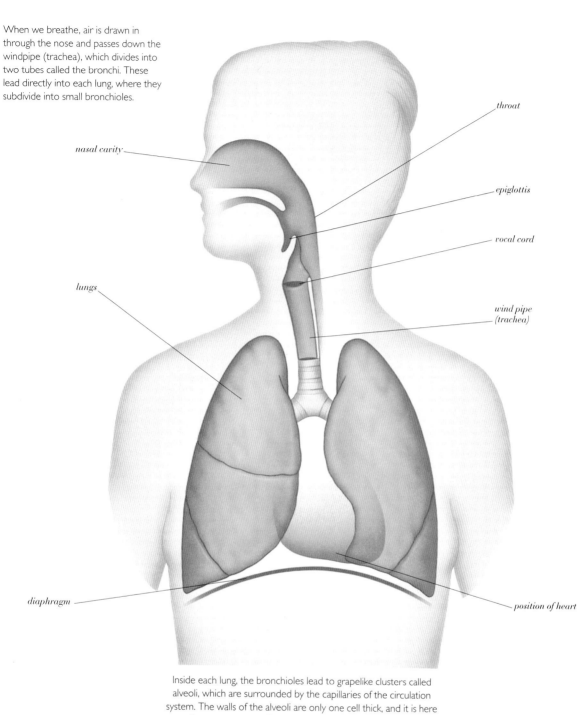

throat

nasal cavity

epiglottis

vocal cord

lungs

wind pipe (trachea)

diaphragm

position of heart

Inside each lung, the bronchioles lead to grapelike clusters called alveoli, which are surrounded by the capillaries of the circulation system. The walls of the alveoli are only one cell thick, and it is here that oxygen passes from the lungs into the bloodstream.

eventually dizziness, faintness, and a sensation of pins and needles caused by metabolic changes in the body. Overbreathing causes the concentration of carbon dioxide in the alveoli of the lungs to fall, leading to a buildup of alkali in the bloodstream and tissue fluid. This alkalosis produces the symptoms outlined above.

When we breathe normally, and efficiently, we use our diaphragm, which contracts and becomes flat, increasing the space in the chest into which the lungs can expand. When lungs are able to expand to their full capacity, all residual carbon dioxide is expelled and more oxygen can be inhaled. Many adults have to relearn breathing because of lifelong bad habits.

A variety of disorders – physical injury, infections, viruses, allergies, and diseases – can disrupt and endanger the normal breathing processes.

ALLERGIES *see page 158*

DIAPHRAGMATIC BREATHING *see page 25* ● INFECTIONS *see page 130* ● VIRUSES *see page 130*

Common Breathing Problems

Breathing problems are becoming more common as air becomes more polluted. Many alternative therapies, especially herbal medicine and homeopathy, can help in many of the more common conditions that affect the respiratory system.

COUGHS

Coughing is the body's natural way of clearing irritation and congestion from the lungs and airways. A dry cough is reacting to an irritant, a productive cough helps to expel congested phlegm. A common cold or influenza is usually accompanied by a cough. But coughs can be a sign of other respiratory problems (a hoarse cough may indicate laryngitis in an adult and croup or whooping cough in a child), or more serious breathing disorders *(see Pleurisy, Pneumonia, Tuberculosis, Emphysema, and Asthma)*.

❧ TREATMENT

HERBAL MEDICINE Make infusions of the following:
* for most coughs white horehound is effective
* for a hard cough use mullein
* for an irritating cough in adults use wild lettuce, and in children wild cherry bark (a mild sedative)
* for a cough with a fever use yarrow or angelica
* for a catarrhal cough use elecampane or elderflower.

DIET AND NUTRITION Biochemic tissue salts, taken in tablet form:
* for a hard, dry cough with fever – Ferrum phos.
* for a cough with thick, white phlegm – Kali mur.
* for a cough with yellow phlegm that is worse at night – Kali sulf.
* for a spasmodic painful cough – Magnesia phos.
* for a loose, rattling cough with watery phlegm – Calcarea, alternating with Ferrum phos.

CAUTIONS AND CONTRAINDICATIONS

Coughs that last for more than a week, or are accompanied by fever, difficulty in breathing, blue tongue or lips, drowsiness, or difficulty speaking should be treated by your physician.

SELF-HELP

Hot lemon and honey drinks will soothe a sore throat and ease coughing. Ensure that rooms are humidified and that the patient does not come into contact with smoke.

AROMATHERAPY Massage chest and back with essential oils – eucalyptus, sandalwood, frankincense, and myrrh are recommended. Add essential oils to hot water and inhale to help expel phlegm. For a dry, hard cough, try cypress, hyssop, bergamot, or camomile oil used as steam inhalations.

HOMEOPATHY

A homeopath might suggest the following

❧ ESSENCE	❧ USE
Bryonia	for dry coughs: painful bouts, worse on movement, accompanied by thirst
Aconite	for frequent, hard sounding coughs: particularly after exposure to cold, with fever
Pulsatilla	for persistent coughs: worse when taking breath
Phosphorus or Drosera	for tickly throat leading to coughing fit: retching, worse when lying down
Rumex	for tickly coughs: set off by cold air
Antimonium tart.	for noisy, rasping, hoarse coughs: with breathing difficulties
Spongia	for rasping but without wheeze: violent at night – (also remedy for croup)
Hepar sulf. Corallium, or Antimonium tart.	for coughs producing phlegm: with spasms, yellow mucus
Arsenicum alb.	for coughs producing phlegm: with frothy mucus, and wheeze

NOTE Doses of the above remedies will vary. Consult your practitioner.

Consult a qualified practitioner/therapist for:

ACUPRESSURE Coughing spasms in the upper back can be relieved by pressure on the point between the shoulder blade and spine, at heart level.

ACUPUNCTURE An imbalance in the flow of energy to the lungs can be treated by inserting needles into the Lung meridian on the arms, or into the meridian of another organ with a related rhythm.

Acupuncture is helpful in rebalancing the energy flow to the lungs. These are Japanese acupuncture needles.

ACUPRESSURE *see page 94* ❧ ACUPUNCTURE *see page 90* ❧ AROMATHERAPY *see page 50* ❧ DIETARY THERAPY *see page 74* ❧ HERBAL MEDICINE *see page 67*

HAY FEVER

Hay fever is an extreme reaction to pollen from flowers, grass, and trees in the spring and summer *(see also Asthma, Eczema, and Allergies)*. Symptoms may include headache, congested runny nose, sneezing, itchy watery eyes, sore throat.

TREATMENT

🖙 **DIET AND NUTRITON** *Cut down on mucus-forming dairy products such as cheese and milk. Take vitamin B. Large doses of vitamin C supplements with bioflavonoids (found in citrus fruits) act as natural antihistamine.*

🖙 **HOMEOPATHY** *Allium cepa, Arsenicum album, and Sabadilla relieve running eyes and painful sneezing.*

🖙 **AROMATHERAPY** *Massage sinuses with essential oils of lavender, elecampane (with jojoba cream), and sweet almond oil, in order to ease congestion.*

🖙 **ACUPRESSURE** *Pressure on the webbing that is found between thumb and index finger, together with vigorous exercise, can help to control hay fever, which is often aggravated by stress.*

Essential oils massaged into the sinuses can help hay fever; used in a steam inhalation they can benefit bronchitic wheezing, although they are not recommended for asthmatic conditions.

BRONCHITIS/WHEEZING

Bronchitis is an inflammation of the airways that connect the windpipe to the lungs (bronchi). Acute bronchitis lasts up to two weeks and is caused by a variety of viruses and bacteria. It can be dangerous in the elderly and those with heart disease. Chronic bronchitis is more serious and can last for months, getting progressively worse. It is usually caused by breathing polluted air or smoking. Coal miners and construction workers, for example, are particularly susceptible.

Symptoms of bronchitis include a persistent cough producing phlegm, breathlessness, chest pains, fever, and headache.

🖙 **TREATMENT**
AROMATHERAPY Take deep inhalations of eucalyptus and sweet thyme.

The fluffy seeds of dandelion "clocks" can trigger a bout of hay fever.

HERBAL MEDICINE A cupful of elecampane infusion, three times daily, can be helpful in clearing mucus and easing a bronchial cough. And taking garlic capsules every night in winter and herbal teas cold twice daily may help prevent a recurrence of acute bronchitis.

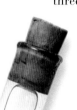

Consult a qualified practitioner/therapist for:
HOMEOPATHY Remedies will be prescribed for the individual case but may include the following: Aconite 6c for fever, tight chest, tickly cough, and thirst might be recommended; Kali bich. 6c when there is loose white sputum, a rattling cough, and irritability; Phosphorus 6c for voice loss, burning throat, cough, and thirst; Pulsatilla for dry cough at night when lying down, lack of thirst, and loose green sputum in the morning.

TRADITIONAL CHINESE MEDICINE This treatment aims to improve lung energy with remedies such as plantain seed, balloon flower root, honeysuckle flowers, or gardenia fruit.

SELF-HELP

Cover windows with net curtains; wear sunglasses. Use an ionizer to reduce airborne irritants. Control household dust and mites with special quilt and mattress covers.

CAUTIONS AND CONTRAINDICATIONS

Chronic bronchitis should be brought to the attention of your physician. If there are signs of respiratory failure (characterized by severe shortness of breath and blue lips), seek emergency medical attention.

SELF-HELP

Stop smoking and use steam inhalations whenever possible. Bedrest is suggested for attacks, with hot drinks and a hot water bottle placed on the chest. Avoid cold and damp air, and avoid contact with people suffering from colds.

🖙 ACUPRESSURE *see page 94* 🖙 AROMATHERAPY *see page 50* 🖙 DIETARY THERAPY *see page 74* 🖙
HERBAL MEDICINE *see page 67* 🖙 HOMEOPATHY *see page 83* 🖙 TRADITIONAL CHINESE MEDICINE *see page 30*

Allergies

AN ALLERGY is an abnormal reaction of the immune system to substances that cause no symptoms in the majority of people *(see page 131)*. One in eight people has one or more allergies, and allergic conditions tend to run in families. The condition is described as atopy, and people with classic allergic symptoms are described as atopic. As atopy is often inherited, it may be that the genes responsible for immune control are acting abnormally. Many common conditions such as hay fever, asthma, and eczema are caused by allergic reactions.

Allergic responses are triggered by the immune system, whose job it is to recognize foreign proteins (antigens) such as bacteria and viruses, and produce antibodies to fight them. The immune system also sensitizes the lymphocytes (white blood cells) to interact with the antigens to destroy them.

In allergies, the immune system mistakes harmless substances (allergens) for antigens and forms antibodies and sensitized lymphocytes to fight them. For example, in hay fever (also called allergic rhinitis) the allergy is the result of breathing in allergens such as dust, pollen, or house mites. Allergies can also be caused by exposure of the skin to chemicals, or an adverse reaction to certain foods.

Wheat and wheat products are common allergy triggers.

There are several mechanisms involved in allergies, or hypersensitivity reactions as they are also called. Most common allergies are caused by Type 1 hypersensitivity reactions, which cause immediate symptoms. The allergen causes the immune system to produce specific antibodies called immunoglobulin E (IgE), which coat mast cells present in the lungs and respiratory tract, skin, and stomach. Once activated the mast cells release powerful substances, including histamine and prostaglandins, which cause the immediate and familiar symptoms. An adverse reaction can occur in minutes, or develop over several hours. Typical symptoms include swollen eyes and lips, tingling mouth, sneezing, rashes, red watery eyes, runny nose, abdominal distention and pain, diarrhea, and vomiting. In a severe allergic reaction a sudden drop in blood pressure can occur, resulting in life-threatening anaphylactic shock.

If you suspect an allergy consult a physician for help with diagnosis. First, find out if any other members of your family suffer from allergies (asthma, hay fever, eczema). Also, write a diary of your symptoms and try to detect what food, substances, or situations trigger your symptoms.

Some physicians will arrange scientific diagnostic tests for allergies. In the usual test, patches soaked with the substances suspected of causing the allergy are taped to the skin (often on the back). Alternatively, the substances may be injected just below the surface of the skin. The reactions are then monitored to identify the allergens. When the patches are removed the allergy-producing substances leave an inflamed red area (the same happens on the sites of the skin pricks). The test is not infallible, and red areas may occur with substances to which you are not allergic. With suspected food allergy an exclusion diet *(see page 75)* may be suggested.

The tiny house dust mite, found in upholstery, bedding, and carpets, triggers an allergic response in many people.

Some people cannot live with the allergens produced by cat fur, which can provoke an asthmatic response or an itchy skin rash.

COMMON ALLERGIES

ALLERGIES	ALLERGENS
Asthma	Pollen, dust, (exercise, infections), tobacco smoke, pollutants
Eczema	Silk, synthetic fabrics, wool, foods *(see below)*, detergents, skin and bathing products
Food allergies	Chocolate, nuts, oranges, eggs, cow's milk and other dairy produce, wheat (flour, cereal, bread, and other baked items), strawberries, fish, and shellfish
Hay fever	Pollens from grass, trees, flowers

ASTHMA *see page 160*
ECZEMA *see page 203*

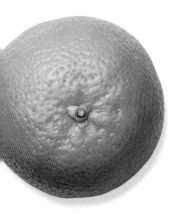

Oranges are just one of the many fruits that can cause an allergic reaction.

If you suspect food allergy or intolerance in a child, seek help from your physician or dietitian before excluding foods. A restricted diet for children might leave them short of essential nutrients for growth and health.

❧ TREATMENT

The best treatment is to avoid the allergen. One of the drugs available is antihistamine, which relieves symptoms such as itching from insect bites and stings. However, it can make people drowsy, which is disadvantageous at work, although it may help eczema sufferers to sleep better and therefore reduce scratching. Corticosteroid creams (for eczema) and inhaled corticosteroids (for severe asthma) have side effects. Desensitization or hyposensitization is no longer very popular due to side effects and the lowish success rate. Hyposensitization takes two to three years and involves giving gradually increasing doses of the allergen to increase antibody formation, which is alleged to promote tolerance.

Eggs can trigger nausea and hot swelling on the skin, especially in people who suffer from asthma.

Consult a qualified practitioner/therapist for:
RELAXATION TECHNIQUES AND ALEXANDER TECHNIQUE These will help to reduce stress levels.

HOMEOPATHY Treatment will be prescribed according to the individual case but will include desensitization.

CAUTIONS AND CONTRAINDICATIONS

Elimination dieting can be very dangerous; always check with your physician before altering your diet in any way. Remember that an untreated allergy can lead to an acute reaction, which is life-threatening.

ACUPUNCTURE This can be extremely effective in treating allergies, balancing the organ energies so that they are able to cope.

REFLEXOLOGY AND HERBAL MEDICINE Both have a good success rate in working with allergies. A herbal practitioner will be able to advise on diet and individual remedies.

ANAPHYLACTIC SHOCK

Anaphylactic shock is a severe generalized reaction that causes breathing difficulties and swelling inside and around the mouth and throat, carrying a risk of suffocation. Appropriate first aid is vital, and conventional medical assistance must be called immediately. Until help arrives support the person in the position that most aids their breathing. Loosen clothing at the neck and waist. If the person loses consciousness put them in the recovery position and be prepared to resuscitate them *(for instructions see page 259)*.

Where it is known that a person is in danger of a severe allergic reaction (for example, to peanuts) a physician may provide them with a syringe of adrenaline for use in emergencies.

TEN TIPS FOR BEATING ALLERGIES

❧ The best way is to avoid the allergen.

❧ Learn to live with your allergy: it may be lifelong.

❧ Think ahead. If, for example, you are allergic to cats, ask hotels, restaurants, and friends whether they have cats before you make a booking or agree to stay.

❧ If pollen is your allergen, keep car windows closed and close bedroom windows at night.

❧ If you suffer from hay fever, take your vacation abroad during the season that gives you most problems at home.

❧ Learn all the synonyms for the food or other substance to which you are allergic, and get into the habit of reading packaging and food labels.

❧ Be assertive. Question staff in stores where goods are unlabeled and do not buy them if the exact ingredients are not known.

❧ When eating out, ask if a particular dish contains the food to which you are allergic. Remember, it may not be in the description of the dish but it may be used as a garnish or decoration.

❧ Write to your supermarket, health food store or pharmacy for a list of foods free from the ingredient(s) to which you are allergic, or for details of egg replacers, wheat-free pasta and bread, and gluten-free bread mixes.

❧ Be your own expert. Join an appropriate organization/support group (for asthma, eczema, hay fever, for example) to keep up to date on the latest research/products and get moral support.

ACUPUNCTURE *see page 90* ❧ ALEXANDER TECHNIQUE *see page 57* ❧ ELIMINATION DIETS *see page 28* ❧
HERBAL MEDICINE *see page 67* ❧ HOMEOPATHY *see page 83* ❧ REFLEXOLOGY *see page 52* ❧ RELAXATION *see page 116*

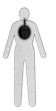

Asthma

The Ailments

Asthma is a chronic inflammatory condition that results in wheeziness and breathing difficulties. The air tubes in the lungs become extremely sensitive, and irritants, such as pollen, house dust, mites, animal fur, cold air, exercise, and emotional upset, can all trigger an attack. When this happens, muscle spasms in the walls of the airways cause them to narrow: the secretion of mucus adds to the problem, and the flow of air is considerably hampered.

It is important to breathe correctly so that the diaphragm rises and falls and the lungs fill and empty properly.

Symptoms may include wheezing, coughing, breathlessness, and tight chest. A bad attack can cause sweating, rapid heartbeat, and extreme gasping for breath.

☙ TREATMENT

The condition and its trigger factors are still not fully understood. All asthma sufferers are deficient in magnesium. Naturopaths believe that magnesium, given intravenously, is the most effective remedy to stop an attack.

DIET AND NUTRITION Stick to naturally- and organically-grown foods. Avoid additives, which can trigger allergic reactions, and cut down on dairy products (see *Allergies, Hay fever*). Eat plenty of fruit and vegetables: garlic and onions are said to deter mucus production.

Keeping an asthma diary to record where and when attacks take place and what circumstances may have triggered them can help asthmatics to organize their lives so that they can live with the condition rather than let it dominate their lives.

HERBAL MEDICINE Infusions of elecampane, euphorbia with thyme, grindelia or senega, ephedra (alone or with grindelia), and skunk cabbage help relax muscular spasms, loosen phlegm, and relieve tension. Inhalations of camomile or eucalyptus have a similar effect. A tincture of fiery cayenne desensitizes airways.

Consult a qualified practitioner/therapist for:

HOMEOPATHY A homeopath will prescribe according to the individual case but might recommend the following:

❋ for difficulties in breathing, where the sufferer has to bend forward to breathe, feels restless and exhausted, and worse between midnight and 2 a.m. – Arsenicum alb. for both adults and children

❋ for a sudden attack after exposure to cold or dry wind – Aconite

❋ for coughing, gasping for air, vomiting mucus, worse at night and when humid – Carbo veg.

❋ if sufferer is pale, lethargic, worse at night, particularly in warm climate – Kali carb.

❋ for wakefulness in early hours in damp atmosphere, where sufferer holds chest while coughing, shows symptoms of fluid retention, and has morning diarrhea – Natrum sulf.

❋ where a child coughs green phlegm and craves fresh air – Pulsatilla

❋ for acute breathlesssness, excess mucus production, and vomiting – Ipecacuanha

❋ for a choking cough accompanied by asthma that is better in damp but worse in dry, cold conditions – Hepar sulf.

❋ for noisy wheezing, coughing and gasping – Antimonium tart.

❋ for asthma that follows on from childhood eczema – Psorinum

❋ for asthma following a cold – Silica.

REFLEXOLOGY, MASSAGE, HYDROTHERAPY, AROMATHERAPY, ACUPUNCTURE, BACH REMEDIES, OSTEOPATHY, ALEXANDER TECHNIQUE, AND CHIROPRACTIC. All of these can be helpful. Consult a qualified practitioner who will be able to assess your particular case properly.

SELF-HELP

Avoid smoking and smoky environments. Check for allergies to pollen, food, drinks, and pollutants. Keep your bedroom as dust free as possible, removing, for instance, carpets, books, soft toys and furnishings, and some bedding. A humidifier will reduce the incidence of attacks.

SELF-HELP

If the sufferer turns blue, pale, or clammy, seek emergency medical attention. Always see your physician if your asthma does not respond to the prescribed drugs — conventional or complementary. All asthma sufferers should be kept under regular medical review.

DIETARY THERAPY *see page 74* ☙ **HERBAL MEDICINE** *see page 67* ☙ **HOMEOPATHY** *see page 83*

Pleurisy

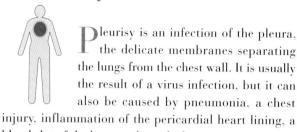

Pleurisy is an infection of the pleura, the delicate membranes separating the lungs from the chest wall. It is usually the result of a virus infection, but it can also be caused by pneumonia, a chest injury, inflammation of the pericardial heart lining, a blood clot of the lung, and, rarely, lung cancer.

Symptoms of pleurisy may include sharp, stabbing pains in chest or shoulder, which can be felt with every intake of breath, and usually a high fever.

⁓ TREATMENT

FOLK REMEDY Make a warming drink from oven-dried, homemade wheat bread, toasted and broken into a powder, in hot water with added salt and butter.

HYDROTHERAPY Chest and back compresses help to reduce inflammation.

DIET AND NUTRITION A daily dose of 2–3g of vitamin C and 50iu vitamin A should boost the immune system and help to speed recovery.

Consult a qualified practitioner/therapist for:

HOMEOPATHY A homeopath might recommend the following remedies:

❋ for pain worse on moving, where sufferer is irritable and thirsty – Bryonia each hour for a maximum of 12 hours

❋ for a sudden attack after exposure to cold wind, where sufferer is anxious, restless, and frightened of dying – Aconite once an hour for up to 12 hours

❋ where the sufferer is flushed in the face, with dilated pupils, and is hot, excitable, and thirsty – Belladonna

❋ when there is fluid on the lung, causing breathlessness and burning pains; mild fever, rapid heartbeat, irregular dry cough – Cantharis

❋ when there is fluid pressing on the affected lung with severe pain – Sulfur

❋ when pain comes on quickly, hot face, flushing, profound thirst, confusion – Belladonna

❋ when recovery from pleurisy is slow – Hepar sulf.

NATUROPATHY A naturopath may suggest hydrotherapy, in particular back and chest compresses, which will help to reduce inflammation and ease breathing.

Vitamin C may be recommended in order to boost immunity.

ACUPUNCTURE Treatment will be aimed at reducing inflammation, building up the immune system, and providing relief from the pain.

The flower of pleurisy root Asclepias tuberosa, long recognized by herbalists as a remedy for lung complaints.

AROMATHERAPY Treatment would be aimed at the individual symptoms, but some of the following oils may prove useful, for a compress, massage, or inhalation: angelica, star anise, French basil, silver fir, myrrh, naiouli, black pepper, pine, rosemary, sage, tea tree oil.

A traditional folk remedy is a soothing drink that can easily be made at home. Crumble dried, toasted wholewheat bread into a powder and mix it with hot water, a pinch of salt, and a knob of real butter.

CAUTIONS AND CONTRAINDICATIONS

Always consult a physician first if pleurisy is suspected.

SELF-HELP

Bedrest is recommended, as well as drinking plenty of fluids. Take extra vitamin C to encourage the body to fight off the infection.

ACUPUNCTURE *see page 90* ⁓ AROMATHERAPY *see page 50* ⁓ DIETARY THERAPY *see page 74* ⁓ HOMEOPATHY *see page 83* ⁓ HYDROTHERAPY *see page 26* ⁓ NATUROPATHY *see page 24*

The Ailments

Pneumonia and Emphysema

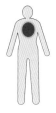

Pneumonia is an infection of one or both lungs by a virus, or a bacterial infection. It may be mild in healthy people but can be life threatening to the elderly and the very young. Pneumonia is sometimes a feature of Aids *(see page 136)*.

Symptoms include fever, chills, breathlessness, chest pain, a cough that produces yellow or green phlegm, and sometimes blood.

✌ TREATMENT

HERBAL MEDICINE Natural expectorants such as lobelia or thyme, with anti-infective herbs such as echinacea or garlic may be used to loosen phlegm. Treat fever with elderflower and yarrow. Make a soothing infusion of coltsfoot. You can add motherwort to the infusion if the sufferer has a weak heart.

Consult a qualified practitioner/therapist for:
HOMEOPATHY A homeopath will prescribe according to the individual case but might recommend the following:
❊ for rapid onset in cold, dry weather, accompanied by fever – Aconite
❊ for sharp, stitching chest pains that worsen on movement and when coughing – Bryonia
❊ for chest pains with dry cough, blood in sputum, and symptoms that worsen when the person is lying on left side – Phosphorus
❊ where sufferer is pale and weak, with bloody phlegm and nosebleeds – Ferrum phos.

> **SELF-HELP**
>
> Take plenty of fluids and eat small, nutritious wholefood meals and lots of fresh fruit. Drink fresh vegetable juices. Avoid mucus-making dairy products and sweet foods. Use vitamin C and A supplements to boost immune system.

EMPHYSEMA

Emphysema is a progressive and incurable disease. Heavy smokers and those living or working in polluted atmospheres are most at risk, as are sufferers from asthma and bronchitis. It occurs when tiny air sacs (alveoli) in the lungs become damaged and then enlarge and burst. This reduces the oxygen intake and can lead to heart failure. Breathlessness and blue lips are symptoms of emphysema.

TREATMENT

✌ **LIFESTYLE** *Studies have shown that exercise that concentrates on controlled breathing, such as cycling, walking, swimming, and yoga, can greatly relieve symptoms.*

✌ **AROMATHERAPY** *Massage chest with Atlas cedarwood, peppermint, and eucalyptus. Inhale basil, cajeput, eucalyptus, hyssop, and thyme – in a diffuser or an essential-oil burner.*

✌ **HERBAL MEDICINE** *Licorice root and comfrey are natural expectorants (see Bronchitis).*

Consult a qualified practitioner/therapist for:

✌ **ACUPUNCTURE** *This can improve blood circulation in the lungs and promote easier breathing.*

✌ **REFLEXOLOGY** *Gentle massaging of the lung area on the upper surface of both feet eases breathing (see page 52).*

✌ **HOMEOPATHY** *A homeopath might recommend the following remedies:*
✌ *for noisy and suffocative wheezing without producing phlegm – Antimonium tart.*
✌ *where condition is worse on cloudy days, in warm rooms, and in the early morning – Ammonium carb.*
✌ *where condition is worse in cold air and in drafts in the late evening – Hepar sulf.*

Garlic Allium sativum is a very powerful herbal treatment, acting on bacteria, viruses, and parasites. It is useful in all chronic respiratory disease.

> **CAUTIONS AND CONTRAINDICATIONS**
>
> **PNEUMONIA**
> If pneumonia is suspected, consult a physician before undertaking any alternative therapies.

> **CAUTIONS AND CONTRAINDICATIONS**
>
> **EMPHYSEMA**
> If there are signs of respiratory failure (characterized by severe shortness of breath and blue lips), seek emergency medical attention and begin artificial respiration until help arrives.

ACUPUNCTURE *see page 90* ✌ AROMATHERAPY *see page 50* ✌
HERBAL MEDICINE *see page 67* ✌ HOMEOPATHY *see page 83* ✌ REFLEXOLOGY *see page 52*

Tuberculosis (TB)

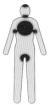

Tuberculosis (TB) is an infectious disease that can be controlled by immunization. It was becoming rare in developed countries but, since Aids can predispose to TB, more cases are now being seen. Tuberculosis is endemic in countries where there is overriding poverty, malnutrition, and overcrowding but is rapidly increasing elsewhere. The rise of HIV *(see page 136)* means more people are susceptible to TB, which thrives where the immune system is debilitated. Migration, tourism, and international air travel have helped to transmit the bacillus *Mycobacterium tuberculosis* with frightening efficiency. TB is highly infectious and easily spread through moisture droplets in the air. Bodily contact is not necessary.

The most commmon site of infection is the lungs, but it can also be found in the lymph glands and membranes covering the brain.

The symptoms of TB are weight loss, fever, and night sweats; persistent cough with yellow or bloodstained phlegm, chest pain, breathlessness; swelling of lymph glands, sometimes with discharge through skin; soft bones and collapse of bones leading to deformity; destruction of kidneys and inflammation of bladder.

> **SELF-HELP**
>
> Increase your intake of foods rich in magnesium (or take a supplement) and protein. Rest and fresh air will also encourage healing.

> **CAUTIONS AND CONTRAINDICATIONS**
>
> It is vital to get conventional medical help if TB is suspected – to prove the diagnosis, to set up long-term antibiotic treatment, to procure hospitalization in severe cases, to prevent the spread of the disease, and to trace infected contacts.

❧ TREATMENT

NATUROPATHY Garlic is particularly effective. A high-altitude cure used to be recommended: good diet, rest, relaxation, freedom from stress, sun, and clean, clear fresh air.

Consult a qualified practitioner/therapist for:
HOMEOPATHY AND AROMATHERAPY Both can be very helpful in easing symptoms. A homeopath may offer a "nosode" (a remedy made from a sample of diseased tissue) as a preventive.

PASTEUR, GARLIC, AND TB

The great 19th-century French chemist Louis Pasteur discovered that garlic had antiseptic properties. Garlic was first used to treat TB in the early part of the 20th century, and studies since have established it as effective on bacteria, fungi, viruses, and parasites. Herbalists regard garlic as an effective preventive.

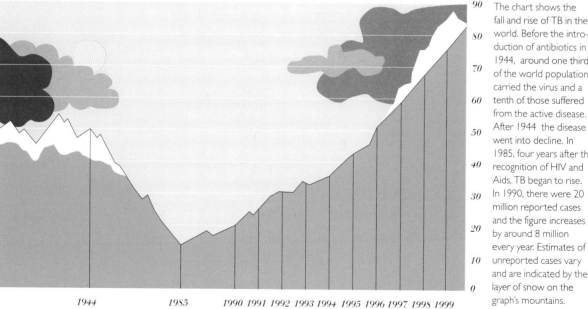

The chart shows the fall and rise of TB in the world. Before the introduction of antibiotics in 1944, around one third of the world population carried the virus and a tenth of those suffered from the active disease. After 1944 the disease went into decline. In 1985, four years after the recognition of HIV and Aids, TB began to rise. In 1990, there were 20 million reported cases and the figure increases by around 8 million every year. Estimates of unreported cases vary and are indicated by the layer of snow on the graph's mountains.

AROMATHERAPY *see page 50* ❧ HOMEOPATHY *see page 83* ❧ NATUROPATHY *see page 24*

Problems of the Heart and Blood

Diseases of the heart and blood vessels (particularly the arteries) are not only the single biggest cause of death in the modern world, particularly the Western world, but the most preventable. Together they kill almost as many people as all other diseases together, including cancer, particularly in northern Europe and North America.

Most heart and arterial disease is caused by poor eating and living habits (including smoking), stress, lack of exercise and excess weight. More than half the people who are overweight die of heart disease or related problems such as stroke, for example, while in most Western countries an increasing number of quite young people, even teenagers, are suffering from advanced arterial disease.

Yet both conditions seem to be almost unknown among primitive societies – which is why they are often called "the classic diseases of civilization" and why they are variously estimated to be about 95 percent preventable. Recent research, particularly in the United States, has shown that the same factors that can cause disease can also reverse it if turned around.

Balanced diet, exercise, relaxation, and healthy living generally have now been shown to be capable of unclogging arteries and reenergizing the heart. For this reason, alternative medicine has moved to the forefront in many countries in the treatment of heart and arterial disease, and could become more important than conventional management drugs in the years ahead.

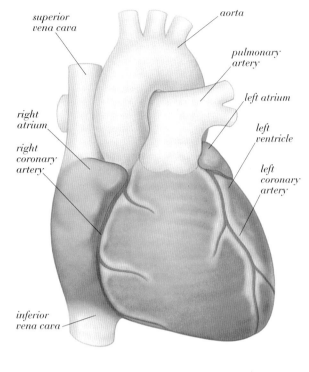

The heart consists of four chambers (two atria and two ventricles), which are separated from each other by one-way valves so that the blood does not flow backward.

Heart, blood vessels, and blood make up the circulatory system, which circulates blood around your body.

Blood carries oxygen from the air to "fuel" the cells, nutrients to feed the body, and other chemicals, such as hormones, essential for the body's function, repair, and maintenance as well as protection against disease.

POOR CIRCULATION

The heart pumps the blood, arteries carry it from the heart, and veins return it to the heart. Normally, the heart pumps about 10pt/5l of blood per minute around the body. However, if the blood flow is restricted for some reason, circulation is slowed down. Poor circulation occurs mainly in the elderly and most often affects the areas farthest from the heart. Medically the condition is known generally as peripheral ischemia and can result in a wide range of symptoms, from cold hands and feet and cramp, to gangrene in extreme cases, where an area of tissue dies and starts to decay. Poor circulation is usually the result of the combined effect of a less healthy heart and narrowed and hardened arteries *(see page 169)*, normally as a result of age. Smoking is the most common cause but it can also be a concomitant symptom of diabetes *(high blood sugar – see pages 218–19)*, infection *(see pages 132–3)*, and long exposure to cold.

HEART FACTS

Your heart:

✺ beats roughly 100,000 times a day, or 3 billion times during a lifetime

✺ pumps about 10pt/5l of blood every minute when you rest – but up to six times more when you exercise

✺ pumps nearly 6,000 gall/23,000l of blood per day

✺ pumps your entire blood supply around your body about once every minute, but more quickly if you rush around

✺ weighs about 8–10oz/230–80g in the average adult female and between about 10–12oz/280–340g in the average adult male

✺ is about the size of your fist.

DIETARY THERAPY *see page 74* ✺ EXERCISE *see page 170* ✺
RELAXATION *see page 116* ✺ STRESS *see page 223* ✺ WEIGHT *see page 215*

✄ TREATMENT

Treatment should concentrate on stopping smoking and increasing the supply of blood to the area by helping the blood vessels to expand and the heart to pump more effectively. Improvement in the quality of the blood, particularly its red cell count, should also be sought.

MASSAGE This is a good way to stimulate the circulation in any condition. Do not massage directly over injuries (cuts, bruises, or breaks), inflamed veins (phlebitis), varicose veins, or tumors. Alternatives to massage are reflexology and aromatherapy with black pepper and rosemary essential oils.

HYPNOSIS/BIOFEEDBACK Temperature biofeedback training *(see page 170)* may help to raise the temperature of the extremities.

DIET AND NUTRITION In addition to a generally healthy diet *(see pages 170–1)*, eat plenty of oily fish such as mackerel, herring, salmon, and tuna. Food supplements recommended are vitamin A, C, E, selenium, zinc, manganese, and the essential fatty acids EPA and GLA.

HERBAL MEDICINE The following herbs are widely believed to act as tonics on the blood: garlic, hawthorn berries (crataegus), echinacea, ginger, cayenne, chili and black pepper, prickly ash, and hops.

RAYNAUD'S DISEASE (OR SYNDROME)

This is an uncommon condition caused by nervous spasm in the small arteries, especially of the fingers, resulting in their going cold, white, and often numb. It most often affects young women.

✄ TREATMENT

Keep affected parts well-covered in cold weather and avoid drinking coffee and smoking since both constrict blood vessels.

DIET AND NUTRITION Eat iron-rich food *(see Anemia p.166)* and cut out tea, which inhibits iron absorption.

TRADITIONAL CHINESE MEDICINE Cinnamon twigs and angelica are recommended.

Consult a qualified practitioner/therapist for:
HOMEOPATHY Arsenicum alb. 6c, Pulsatilla 6c, and Carbo veg. 6c can be helpful.

CHILBLAINS

Chilblains are caused by exposure of extremities such as fingers, ears, nose, and, especially, feet and toes to cold and damp, causing the skin to become tender, painful, and intensely itchy. People with sensitive skin or poor circulation are most vulnerable, especially those who smoke (nicotine reduces circulation in the skin).

✄ TREATMENT

HERBAL MEDICINE Rub in calendula (marigold) ointment if the skin is broken.

TRADITIONAL CHINESE MEDICINE Herbs said to help are cinnamon twigs, red sage, ginger, and angelica.

NATUROPATHY Stimulate circulation by putting affected feet or hands first into warm water for half a minute and then into cold water. Repeat for about 15 minutes. Spread a paste of honey and glycerin mixed with egg white and flour on the affected part, bandage, and leave for 24 hours.

DIET AND NUTRITION Take extra vitamin C, E, and B complex, and also increase your calcium intake.

Consult a qualified practitioner/therapist for:
HOMEOPATHY Tamus 6c ointment, Rhus tox. 6c, Agaricus 6c, Petroleum 6c, and Carbo veg. 6c may be recommended.

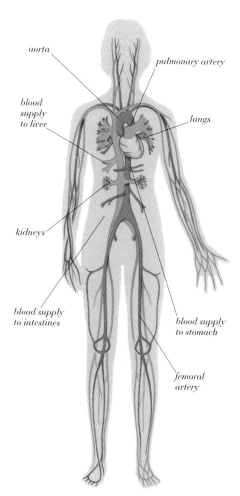

aorta
pulmonary artery
blood supply to liver
lungs
kidneys
blood supply to intestines
blood supply to stomach
femoral artery

Blood enters the right side of the heart, then is pumped to the lungs where it picks up oxygen. Then it flows back to the left side of the heart, from where it is pumped out to circulate the body once more.

BIOFEEDBACK *see page 117* ✄ DIETARY THERAPY *see page 74* ✄ HERBAL MEDICINE *see page 67* ✄
HOMEOPATHY *see page 83* ✄ HYPNOSIS *see page 112* ✄ MASSAGE *see page 48* ✄ NATUROPATHY *see page 24* ✄
TRADITIONAL CHINESE MEDICINE *see page 30*

The Ailments

Blood Problems

Problems with the blood, as opposed to the supply or circulation of blood, are normally the result of something wrong in the chemical composition of the blood so that either it does not flow as it should (it may clot too quickly or not fast enough) or it does not have the right amount of chemicals to nourish and protect the body or itself properly.

Serious blood problems such as hemophilia (an inherited deficiency in which blood will not clot properly, resulting in excessive bleeding), agranulocytosis (which is the result of a white blood cell deficiency), leukemia (cancer of the blood's white cells, *see Cancer, pages 140–1*), polycythemia (high altitude or mountain sickness, from having too many red blood cells), and septicemia (blood poisoning, the result of an overload of disease-causing bacteria in the bloodstream) are relatively rare but need medical help, mostly urgently. They are really not suitable subjects for treatment by alternative therapies.

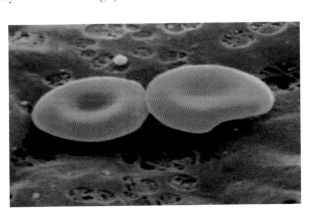

Red blood cells, erythrocytes, make up just under half of the blood by volume. They contain hemoglobin, which carries the oxygen collected from the lungs into the bloodstream.

ANEMIA

Anemia, which simply means lack of blood, is not a disease so much as a disorder. It is caused by a deficiency of the red oxygen-carrying pigment in blood (hemoglobin), often from lack of iron in the diet. It is more common among women than men and can be a particular problem for women with heavy periods *(see Women's Problems, pages 238–45)*. Iron-deficiency anemia may also be caused by blood loss into the gut in conditions such as peptic ulcer and stomach cancer.

Symptoms of anemia are a "tired-all-the-time" feeling, pale skin, shortness of breath, dizziness, poor concentration, recurrent colds and infections, and white eyelid linings.

SICKLE CELL ANEMIA

Several blood disorders are the result of a single gene. Sickle cell anemia causes a distortion of the red blood cells into sickle shapes (a sort of half-moon shape), slowing the blood flow and decreasing the amount of oxygen the red cells are able to carry. It is much more common in Africans, Caribbeans, and people of Middle Eastern descent; in the United States, 1 in every 400 Afro-Americans has this disease. There are several forms of sickle cell anemia, ranging from mild to severe. Symptoms of the severe form, which usually begins at about six months of age, include organ dysfunction, pain, and jaundice, eventually leading to fever and extreme lethargy.

Sickle cell anemia cannot be cured, but most sufferers maintain a good lifestyle with regular transfusions. It is often suggested that sufferers take specific inoculations in order to avoid infection. Dehydration and coldness may cause painful sickle cell crises in the sufferer and should be avoided.

☙ TREATMENT

DIET AND NUTRITION The treatment of iron-deficiency anemia is to take more iron in food or as food supplements, ideally in a multimixture that includes a complex of B vitamins, especially B12 and folic acid, vitamins C, E, copper, and selenium. Supplements may be taken as tablets or liquid tonic. Iron-rich foods include liver, beef, and chicken. The best non-animal sources are soybeans, corn flour, spinach, black kidney beans, rhubarb, dried fruits, and dark green leafy vegetables. Biochemic tissue salts may also help. Avoid tea: it cuts down the amount of iron the body can absorb.

Consult a qualified practitioner/therapist for:
TRADITIONAL CHINESE MEDICINE Chinese herbs (*gui pi wan* or "Return spleen tablets") may help.

ACUPUNCTURE Some find this therapy helpful.

CAUTIONS AND CONTRAINDICATIONS

There are several types of anemia. Anyone who suspects that they may be anemic should visit their physician for blood tests to determine its type, and possible investigation of any underlying cause. Iron deficiency should always be investigated further in people over 45. Iron supplements are dangerous in overdose and should generally only be taken after medical advice. Pernicious anemia is an old term for anemia caused by failure to absorb vitamin B12.

Blood Pressure Problems

Blood pressure is the pressure that blood is under while it is being pumped around the body. It normally rises when we are active, excited, angry or afraid – part of the normal "fight-or-flight" response – and drops when we are relaxed. Blood pressure is related to pulse rate and the normal range for both in a healthy adult of either sex is shown in the table opposite, although athletes normally have slow pulse rates and young women normally have low blood pressure.

GUIDE TO BLOOD PRESSURE AND PULSE READINGS

❧ BLOOD PRESSURE		❧ PULSE (AT REST)	
"Normal" range	100/60–140/90	"Normal" range	60–80 beats a min
High risk	Under 100/60 Over 160/100	High risk	Under 50 beats a min Over 100 beats a min

LOW BLOOD PRESSURE

Low blood pressure (hypotension) is common in young people, especially women. However, it may also be a sign of a serious underlying condition, after an accident resulting in severe internal or external bleeding, a heart attack, or severe allergic reaction.

Symptoms are lack of energy, dizziness on getting up suddenly, headaches, a weak pulse, cold hands and feet, and poor concentration. Very rarely symptoms such as dizziness on standing upright may signify adrenal failure, which requires medical advice.

❧ TREATMENT

DIET AND NUTRITION Vitamins C and E and minerals zinc and selenium are helpful.

SELF-HELP

Rest and relaxation in the short term is recommended, coupled with treatment to improve the stamina of the heart and "tone" of the blood vessels in the longer term. Take regular gentle exercise, especially yoga.

CAUTIONS AND CONTRAINDICATIONS

The consequences of untreated hypertension, and to a lesser extent hypotension, are serious, including kidney failure, stroke, heart attack, or a burst aneurism, so consult your physician at once if you suspect them.

MASSAGE, REFLEXOLOGY, AND AROMATHERAPY These are beneficial.

HERBAL MEDICINE Broom, gentian, ginseng, hawthorn berries, kola, oats, skullcap, and wormwood are said to help.

BACH FLOWER REMEDIES These can benefit any underlying psychological problem.

HIGH BLOOD PRESSURE

High blood pressure – or hypertension – is a risk factor for heart disease and stroke and can be a symptom of both. It can lead to stroke and heart attack as well as kidney failure and, sometimes, eye damage.

Symptoms are flushing in the face and giddiness linked to a "loud" heartbeat on exertion, but often there are no obvious symptoms.

❧ TREATMENT
(See page 170.)

TRADITIONAL CHINESE MEDICINE Useful herbs include chrysanthemum, peony root, and astragalus.

AROMATHERAPY Essential oils of lavender, lemon, clary sage, marjoram, melissa, or ylang-ylang used in massage or added to a bath are helpful.

Consult a qualified practitioner/therapist for:
ACUPUNCTURE AND ACUPRESSURE Work on points on the back, knee, ankle, stomach, head, and wrist is said to be effective.

HERBAL MEDICINE Crataegus, garlic, onion, buckwheat, cramp bark, lime blossom, mistletoe, yarrow, and strawberries are recommended.

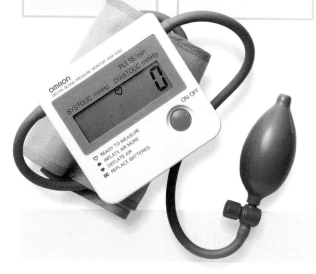

A blood pressure gage that can be used at home helps people with blood pressure problems monitor their status.

Red wine (above), when it is taken in moderation, is said to help keep blood pressure levels down.

ACUPRESSURE *see page 94* ❧ ACUPUNCTURE *see page 90*
DIETARY THERAPY *see page 74* ❧ HERBAL MEDICINE *see page 67* ❧ TRADITIONAL CHINESE MEDICINE *see page 30*

Heart Disease

Heart disease is not really disease of the heart itself, but of the blood vessels supplying it. Conditions such as "hole-in-the-heart" and problems with heart valves (sometimes a consequence of rheumatic fever) can occur, but most problems with heart valves are now the result of their becoming hardened and leaky with age. Heart valve disorders, especially of the main aortic and mitral valves, can cause stress in the heart muscle resulting in heart failure and are best corrected by surgery.

The wide variety of medical names used to cover what most people call "heart disease" – cardiovascular disease (CVD), coronary artery disease (CAD), coronary heart disease (CHD), and ischemic heart disease (IHD) – reveals that the main source of the problem is the arteries that surround and feed the heart (the "coronary arteries"). The real cause of "heart disease" is clogged and hardened arteries, a condition known as arteriosclerosis *(see page 169)*.

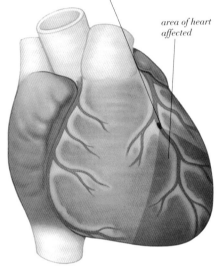

blocked coronary artery

area of heart affected

A diseased heart is often enlarged.

HEART ATTACK

A heart attack is the most dramatic outcome of heart disease. Known medically as a coronary thrombosis or acute myocardial infarction, it is the result of blockage in the coronary arteries feeding the heart. A heart attack invariably comes on suddenly and is often fatal. Symptoms are a vicelike pain in the chest and pains down the left arm and up the left side of the neck to the jaw, sweating, and breathlessness. A heart attack is a serious medical emergency.

ANGINA

Angina (*angina pectoris* in full) is a severe chest pain caused by a lack of blood to the arteries around the heart (coronary ischemia in medical terms) and is a clear symptom of heart disease. More common in middle-aged and older men than women, it usually comes on during or immediately after physical exercise or a period of mental and emotional strain. The main symptom is an aching or crushing pain in the center of the chest, sometimes mistaken for heartburn.

⋅≋ TREATMENT

Emergency medical treatment is with nitroglycerine but acupuncture can be an effective alternative for some people. *(See also Atherosclerosis, page 169.)*

STROKE

A stroke is caused by damage to blood vessels supplying the brain. A clot (thrombosis) in one of the cerebral arteries causes part of the brain to die from failure of its blood supply (infarction). Another type of stroke is a cerebral hemorrhage or burst blood vessel. Both cause a similar picture clinically – the affected part of the brain ceases to work. This may lead to weakness in the limbs, blindness, or loss of higher functions such as speech. Many strokes are immediately fatal, but partial or complete recovery is possible, with skillful rehabilitation, for those who survive the first few weeks after the initial stroke.

⋅≋ TREATMENT

This concentrates on maintaining a healthy blood flow and keeping muscles and ligaments strong and flexible.

DIET AND NUTRITION Follow the advice on eating for a healthy heart given on pages 170–1.

HERBAL MEDICINE Yarrow tea (two teaspoons of dried herb in hot water three times a day).

Consult a qualified practitioner/therapist for:
TRADITIONAL CHINESE MEDICINE Lovage tuber can be helpful.

ACUPUNCTURE Should be used as soon as possible to counter the effects of paralysis.

HOMEOPATHY Arnica 6c and the biochemic tissue salt Kali mur. 6x twice daily may be helpful.

MASSAGE, OSTEOPATHY, CHIROPRACTIC, HYDROTHERAPY, AND YOGA These manipulation and balance therapies can safely be used to maintain muscle tone and flexibility.

ACUPUNCTURE *see page 90* ⋅≋ DIETARY THERAPY *see page 74* ⋅≋ HERBAL MEDICINE *see page 67* ⋅≋ HOMEOPATHY *see page 83* ⋅≋ TRADITIONAL CHINESE MEDICINE *see page 30*

Atherosclerosis

Atherosclerosis is the result of smoking, too much fat in the diet (including cholesterol, see box "Ideal cholesterol levels"), and lack of proper exercise, coupled with excessive mental and emotional stress and strain. This causes a gradual buildup of fatty deposits – or atheroma – on the walls of the arteries, which gradually hardens or calcifies with time and prevents the arteries from expanding and contracting as they should. Hardening of the arteries is called arteriosclerosis.

Arteries that become "furred up" and hardened restrict the vital flow of blood to other parts of the body, so the organs and tissues there become affected and stop working as well. Eventually, if no action is taken, the arteries become blocked, cutting off the blood supply completely. When this happens to the arteries around the heart the result is a heart attack. In the brain it is a cause of a stroke.

Common signs and symptoms of atherosclerosis are chest pain (angina), leg cramps (intermittent claudication), poor circulation (peripheral ischemia), leg ulcers, dizziness, weakness, breathlessness, mental feebleness (poor memory, mental confusion), weak pulse (or "wide" pulse pressure), increasing clumsiness, lack of coordination, dexterity, or agility.

❧ TREATMENT

Alternative therapies combining a range of physical and psychological approaches have been shown by Dr. Dean Ornish in the United States to halt and even reverse atherosclerosis. Particularly successful seem to be those

IDEAL CHOLESTEROL LEVELS

❧ HDL CHOLESTEROL	❧ INTERNATIONAL	❧ USA
Men	Minimum 0.8–1.9	30–75
Women	Minimum 0.9–2.2	35–85
❧ LDL CHOLESTEROL	Maximum 4.9	160
❧ TOTAL CHOLESTEROL		
Under 60	Maximum 6.0	200
Over 60	Maximum 7.0	235

International measurements in mmol per liter; US in mg/100ml.

NOTE *The role of cholesterol is largely misunderstood and misrepresented in heart disease. Cholesterol is essential to life. The important distinction is between HDL and LDL cholesterol. HDL is "good" and LDL "bad". The higher the HDL reading (ideally over 20 percent of total cholesterol) and the lower the LDL (ideally zero) the better. So it is important to ask for a test that shows the two readings separately.*

involving a healthy diet with food supplements, exercise, yoga, massage, and relaxation therapy, counseling and other "talking therapies" linked to close social support. In other words, most of the ways of preventing heart disease are also effective for treating it *(see pages 170–1)*. Other therapies can also help.

DIET AND NUTRITION All dietary fiber is beneficial to the body, but particularly the water-soluble type that is found in oats and pulses, because it reduces excess cholesterol. Ginger can be added to many dishes with the same effect. *(See also box "Supplements for Heart Health" page 171.)*

HERBAL MEDICINE Garlic, ginger, hot red, or chili, peppers, yarrow herb, and alfalfa have been shown to reduce the "stickiness" of blood and help prevent clotting. They may also help dissolve atheroma already in arteries, as may hawthorn berries.

CHELATION THERAPY This is a controversial therapy, popular mainly in the United States, that uses a synthetic amino acid ethylenediaminetetracetic acid (or EDTA) as part of a cocktail of anticoagulant drugs and nutrients to dissolve atheroma and flush it away through the kidneys. The treatment is by long-term injection and can only be carried out by a conventional medical doctor. There is some evidence of efficacy, but there are doubts about safety and the therapy is still under investigation.

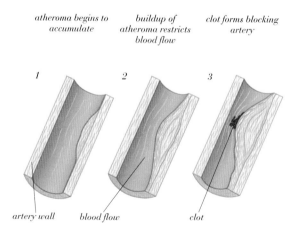

atheroma begins to accumulate

buildup of atheroma restricts blood flow

clot forms blocking artery

1   *2*   *3*

artery wall   blood flow   clot

Blood vessels can be clogged by the gradual buildup of a fatty deposit called atheroma. As blood flow is restricted, the heart has to work harder to push blood through, and blood pressure rises. Complete blockage results in stroke or heart attack.

DIETARY THERAPY *see page 74* ❧ **HERBAL MEDICINE** *see page 67*

Preventing and Treating Heart Disease

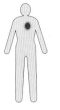

HEART DISEASE can be prevented as well as treated by adopting a four-pronged approach: stopping smoking; reducing and managing stress; altering and improving the quality of your diet; taking more exercise. You should also take steps to control high blood pressure if you have it.

STRESS REDUCTION

Learn how to handle your stress levels and take time to relax. New research has shown that relaxation is far more important in heart disease than was once realized.

Relaxation therapies (including self-help):

• *Physical therapies (massage, aromatherapy, reflexology, flotation therapy)*

• *Meditation and visualization (autogenic training, self-hypnosis, biofeedback)*

• *Balance and movement therapies (yoga, t'ai chi)*

• *Talking therapies (counseling, psychotherapy, hypnotherapy/hypnosis)*

• *Expression therapies (art, music, dance, sound, color, and drama therapies)*

• *Energy therapies (polarity therapy, acupuncture/acupressure, healing, homeopathy, flower remedies, Ayurvedic medicine).*

EXERCISE

Take regular exercise, enough to raise your heartbeat for at least 20–30 minutes three or four times a week. This is usually known as aerobic exercise. Remember, fitness cannot be stored. It has to be worked at constantly. Also, aerobic exercise is an excellent way to unwind emotionally and mentally as well as physically. Good ways to exercise for a healthy heart are walking, cycling, swimming, and jogging. Or join a regular exercise class at your local fitness center or gym.

CONTROLLING BLOOD PRESSURE

Blood pressure is usually measured in millimeters of mercury (mm/Hg). The average is 130/80 but there is no such thing as an "ideal" reading. Blood pressure and pulse both naturally vary with age, sex, and between individuals of the same age and sex. Pressure is normally higher in men than women and with age.

✍ TREATMENT

High blood pressure responds best to significant changes in lifestyle habits, particularly reducing weight, managing stress, taking regular exercise, eliminating smoking, and cutting down on alcohol.

DIET AND NUTRITION

Cutting down salt intake and alcohol are important. Green buckwheat tea (rutin), fruit and vegetable juices (orange, grapefruit, pear, pineapple, celery), supplements (vitamins A, C, E, minerals magnesium, selenium, and zinc; also lecithin and calcium) are all helpful. (*See Food and Diet, page 28, and Dietary Therapy, pages 74–5.*)

Regular gentle exercise is one of the best ways to a healthy heart at any age.

TEMPERATURE BIOFEEDBACK The American Dr. Elmer Green has shown that 80 percent of people with hypertension can bring it under control by learning to warm the temperature of the feet to 96°F/36°C by using temperature biofeedback. Tape an ordinary household thermometer to the feet and raise its temperature by "thinking" the feet warm with mental pictures of heat, or repeating to yourself "my feet are getting warmer and warmer...."

CAUTIONS AND CONTRAINDICATIONS

Sudden strenuous exercise by very obese people or people over 50 who have done no exercise for many years is dangerous and can lead to a heart attack. Work into it gradually – and get a proper medical checkup before beginning.

BIOFEEDBACK *see page 117* ✍ **DIETARY THERAPY** *see page 74* ✍ **STRESS** *see page 223* ✍

Feeding the Heart

A LONG-TERM preventive measure against heart disease – and stroke and high blood pressure – is to review your eating and drinking habits, take advice from a nutritionist, and compile a healthy eating program that includes enjoyable food and moderate alcohol if you like it. Try to establish a routine of eating for a healthy heart so that you automatically choose the healthier option; if you do this slowly and gradually, eventually your body will no longer crave salt, sugar, and fats. Try the Mediterranean diet advocated below.

Here are some easy-to-follow guidelines:

❊ get down to (or make sure you stay at) your "ideal" weight *(see table on page 215)*

❊ don't smoke

❊ control what you eat and drink, in particular: avoid sugar, salt, saturated fats, and processed food as much as possible; eat plenty of fresh (preferably organic) fruit and vegetables, particularly those known to "tone up" the blood and blood vessels, oily fish, and fiber; reduce consumption of dairy products (especially full-fat cow's milk and cheese); drink plenty of good, clean water (at least 4pt/2l a day)

❊ drink alcohol in moderation if you like it and it is part of your lifestyle.

THE "MEDITERRANEAN DIET"

Statistics produced by the World Health Organization in Geneva have shown consistently that the levels of heart disease in southern Europe are not nearly as high as those in northern Europe. In France, Greece, Italy, Portugal, and Spain, for example, only half as many people overall die of heart disease as in Denmark and Holland – and the figure is well under a third when compared with Scotland and Northern Ireland in the United Kingdom, which has one of the worst records anywhere in the world.

This has given rise to the idea that it is the Mediterranean diet that provides protection, particularly the regular consumption of salads, fish, rice, fruit, and red wine. Other contributory factors, equally strong, include the natural thinning effect of hot weather on the blood, coupled with the slower and more relaxed pace of life (the afternoon siesta, for example) and a close network of social support among many families.

TEETH AND THE HEART

It is important to visit a dentist regularly and keep teeth and gums healthy. Poor dental hygiene can lead to a dangerous heart condition known as infective endocarditis. Bacteria enter the bloodstream through bleeding gums and cause infection of the heart valves. It is particularly dangerous for people who already have defective or artificial valves. They are usually recommended to have short-term antibiotic cover whenever they have dental work done. Efficient and regular brushing with a good, natural toothpaste (such as baking powder) and an occasional massage of the gums with a finger is the best prevention.

SUPPLEMENTS FOR HEART HEALTH

Recommended daily amounts

Vitamins	Prevention	Treatment
Beta carotene	20,000iu	20,000–40,000iu
Vitamin B3	30mg	50–250mg
Vitamin B6	25mg	50–100mg
Vitamin C	1000mg	2000–10,000mg
Vitamin E	200iu	400–1000iu
Biotin (vit H)	50mcg (a coenzyme of vitamin C)	
CoenzymeQ10 (vit Q)	40mg	60–150mg
Folic acid (vit M)	100mcg	200–450mcg
Minerals		
Calcium	350mg	350–800mg
Magnesium	175mg	175–500mg
Manganese	2.5mg	10–20mg
Selenium	100mcg	100–200mcg
Zinc	20mg	20–50mg
Amino Acids		
Carnitine	250–1500mg	1500–3000mg
Histidine	250–1000mg	1000–3000mg
Lysine	3000mg	3000–6000mg
Methionine	250–1500mg	1000–3000mg
Serine	250–1000mg	1000–3000mg
Taurine	250–1000mg	6000mg
Tryptophan	Currently banned in USA and UK	
Fatty acids and fats		
EPA	180mg	300–3000mg
GLA	80–100mg	200–240mg
Lecithin	15000mg	45000mg

Note: Dosage figures are given for guidance only. Treatment is best carried out under the guidance of an experienced practitioner.

DIETARY THERAPY *see page 74* ❧ TEETH *see page 152*

Problems of the Muscles, Bones, and Joints

THE STRUCTURES that form the human frame are collectively known as the neuromusculoskeletal system. This is the largest system in the body, using the most energy and producing the most waste.

The bones that make up the human frame meet at the joints, which are linked together by ligaments and are moved by muscles. The joints are lubricated by the synovial fluid and the membranes that line them. Cartilage cushions them from impact. The muscles are attached to the bones by tendons, and the fabric of the body is held together by "connective tissues" or "fascias," forming a continuous sheath covering the muscles and organs throughout the entire body.

Arteries run throughout the body, and through the blood they supply nourishment to the neuromusculo-skeletal system. The waste products are washed away by the venous and lymphatic channels (the lymphatic system runs parallel to the circulatory system). All activities and functions are governed by the nerves connecting the joints to the spinal cord and brain.

WHAT CAN GO WRONG?

The internal systems of the body are there to serve the needs of the body framework: that is, to nourish, repair, maintain, and organize it. When all the systems are working together in harmony, automatically adapting to the constantly changing needs, the body is healthy. When these break down ill-health or "dis-ease" sets in.

The body framework is the system in the body responsible for most aches and pains, as well as stiffness and restricted mobility. There may be injuries to bones, strains and cramps in muscle, stiffness and general wear and tear on joints. It can be affected greatly by internal ill-health, and when the framework itself becomes dysfunctional, it can alter the health of the internal organs and the whole body system.

Pain in the body framework may be due to many causes. Organic pathologies such as secondary cancer, prostate cancer, infections, gynecological, and kidney problems, among others, must first be eliminated before treatment is undergone.

It must be stressed that although the treatments described will deal with the presenting complaint, alternative medicine does not work on a symptomatic "formula" basis. There are invariably underlying factors to the presenting symptoms that must be addressed to enable full recovery. Professional advice must be sought for a correct diagnosis and overall constitutional treatment, which will always be individually tailored.

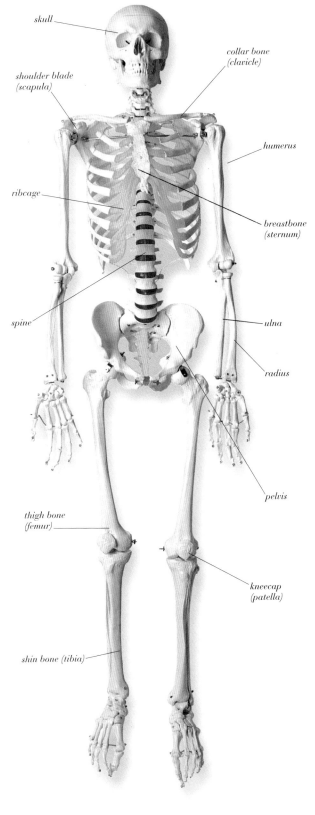

skull

collar bone (clavicle)

shoulder blade (scapula)

humerus

ribcage

breastbone (sternum)

spine

ulna

radius

pelvis

thigh bone (femur)

kneecap (patella)

shin bone (tibia)

The human skeleton contains 206 bones connected by ligaments and joints.

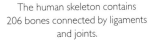CIRCULATION *see page 164* ❧ PAIN *see page 186*

Muscular Dystrophy

uscular dystrophy (MD) is a group of hereditary muscular disorders, characterized by progressive weakness and wasting of various groups of muscles. There are several types, which affect different groups of muscles and arise at different ages. The three major types are listed below.

DUCHENNE

In this case, the first signs usually appear before the age of three and in most cases the muscles appear bulkier than normal. The bulk of actual muscle tissue is not, however, increased and there is progressive weakening. This initially affects the buttocks and leg muscles, causing a characteristic waddle in walking. The weakness causes the child to get up from lying in a typical way – by rolling on his face and using the arms to push himself. Unfortunately, nothing can stop the progress of the disease, which is usually fatal by the teenage years. It affects boys, because the gene that carries the disease is linked to the male X chromosome.

LIMB GIRDLE

This form of muscular dystrophy affects the shoulders, pelvic, and uppermost limb muscles, has a recessive inheritance, and affects both sexes. It usually causes severe disablement within 20 years of onset.

FACIO-SCAPULO-HUMERAL

This type of muscular dystrophy affects the muscles of the face, upper back, and upper arm and is caused by a dominant gene. It progresses very slowly and does not necessarily shorten life. It can occur at any age and may affect several children in one family.

❧ TREATMENT

MASSAGE Relaxing and full-body massage will stimulate the muscles.

HYDROTHERAPY Swimming and exercise in water encourages mobility and builds up strength without excess strain on the muscles themselves.

Consult a qualified practitioner/therapist for:
OSTEOPATHY Treatment will be aimed at improving musculoskeletal function.

THE TRAGER APPROACH The treatment may improve general health, enhance self-image and increase mobility.

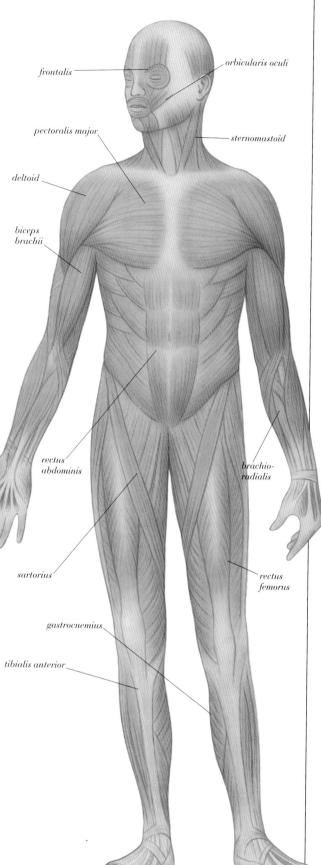

frontalis
orbicularis oculi
pectoralis major
sternomastoid
deltoid
biceps brachii
rectus abdominis
brachio-radialis
sartorius
rectus femorus
gastrocnemius
tibialis anterior

The human body contains over 650 muscles to coordinate movement and posture.

HYDROTHERAPY *see page 26* ❧ MASSAGE *see page 48* ❧ OSTEOPATHY *see page 42* ❧ TRAGER APPROACH *see page 58*

Back Problems

Back pain is the most common problem for the majority of the population. If back pain is unrelenting, unaffected by movement or accompanied with fever, malaise, reduced appetite, sudden weight loss, or severe headache (especially when accompanied by nausea and vomiting), medical treatment must be sought immediately. A medical doctor must always be consulted if the spine is damaged as a result of a fall or accident, if there is suspected fracture, or when there is serious illness, such as a heart attack.

LUMBAGO OR LOWER BACK PAIN

Lower back pain may range from being an occasional dull ache below the waist level to a constant, severe pain causing the back to "lock". The pain may remain in the lower back, be one-sided, or both, or may spread into the buttock or the leg, as far as the knee and foot. There may be accompanying pins and needles and aching in the leg (sciatica). It is made worse by bending, menstruation, changing positions, or by turning over in bed.

❧ TREATMENT

MASSAGE This can help to reduce muscular tension and pain, although it is important not to massage over the vertebrae.

ACUPRESSURE This may help.

BACH FLOWER REMEDIES Try Agrimony and Hornbeam, which may help when there are sleep problems caused by the condition.

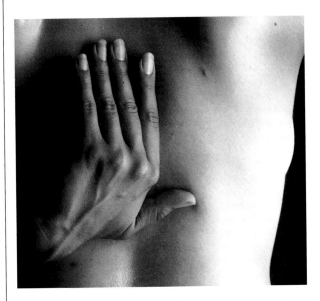

CAUTIONS AND CONTRAINDICATIONS

Any back pain that is accompanied by the following symptoms, requires urgent medical attention:
loss of bladder or bowel control;
pins and needles in uro-genital area;
progressive weakness in legs associated with uncontrollable foot drag/drop;
muscle wasting.

---

muscle spasm. It will be worse after rest, coughing, sneezing, or bending, and may be accompanied by pins and needles and numbness in the leg or foot.

❧ TREATMENT

A prolapsed disk must be seen by a medical professional before any treatment is undergone.

TENS (TRANSCUTANEOUS ELECTRICAL NERVE STIMULATION) This uses electrodes to block nerve impulses and stimulate the release of endorphins, the body's natural pain-relief hormones.

HOMEOPATHY Arnica every 30 minutes for up to six doses, then four-hourly for up to five days.

BACH FLOWER REMEDIES Rescue Remedy is appropriate for the shock accompanying pain.

HYDROTHERAPY Hot and cold compresses.

Consult a qualified practitioner/therapist for:
OSTEOPATHY, CHIROPRACTIC, AND ACUPUNCTURE.

Aches and pains in the back may be the legacy of minor mechanical strain in the past.

Consult a qualified practitioner/therapist for:
OSTEOPATHY, CHIROPRACTIC, ALEXANDER TECHNIQUE, AND ACUPUNCTURE All can be extremely effective.

SLIPPED DISK

A slipped disk occurs when one of the fibrous disks that separate the vertebrae ruptures and presses against the nerves in the spinal canal.
There will be sudden, severe, aching pain, with

SELF-HELP

Care must be taken when lifting, carrying, and getting in and out of chairs and bed. Avoid soft chairs and mattresses. It is important to keep active, although regular rest is recommended. Later, exercise to strengthen the abdominal and thigh muscles will be recommended, together with swimming, cycling, and yoga.

ACUPRESSURE *see page 94* ❧ BACH FLOWER REMEDIES *see page 86* ❧
HOMEOPATHY *see page 83* ❧ HYDROTHERAPY *see page 26* ❧ MASSAGE *see page 48* ❧
TRANSCUTANEOUS ELECTRICAL NERVE STIMULATION (TENS) *see page 101*

Neck Injuries

Pain that is experienced in the nape of the neck may spread into the shoulder blades or upward into the neck to give "tension" headaches, tired eyes, or jaw pain. Whiplash injury and stiff neck are the two most common forms of neck injury.

WHIPLASH INJURY

Whiplash is the result of any accident producing an unexpected rapid shunt forward and back from behind. The spine is briefly flicked forward, reacting by snapping backward like a cracking whip. The head is the end of the whip so maximum strain is absorbed by the soft tissues of the neck. The whole spine, including the pelvis, is affected. Whiplash commonly occurs when a stationary car is struck from behind.

Symptoms may occur immediately or may be delayed for some time; they include pain, stiffness in the neck, headaches, impaired vision, vague aching, weakness, and pins and needles in the shoulder blades, arms, and hands. Depression and anxiety may also result from whiplash injury.

❧ TREATMENT

It is important to see a conventional medical doctor to ensure that no long-term damage has been done to the spine and/or neck. Following diagnosis of whiplash, a number of alternative therapies may be useful.

DIET AND NUTRITION High doses of calcium pantothenate may relieve stiffness. A good vitamin and mineral supplement can encourage healing.

AROMATHERAPY Sweet marjoram and rosemary may be used to relieve pain, through massage, or by drops added to the bath.

HOMEOPATHY Arnica can be taken for up to six doses, every five minutes following the accident, and then Hypericum, four-hourly, for up to three days.

HYDROTHERAPY Ice packs alternated with hot compresses will encourage healing and relieve pain.

Consult a qualified practitioner/therapist for:
OSTEOPATHY, CHIROPRACTIC, MASSAGE, ACUPUNCTURE, AND ALEXANDER TECHNIQUE These treatments can help to alleviate pain and restore normal movement as quickly as possible. However, they should not be used if there is a fracture of the vertebrae.

STIFF OR "CRICKED" NECK

A stiff neck is characterized by spasm of the neck muscles. Pain may be constant, and particularly severe upon twisting the neck and drawing the head to one side. The acute pain and stiffness may be caused by injury, sleeping awkwardly, or stress. Acute stiffness may be a symptom of meningitis (*see page 139*).

❧ TREATMENT

HYDROTHERAPY Use hot and cold compresses to encourage healing and relieve discomfort.

REFLEXOLOGY Address treatment to the point where the big toe joins the foot, on the sole of the left foot. Rotation of the big toes may help.

Consult a qualified practitioner/therapist for:
HOMEOPATHY, ALEXANDER TECHNIQUE, OSTEOPATHY, CHIROPRACTIC AND ACUPUNCTURE Manipulation therapies are invaluable for the treatment of the majority of back pain, relieving nerve pressure and generally improving body mechanics.

STIFF NECK EXERCISES

If you have a stiff neck after driving too far or staring at a computer screen for too long, try these self-help exercises to loosen up.

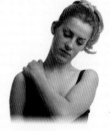

Use one hand to hold the opposite shoulder. Lean your head away from your hand, to stretch the neck muscles.

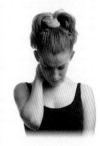

Gently push your head forward, to stretch the muscles and cervical vertebrae in the neck.

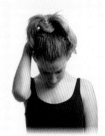

Push head down to feel the full stretch. Repeat on other side of neck. Then roll your head in a full circle.

AROMATHERAPY *see page 50* ❧ DIETARY THERAPY *see page 74* ❧
HOMEOPATHY *see page 83* ❧ HYDROTHERAPY *see page 26*

Body Systems

Posture

Good posture is an effortless, non-tiring stance that can be maintained for a long time. Your posture can be a reflection of your body attitude. A curvature is any deviation of the spine from its normal direction or position.

There are two basic spinal curves, which can be viewed from the side. When the posture is faulty, these curves become exaggerated or reduced. Lordosis exists when the neck and lower back dips in to display a C-curve. Seen from behind, lordosis is an exaggerated hollowing of the back. After time, this may result in a hollow, saddle, or sway back. Kyphosis occurs when the curve dips in the opposite direction, from the nape of the neck to the waist. Seen from behind, kyphosis is an exaggerated rounding or hump. After time, this may result in a humpback.

Viewed from the back, the shoulders and pelvis should be parallel and the head in line above the tail, displaying a straight vertical line. Scoliosis is a deviation from that straight line, where the spine curves from its central axis from side to side, resembling an S.

Poor posture results in a multitude of symptoms, such as back pain, headaches, general breathing and digestive difficulties, malaise, and feet problems.

Causes of bad posture include

❋ training (children copy parental posture)
❋ asymmetrical body use (maintaining the same stance for long periods)
❋ fatigue (insufficient energy to maintain constant good body posture)
❋ poor seating habits
❋ illness (which may also cause fatigue and through that poor posture)
❋ psychological problems (which are often manifested as introverted posture and hunched shoulders)
❋ birth abnormalities (such as dislocated hips)

> ### SELF-HELP
>
> Sleep on your back with a single pillow. If you need to sit for long periods of time, get a chair that has a forward sloping seat. Sit as erect as you can. Gentle exercises will help to improve posture.

> ### CAUTIONS AND CONTRAINDICATIONS
>
> Postural problems will take some time to rectify, and some stiffness and discomfort is to be expected; however, any sharp or recurrent pain should be addressed by your physician.

❋ disease (such as polio and arthritis)
❋ mechanical faults (including problems with the back, pelvis, knees, or feet).

❧ TREATMENT

The conditions that are causing the postural problems must always be diagnosed and addressed in the first instance. When illness, disease, or congenital defects have been ruled out, the following treatments may be found appropriate.

ALEXANDER TECHNIQUE This will involve retraining with exercises. It is the most useful therapy for long-term postural improvement.

DIET AND NUTRITION Where energy problems or disease are at the root of the postural problems, vitamin and mineral supplements may be appropriate.

OSTEOPATHY AND CHIROPRACTIC The manipulative therapies are excellent for overall postural treatment and retraining.

FELDENKRAIS Treatment will involve the restoration of natural energy flow, breathing, and less stressful patterns of alignment.

ROLFING Structural treatment breaks the cycle that can exist between pain/muscle tension/worse posture.

YOGA This is appropriate for mental and physical integration.

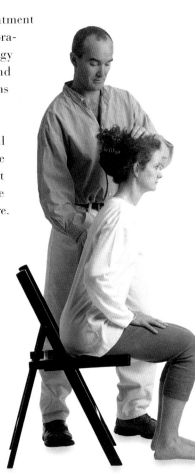

The Alexander teacher's gentle touch helps maintain a sense of poise and body/mind unity in the act of standing.

ALEXANDER TECHNIQUE *see page 57* ❧ CHIROPRACTIC *see page 39* ❧ DIETARY THERAPY *see page 74* ❧
OSTEOPATHY *see page 42* ❧ ROLFING *see page 46* ❧ YOGA *see page 61*

Osteoporosis

Osteoporosis, or "brittle bones," occurs when the bone density is reduced, resulting in thin, weak, and porous bones. The bone becomes thin due to a loss of calcium, causing persistent backache, in the neck, rib, and hip area. The back gradually becomes stooped, reducing height. The causes of osteoporosis are varied, and include

❋ menopause, when the female hormone estrogen is no longer produced (estrogen has a protective effect on the bones)
❋ deficiency in calcium and vitamins C and D
❋ malabsorption
❋ long-term use of corticosteroids
❋ rheumatoid arthritis
❋ immobilization
❋ lack of sunshine.

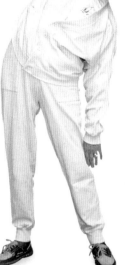

A gentle stretching exercise regime can help you stay mobile and keep weight down, both of which can help in osteoporosis.

✇ TREATMENT
DIET AND NUTRITION
Increase your intake of dark green, leafy vegetables, sesame seeds, fish, beans, peas, dark blue-black berries, cherries, raspberries, citrus-rinds, and colorful fruits. Reduce your intake of refined carbohydrates, fat, animal products, and fizzy drinks. Dietary supplements include vitamins B6 100mg, folic acid 1mg, B12 1mg, calcium citrate 1g, and magnesium citrate 500 mg daily *(see pages 78–9)*. An alternative treatment is natural progesterone cream, with added vitamin D, calcium, and magnesium.

Consult a qualified practitioner/therapist for:
ACUPUNCTURE This can restore the balance of energy in the body and provide relief from pain. Malabsorption may also be addressed.

NATUROPATHY Biochemic tissue salts Calc. fluor. and Calc. phos. taken four times daily for four weeks.

> **SELF-HELP**
> Exercise should be increased – duration is more important than intensity, and 30 minutes at least three times a week is recommended. Ensure that you are exposed (with suitable sunscreens) to sunshine on a regular basis.

MASSAGE Aromatherapeutic massage, relaxation therapy, and shiatsu may be useful.

HERBALISM Treatment may include the following as teas: dong quai, false unicorn root, black cohosh, licorice, and fennel.

OSTEOPATHY (INCLUDING CRANIAL) Gentle techniques for joint mobility will maintain musculoskeletal integrity.

ANKYLOSING SPONDYLITIS (AS)
AS is a degenerative rheumatic disease where spinal joints become inflamed, stiff, and eventually fused. It develops slowly. Symptoms are usually worse after rest and later may affect the chest, shoulders, hips, and knees, spreading up to the neck in severe cases.

✇ TREATMENT
Seek treatment from a registered practitioner who will prescribe according to your specific symptoms and constitution. Mobility delays fusion, and swimming and stretching may be suggested.

TENS (TRANSCUTANEOUS ELECTRICAL NERVE STIMULATION) This uses electrodes to block nerve impulses and to stimulate the release of endorphins.

HYDROTHERAPY Epsom salt baths may be suggested, or adding aromatherapeutic oils to the bathwater, including lavender, rosemary, and basil. Massage with these oils may also relieve symptoms.

HOMEOPATHY Treatment should be constitutional, but Arnica, Rhus tox. and Bryonia may be appropriate short term remedies.

> **CAUTIONS AND CONTRAINDICATIONS**
> Avoid heavy manipulation if you suffer from osteoporosis, or where there is acute inflammation and a fused spine.

HERBAL MEDICINE Herbal treatment may consist of black willow, devil's claw, and bogbean, taken as teas.

Consult a qualified practitioner/therapist for:
ACUPUNCTURE AND OSTEOPATHY These can be helpful.

ACUPUNCTURE *see page 90* ✇ DIETARY THERAPY *see page 74* ✇ HERBAL MEDICINE *see page 67* ✇
HOMEOPATHY *see page 83* ✇ HYDROTHERAPY *see page 26* ✇ NATUROPATHY *see page 24* ✇
OSTEOPATHY *see page 42* ✇ TRANSCUTANEOUS ELECTRICAL NERVE STIMULATION (TENS) *see page 101*

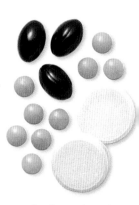

Arthritis and Rheumatism

THERE ARE many different types of arthritis, each of which involves some disorder or inflammation of one or more joints. The two most common forms are osteoarthritis and rheumatoid arthritis.

OSTEOARTHRITIS (OA)

Osteoarthritis is the most common type of arthritis, affecting the middle-aged. It is a degenerative joint disease and is characterized by pain, stiffness, and swelling in spinal joints, hips, knees, and joints of the hand, with progressive loss of function. The cartilage that lines the bones degenerates, becoming inflamed, rough, and hardened, and eventually wears away. Tendons, ligaments, and muscles that are holding the joint together become weaker, causing deformity, pain, and reduced movement.

Osteoarthritis is the result of natural wear and tear, but other causes can include
* repeated strain to joints, ligaments, and muscles
* joint deformation from birth or previous injury
* rheumatoid arthritis
* gout
* nutritional and hormonal influences.

☙ TREATMENT

DIET AND NUTRITION Correct body weight should be maintained to prevent strain from causing osteoarthritis. Tomatoes, potatoes, eggplants, peppers, and simple carbohydrates, such as white flour and refined sugar, should be eaten in moderation. Avoid coffee, red meat, artificial additives, and processed foods. Increase your intake of vegetables, fruits, complex carbohydrates, wheat germ, and oily fish. A nutritionist might suggest daily supplementation with vitamins A (10,000iu), C (2g), E (600iu), and B6 (50mg).

MASSAGE Joints can be massaged effectively with tiger balm, lavender and camomile oils, and with Ruta grav. cream.

YOGA This will help to encourage joint mobility and improved posture.

Consult a qualified practitioner/therapist for:
ACUPUNCTURE With or without using moxibustion, this will act to balance energies and reduce both inflammation and pain.

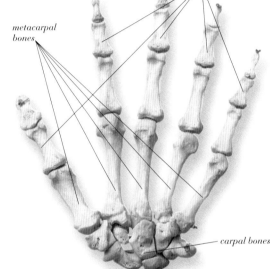

phalanges

metacarpal bones

carpal bones

The hand is a complex arrangement of bones, joints, and tendons, which make it vulnerable to wear and tear.

Regular supplements of iron, magnesium, and vitamin C can help keep joints mobile.

AYURVEDA Treatment is aimed at balancing the elements of air, fire, water, and mindbody connections.

HERBAL MEDICINE Some herbalists might recommend celery seed, yucca leaves, bogbean, and devil's claw, taken daily. Infusions of alfalfa and nettle may be suggested as nutritional supplements. Wild yam root and glucose amine (1500mg per day) are also useful.

HOMEOPATHY Rhus tox. 6c is suitable when the condition is worse with rest and dampness, and Ruta grav. is appropriate when symptoms are relieved by warmth.

OSTEOPATHY AND CHIROPRACTIC These are useful for maintenance of efficient body mechanics and pain relief.

ROLFING Treatment will address postural integration.

CAUTIONS AND CONTRAINDICATIONS

Always see your physician if you suffer from any of the symptoms of arthritis; early treatment can often prevent long-term suffering.

SELF-HELP

Light exercise, such as gentle swimming, may be suggested to retain the range of joint movement and muscle strength as far as possible.

ACUPUNCTURE *see page 90* ☙ AYURVEDA *see page 34* ☙ DIETARY THERAPY *see page 74* ☙
HERBAL MEDICINE *see page 67* ☙ HOMEOPATHY *see page 83* ☙ MASSAGE *see page 48* ☙
ROLFING *see page 46* ☙ YOGA *see page 61*

Rheumatoid Arthritis (RA) and Gout

Rheumatoid arthritis is a systemic disease that begins with severe pain in the small joints of hands and feet, spreading to the wrists, knees, shoulders, ankles, and elbows. Overlying skin appears red and shiny. This condition affects mostly women, often beginning between the ages of 20 and 40, although it can occur at any time. Symptoms include joint pain, swelling, and stiffness, accompanied by fatigue, low-grade fever, and poor appetite.

Rheumatoid arthritis is an autoimmune reaction resulting in a chronic, inflammatory condition affecting the joints and the tissues around them. The joints themselves become painful, swollen, unstable, and then greatly deformed. It varies in severity.

CAUTIONS AND CONTRAINDICATIONS

Heavy manipulation should be avoided in the acute stages of the illness.

SELF-HELP

Light exercise, such as gentle swimming, may be suggested.

TREATMENT

DIET AND NUTRITION *(See Osteoarthritis page 178.)* It is sensible to increase your intake of wholefoods, vegetables, and fiber. Reduce intake of meat, refined carbohydrates, and saturated fats. A qualified nutritional therapist will check for food allergies or intolerance, such as dairy, wheat, corn, and so on, and will, perhaps, suggest daily supplementation with vitamins C (2g), E (400iu), and B complex, along with calcium pantothenate, selenium (100mg), and zinc (30mg).

HYDROTHERAPY Cold compresses are useful when the joints are acutely inflamed, followed by alternating hot and cold compresses.

MASSAGE Joints can be massaged with tiger balm, lavender, and camomile oils, and Ruta graveolens cream.

Consult a qualified practitioner/therapist for:
ACUPUNCTURE This will be aimed at energy balance, and pain relief.

HERBAL MEDICINE Useful herbs include black cohosh, wild yam, willow bark, and licorice.

HOMEOPATHY Specific remedies include Arnica 6c, Bryonia 30c, Rhus tox. 6c, and Ruta grav. 6c, but treatment should always be constitutional.

OSTEOPATHY Treatment will be to address the maintenance of body mechanics.

HEALING This therapy can be beneficial.

GOUT

Gout is caused by the buildup of crystalized uric acid around the joints, causing severe pain, swelling, and redness around them. It affects mainly the big toe, knuckles, knees, and elbows. An attack may be accompanied by a high fever, and repeated attacks damage bones. Gout is usually an indication that the body is not processing and removing uric acid efficiently.

TREATMENT

DIET AND NUTRITION Avoid shellfish, sardines, kidneys, and beans, and increase your intake of water. Biochemic tissue salts include Nat. phos and Nat. sulf.

MASSAGE Oils of peppermint, lavender, camomile and geranium may be massaged into the affected area. Ruta graveolens cream may also be used. Self-mobilize the toe by gently pulling it and moving it around.

ACUPRESSURE Massage of points relating to the feet will be useful.

Consult a qualified practitioner/therapist for:
HERBAL MEDICINE Celery seeds, and wintergreen teas; bladderwrack may be taken internally, or seaweed can be eaten or added to the bath. Burdock and nettle neutralize and eliminate poisons from the body. A poultice of comfrey and marigold may be useful.

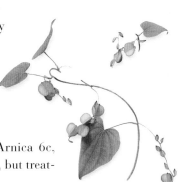

Wild yam *Discorea villosa* is a powerful anti-inflammatory and anti-rheumatic herbal remedy that can help joint pain.

CHIROPRACTIC AND OSTEOPATHY Both provide foot mobilization maneuvers to help the condition.

ACUPRESSURE *see page 94* ACUPUNCTURE *see page 90* DIETARY THERAPY *see page 74*
HERBAL MEDICINE *see page 67* HOMEOPATHY *see page 83* HYDROTHERAPY *see page 26*
MASSAGE *see page 48* OSTEOPATHY *see page 42*

Arms and Hands

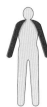

There are a number of causes for pain in the arms and hands. When pain is associated with neck and shoulder blade stiffness, and there is a pins and needles sensation in part of the arm, the pain may be "referred" from the neck or midback. Specific pain in the shoulder, elbow, or joints of the hand may be due to arthritis, especially if accompanied by swelling and reddened skin.

FROZEN SHOULDER

Frozen shoulder is characterized by pain and restriction in the shoulder. Pain is worse when lifting the arm sideways, putting on or removing clothing, and lying on the affected arm.

❧ TREATMENT

Treatment should be given early, before stiffness develops. Light gentle exercise, within the limits of pain, will improve general long-term mobility.

HERBAL MEDICINE Castor-oil packs are very useful.

TENS Transcutaneous electrical nerve stimulation will encourage the body's own natural pain-killers *(see page 101)*.

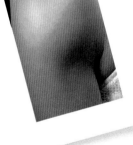
Frozen shoulder makes simple tasks such as brushing the hair very painful ordeals.

HYDROTHERAPY Hot and cold compresses should be alternated.

Consult a qualified practitioner/therapist for:
ACUPUNCTURE Treatment will address the same points as for acupressure and is performed on the shoulder itself. It can help relieve pain and promote mobility of the shoulder joint.

ACUPRESSURE This can relieve symptoms.

AROMATHERAPY Essential oils of rosemary and pine may be used in the bath, in a vaporizer, or for a light massage of the affected area.

CHIROPRACTIC Individual joint adjustment will be necessary.

HOMEOPATHY Treatment will be constitutional, but specific remedies may include Rhus tox. 6c and Bryonia 6c.

MASSAGE Ruta grav. cream, rolfing and shiatsu will all encourage healing, relieve pain, and aid mobility.

OSTEOPATHY Useful in early and chronic stages for reducing inflammation, and maintaining shoulder joint mobility, and trunk and spinal mechanics.

TENNIS ELBOW

Symptoms include pain and tenderness on the outside of the elbow, accompanied by restricted movement.

❧ TREATMENT

ACUPRESSURE This will encourage healing and will relieve symptoms.

HYDROTHERAPY Alternate hot and cold compresses

Consult a qualified practitioner/therapist for:
ACUPUNCTURE Treatment will be aimed at the same points as acupressure.

HOMEOPATHY Constitutional treatment is essential, but specific remedies include Arnica 6c, Rhus tox. 6c and Ruta grav. 6c.

OSTEOPATHY Treatment will include soft tissue re-integration, as well as correction of the mechanics locally, and of the arm in relation to the shoulder and trunk.

MYOTHERAPY Massage of trigger points will generally be undertaken.

SELF-HELP

Hot or cold compresses will help to ease the pain. Rest will encourage healing. Do not continue to use the affected joint until the pain becomes less persistent.
Very gentle movement will help to maintain some mobility.

CAUTIONS AND CONTRAINDICATIONS

Pain will encourage disuse, which will in turn cause further pain and stiffness, until there is very little mobility. If you suffer from the symptoms of these conditions, see your physician at once.

ACUPUNCTURE *see page 90* ❧ AROMATHERAPY *see page 50* ❧ CHIROPRACTIC *see page 39* ❧
HOMEOPATHY *see page 83* ❧ HYDROTHERAPY *see page 26* ❧ MYOTHERAPY *see page 46* ❧
OSTEOPATHY *see page 42* ❧ TRANSCUTANEOUS ELECTRICAL NERVE STIMULATION (TENS) *see page 101*

Repetitive Strain Injury (RSI)

Repetitive strain injury, or RSI, is the name given to the symptom complex of pain in the arm and trunk. It is also called "cumulative trauma disorder," and is characterized by pain, swelling, burning, pins and needles, and numbness of the affected area. Repetitive strain is thought to be caused by activities such as typing, and commonly affects the hand, thumb, neck, shoulder, and trunk.

✑ TREATMENT

Occupational working posture will need to be altered before treatment can be effective.

HYDROTHERAPY Cold compresses will encourage healing and will relieve the symptoms of pain, swelling, and burning.

MASSAGE Local massage with tiger balm and Ruta grav. cream may help.

Consult a qualified practitioner/therapist for:
ACUPUNCTURE
Treatment is aimed at providing pain relief and reducing inflammation.

ACUPRESSURE Specific treatment will be based on individual diagnosis.

ALEXANDER TECHNIQUE Postural integration will encourage resolution of the condition.

BOWEN TECHNIQUE Treatment provides moves for the shoulder and elbow.

CHIROPRACTIC Adjustments for trunk and arm will be undertaken.

HOMEOPATHY Treatment will be constitutional, but specific remedies may well include Rhus tox., Arnica and Bryonia.

MYOTHERAPY Treatment will be addressed to areas around the inflammation.

OSTEOPATHY There will be specific mobilization of the elbow, along with integration of arm and body mechanics.

> **SELF-HELP**
>
> **CARPAL TUNNEL SYNDROME**
> Symptoms may be relieved by hanging the affected arm off the side of the bed at night. Take extra vitamins B2 and B6, which may relieve symptoms.

CARPAL TUNNEL SYNDROME

Carpal tunnel syndrome is a condition in which the median nerve becomes trapped as it passes from the wrist to the hand. It predominantly affects the middle-aged and elderly and is caused by the gradual thickening of the tendons as they pass through the carpal tunnel, taking up greater space and pressing on the nerves, usually through repetitious activity.

Symptoms include pain, numbness, tingling in the thumb, index, and middle fingers, which may spread upward into the forearm.

✑ TREATMENT

Repetitious and painful movements should be avoided.

DIET AND NUTRITION Vitamin B6 deficiency may cause carpal tunnel syndrome, and this will be addressed by your nutritional therapist. It has been discovered that 80 percent of patients have brought it under control with high doses of vitamin B6 plus magnesium. Ferr. phos. and Mag. phos. (both biochemic tissue salts) may also be recommended.

HYDROTHERAPY Hot and cold compresses should be alternated to relieve symptoms.

Consult a qualified practitioner/therapist for:
ACUPRESSURE Specific treatment will be based on individual diagnosis.

ACUPUNCTURE Treatment will be according to individual diagnosis and aimed at the whole body.

OSTEOPATHY Specific mobilization of wrist bones and integration of wrist and arm mechanics will be the main form of treatment.

Cases of repetitive strain injury have risen since the introduction of computers and their keyboards to most occupations.

ACUPRESSURE *see page 94* ✑ ACUPUNCTURE *see page 90*
ALEXANDER TECHNIQUE *see page 57* ✑ HYDROTHERAPY *see page 26*
MASSAGE *see page 48* ✑ OSTEOPATHY *see page 42*

Fibrositis

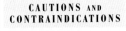

Fibrositis is a painful condition that is characterized by widespread pain with multiple tight and tender spots in the muscles. These are felt as cordlike fibers of muscle in the surrounding, relaxed musculature. Symptoms include pain, fatigue, stiffness, sleep disturbances, an irritable bowel, muscle twitching, frequent urination, premenstrual syndrome, headaches, anxiety, mood swings, poor concentration and memory, and balance problems, among others. The condition appears to be exacerbated by damp weather, intense activity, and stress.

Sufferers are predominantly female Caucasians, and the severity (in this case, the number of tender spots on the muscles) increases with age. The cause is largely unknown, although it is thought to be related to allergies, chemical sensitivities, and toxicity, as well as an individual's stress and anxiety.

❧ TREATMENT

DIET AND NUTRITION Reduce intake of refined carbohydrates, processed foods with artificial additives, and carbonated drinks. Increase your intake of fresh fruit and vegetables, and their juices. A combination of biochemic tissue salts may be appropriate. Supplementation with multivitamins and minerals, especially vitamins C and B complex and zinc may be suggested in order to address any deficiencies that may be causing or exacerbating the condition.

ACUPRESSURE Tender points will be addressed.

Consult a qualified practitioner/therapist for:
ACUPUNCTURE Treatment can be used to control pain; moxibustion will be used for excesses of cold, wind, or dampness.

AROMATHERAPY Lavender, sandalwood, and rosemary oils may be suggested.

CHIROPRACTIC Treatment will be aimed at specific joint adjustments for improved flexibility and muscle release.

HERBAL MEDICINE Your herbalist will treat you according to your individual condition, but suggested herbs may include valerian, bog bean, golden seal, willow and primula, taken as teas, twice daily.

HOMEOPATHY Treatment will be constitutional, but specific remedies may include Rhus tox. 6, Arnica 6, and Bryonia 6.

HYPNOTHERAPY Studies show that this therapy has been useful where others have failed, particularly in reducing pain and inducing sleep.

MASSAGE Shiatsu and massage for relaxation may be undergone. An aromatherapeutic massage might include the essential oils of thyme, lavender, and eucalyptus.

MYOTHERAPY This treatment will be aimed at trigger point release to ease the pain.

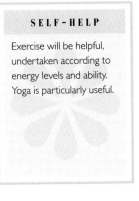

OSTEOPATHY Specific treatment improves general well-being by encouraging the body's own healing processes. Adjustments improve joint mobility, and gentle release techniques work on the musculoskeletal system to reverse fibrotic changes. These in turn help to reduce the fatigue and alleviate associated symptoms.

HEALING Healing provides a mind-body-spirit release.

ROLFING This treatment will include body "expansion" release, and centralization of the body's line of gravity.

Osteopathy is a very useful therapy for fibrositis. Only the gentle adjustments are used.

ACUPUNCTURE *see page 90* ❧ AROMATHERAPY *see page 50* ❧ DIETARY THERAPY *see page 74* ❧
HERBAL MEDICINE *see page 67* ❧ HOMEOPATHY *see page 83* ❧ HYPNOTHERAPY *see page 112* ❧
OSTEOPATHY *see page 42* ❧ ROLFING *see page 46*

CAUTIONS AND CONTRAINDICATIONS

Fibrositis is often caused by occupational or postural habits, and if left untreated can cause muscles to tear.

SELF-HELP

Exercise will be helpful, undertaken according to energy levels and ability. Yoga is particularly useful.

Hips, Legs, and Feet

Pain may occur in part or all of the leg, including the hip, thigh, knee, calf, and foot. When pain is felt within the joint area itself (where two bones join) and is accompanied by swelling, heat, or stiffness, there may be an underlying condition, such as arthritis, or a musculoskeletal dysfunction of the joint. When pain spreads diffusely into the leg, it may be spinal or pelvic dysfunction or "referred" from the back.

HIP COMPLAINTS

Hip complaints are generally felt as pain in the groin, hip, or in the buttock, although it may spread into the thigh and knee. Pain is usually worse when walking, rising from a chair, and lying on the affected side and can be exacerbated by warmth.

The causes of hip complaints and associated pain are manifold and include arthritis and previous joint distortion. Mechanical dysfunction of the pelvis, lower back, or knees can also cause hip problems, and occasionally infection may be at the root.

❧ TREATMENT

It is vital to get sufficient rest, since strain exacerbates the condition. Avoid sitting with your legs crossed.

CAUTIONS AND CONTRAINDICATIONS

The following conditions may cause pain in the hips and should be diagnosed and treated by a conventional medical doctor: abscesses, secondary cancers and infections, severe osteoarthritis and osteoporosis.

DIET AND NUTRITION *(see Arthritis, page 178.)*

HYDROTHERAPY Cold compresses may be used.

Consult a qualified practitioner/therapist for:
ACUPRESSURE This will reduce pain.

ACUPUNCTURE Treatment will aim at balancing the energies.

ALEXANDER TECHNIQUE Postural awareness exercises will be taught.

CHIROPRACTIC Spinal, hip, and pelvic adjustments are common methods of treatent. A practitioner will look at the problem of the whole person.

HOMEOPATHY The following specific remedies may be suggested: Arnica 6c and Rhus tox. 6c.

OSTEOPATHY Specific work into the hip and its surrounding structures, as well as the pelvis and spine, are the best forms of treatment.

ROLFING Treatment consists of expansion of the pelvis and postural integration.

MASSAGE This should be firm and deep with Ruta grav. and Arnica creams, and camphor and ginger oils.

HOUSEMAID'S KNEE

Bursitis of the knee, or Housemaid's knee as it is commonly called, is the inflammation of, and excess fluid over, the kneecap, caused by repeated rubbing or pressure on the knees from kneeling. The inflammation and fluid prevent the free movement of the joint, causing pain, swelling, and heat.

❧ TREATMENT

Knee pads should be worn while kneeling, or a foam rubber mat used to reduce pressure on the kneecaps. After the swelling subsides, exercise, within the limits of pain, is recommended in order to strengthen the thighs.

DIET AND NUTRITION Vitamins A, C, and B complex may be supplemented to reduce the severity of the condition and encourage the body's healing processes.

HYDROTHERAPY Cold compresses should be applied to the affected area when it becomes inflamed.

Consult a qualified practitioner/therapist for:
ACUPRESSURE AND ACUPUNCTURE A practitioner will address specific points.

CHIROPRACTIC Specific joint adjustment, as well as adjustment of the spine and pelvis.

HERBAL MEDICINE Comfrey and slippery elm (used as poultices on the affected area) and infusions of camomile and passionflower, taken internally.

HOMEOPATHY Specific remedies include Ruta grav. 6c, Arnica 6c, and Bryonia 6c.

MASSAGE Local massage with Ruta grav. cream, tiger balm, and ginger and lavender oils is recommended.

OSTEOPATHY This is useful for specific work into the knee and its surrounding structures.

ALEXANDER TECHNIQUE see page 57 ❧ CHIROPRACTIC see page 39 ❧
HERBAL MEDICINE see page 67 ❧ HOMEOPATHY see page 83 ❧ HYDROTHERAPY see page 26 ❧
MASSAGE see page 48 ❧ OSTEOPATHY see page 42 ❧ ROLFING see page 46

Body Systems

Hips, Legs, and Feet • 2

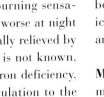

RESTLESS LEGS SYNDROME

This is a surprisingly common condition, characterized by aching, pain, twitching, pins and needles, and a burning sensation in legs. It tends to be worse at night and after prolonged sitting, and is generally relieved by movement. The cause of this syndrome is not known, although evidence points to a possible iron deficiency, especially in women, and reduced circulation to the nerves of the muscle fibers of the legs. Restless legs syndrome is more common in pregnancy, middle age, smokers, and those with a high caffeine intake.

✥ TREATMENT

Exercise, including walking, cycling, and swimming, will improve circulation. Self-massage may help to discourage attacks.

DIET AND NUTRITION

Increase your intake of iron-rich foods, including dried fruits, leafy green vegetables, poultry, fish, parsley, apricots, pumpkin seeds, and red meats. There is some evidence that vitamin E has a therapeutic effect, and foods rich in this vitamin include vegetable oils, seeds, nuts, and wheat germ. Avoid tea within two hours of meals (it inhibits the absorption of iron), and reduce consumption of coffee, cola, and chocolate. Nat. sulf. (a biochemic tissue salt) may be suggested by your nutritionist. A good multivitamin and mineral supplement, including especially vitamins A, C, E, and zinc, should be taken as preventive treatment. (*See pages 76–80 for more information on supplements and megavitamin therapy.*)

Consult a qualified practitioner/therapist for:
ACUPUNCTURE Treatment will be aimed at all points of the leg, and at energy balance.

HERBAL MEDICINE All treatment is individually tailored, and will be constitutional but one of the following herbs, taken as teas, may be suggested: valerian, verbena, ginger, oats, limeflower, and horse chestnut.

HOMEOPATHY Until constitutional treatment is received, try Causticum 30c, and Zinc 6c.

OSTEOPATHY

Your osteopath will improve body mechanics, and nerve and blood flow.

MASSAGE Deep massage, massage for relaxation, rolfing, and shiatsu are all appropriate for treating this syndrome, providing symptomatic relief and frequently curing it completely.

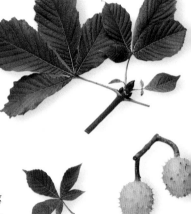

Horse chestnut *Aesculus hippocastrum* drunk as an infusion can help restless legs syndrome.

FOOT PROBLEMS

There are a large number of bones and muscles in the feet, and there are, subsequently, a correspondingly large number of complaints that can affect them. Injury, sprains, poor posture, and arthritis are responsible for the majority of foot problems, causing pain and dysfunction in the ankle, with subsequent difficulty in walking.

SPRAINED ANKLE/ANKLE PAIN

Strains and sprains are usually caused by a wrench, and cause pain, increased by movement or by putting weight on the foot. There will be swelling and perhaps bruising. There may also be damage to the ligaments. Consult a medical practitioner to check that you have not sustained a small fracture if the pain persists for more than a week.

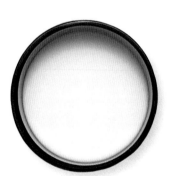

Causticum, the homeopathic remedy made from lime and potassium, is useful for neuromuscular problems.

✥ TREATMENT

Ensure that the foot is rested for a period each day. Recovery will be enhanced by gently exercising the ankle with a wobbleboard, moving the foot in a circular fashion, and stretching the calves.

DIET AND NUTRITION Ferr. phos., a biochemic tissue salt, is recommended for sprains.

HYDROTHERAPY Contrast bathing with hot and cold compresses is recommended.

ACUPUNCTURE *see page 90* ✥ DIETARY THERAPY *see page 74* ✥ HERBAL MEDICINE *see page 67* ✥
HOMEOPATHY *see page 83* ✥ HYDROTHERAPY *see page 26* ✥ MASSAGE *see page 48* ✥ OSTEOPATHY *see page 42*

Consult a qualified practitioner/therapist for:
ACUPUNCTURE AND ACUPRESSURE Stimulation of the relevant points will be undertaken.

HERBAL MEDICINE Your herbalist may suggest a poultice of turmeric, comfrey, and/or ginger.

HOMEOPATHY Specific remedies include Arnica 30c, taken as soon as possible after the injury, and then every hour. Take Rhus tox. 6c, and Ruta grav. 6c four times daily.

OSTEOPATHY Treatment will be aimed at specific mobilization of the ankle and foot, and integration of the leg with the trunk and pelvis.

DROPPED ARCHES/FOOT PAIN
General foot pain, which is not the result of injury, is usually felt in the middle of the foot and can be caused by excess strain on the foot itself, either from overweight, or from standing or walking for long periods of time. Calluses, bunions, and corns may contribute to discomfort. Foot pain can lead to postural problems, and cause the muscles of the calves to ache. (*For more information on posture see page 176.*)

Fallen arches occur when the raised arch of the sole descends, so that the entire foot is flat against the ground (flat feet). This condition may be congenital (some people are born with flat feet, and in others, the arch does not develop properly), or the result of weight gain, ill-fitting shoes, or weakened muscles in the foot.

✍ TREATMENT
Exercise is recommended, including picking up items with the toes, and rocking on the foot, from heel to toe.

HYDROTHERAPY Hot footbaths with essential oils of eucalyptus and rosemary should be alternated with cold footbaths with a few drops of essential oil of peppermint added to them.

Consult a qualified practitioner/therapist for:
MASSAGE Deep massage on the foot, calves, and upper legs will relieve symptoms and stimulate the muscles.

OSTEOPATHY Cranial osteopathy can be used to correct undeveloped arches in babies and children.

CHIROPRACTIC Adults should see a chiropractor for specific joint mobilization.

BUNIONS AND CORNS
Bunions are painful, swollen pads overlying the joint at the base of the big toe. They begin as an inflammation of the joint, which swells so that the overlying skin becomes red, hard, and sore. If left untreated, the ligaments in the toes shorten, pushing them together in what often becomes a permanent deformity. Bunions are caused by wearing ill-fitting shoes, but they can be hereditary.

Corns are painful wedges of hard skin that result from excess pressure on the surface of the skin of the toes or the soles of the feet. Corns are usually caused by wearing ill-fitting shoes, but may also occur when shoes are worn without socks. They are most common in people with high arches, because the arch increases the pressure on the toes when walking.

✍ TREATMENT
It is important to wear comfortable, professionally fitted shoes, and to ensure that your feet are rested every day. A circular corn pad can be worn to reduce pressure on the corn itself. Consult a podiatrist for severe or recalcitrant cases.

DIET AND NUTRITION
Biochemic tissue salts for bunions include Ferr. phos. and Kali mur.

Essential oil of geranium *Pelargonium graveolens* is useful for bruises and inflammation.

MASSAGE To treat bunnions massage your toes with oil of peppermint, blended in a light carrier oil, to stimulate the circulation and prevent swelling. Self-mobilize the toe by gently pulling it and moving it around.

Corns may be massaged with warm oil to soften the hardened skin before removal.

HOMEOPATHY Specific treatments may include Belladonna, Bryonia, Pulsatilla, and Ruta grav.

HYDROTHERAPY Footbaths with mustard, Epsom salts, arnica, and oils of peppermint, lavender, camomile, and geranium will relieve symptoms and discourage swelling.

BIOCHEMIC TISSUE SALTS *see page 81* ✍ CHIROPRACTIC *see page 39* ✍ HERBAL MEDICINE *see page 67* ✍
HOMEOPATHY *see page 83* ✍ HYDROTHERAPY *see page 26* ✍ MASSAGE *see page 48* ✍
OSTEOPATHY *see page 42*

The Ailments

Pain

PAIN is an unpleasant sensation that ranges from mild discomfort to almost unbearable agony, and can be acute or chronic.

Acute pain is short term and can last from a few seconds to a few hours, days or weeks – for instance, pain caused by injections, migraine, burns, and surgery. The pain may be self-limiting, or it may act as a warning that something is wrong and requires immediate treatment.

Chronic pain is persistent, intractable pain that may worsen rather than improve with time. Common examples are arthritic pain, backache, postherpetic pain (after shingles, for instance), neuralgia, and phantom limb pain. Many complementary medical techniques are useful for chronic pain, which is usually more deep-seated than acute and often more distressing, because of its longevity. The prospect of long-term drug therapy to control pain often tips the balance in favor of a decision to try alternative medicine, for this is often gentler, less invasive, and has fewer side effects.

✒ TREATMENT

Exercise helps to stimulate the endorphins, the body's natural painkillers, and also provides distraction from pain. Even a brisk, ten-minute walk can help, but do seek professional advice before undertaking any exercise program.

PSYCHOLOGICAL THERAPY Our thoughts, feelings, and behavior have a considerable impact upon how much pain we feel, regardless of the causes. If we are depressed or anxious, pain is likely to affect us more;

the more we dwell on it or encourage others to treat us as ill, the worse it is likely to become. Psychologists who specialize in pain-relief programs suggest that chronic-pain sufferers take up active hobbies or interests as a distraction from it. They also advise positive thinking, whenever feelings of pain threaten to overwhelm them.

DIET AND NUTRITION

The pain-relieving amino acid DL-phenylalanine (DLPA), which is found naturally in foods such as nuts, cheese, avocados, bananas, sesame, and pumpkin seeds, is available as a dietary supplement, and has proved useful in treating pain. However, consult your physician, since migraine victims and some sufferers of high blood pressure should not use it.

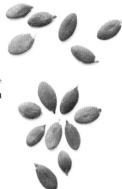

Pumpkin seeds *Cucurbita pepo* contain a natural pain reliever. They are also very nutritious.

AROMATHERAPY

Different oils, either sprinkled in a bath or inhaled from a few drops on a handkerchief, can ease various types of pain. For instance, camphor, lavender, and sage can relax painful muscles. Lavender is also analgesic, and is often used in the treatment of migraine. Bergamot, camomile, and marjoram are used to relieve pain.

VISUALIZATION This is a technique that helps many people. Close your eyes, relax, and choose an image you could believe would soothe your pain, such as a warm golden glow that melts it away, or a gently flowing stream that carries it away. Use whatever works for you.

RELAXATION Pain generally feels worse when you are tired, stressed, and tense, so practicing a relaxation technique on a regular basis should help to relieve it.

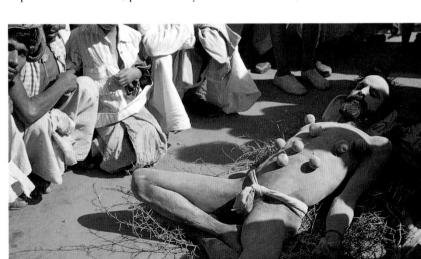

Some fakirs of India can control their perception of pain by vigorous mental application.

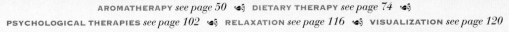
AROMATHERAPY *see page 50* ✒ DIETARY THERAPY *see page 74* ✒
PSYCHOLOGICAL THERAPIES *see page 102* ✒ RELAXATION *see page 116* ✒ VISUALIZATION *see page 120*

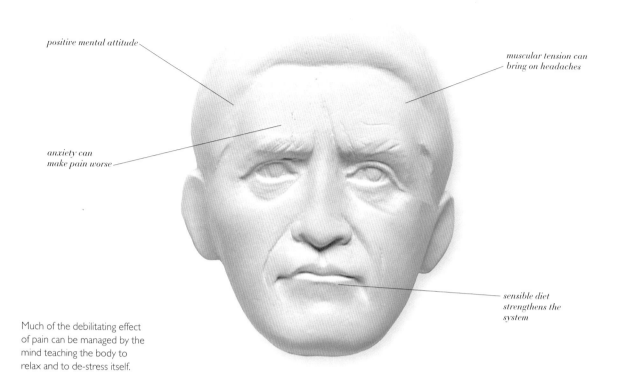

positive mental attitude

muscular tension can bring on headaches

anxiety can make pain worse

sensible diet strengthens the system

Much of the debilitating effect of pain can be managed by the mind teaching the body to relax and to de-stress itself.

Consult a qualified practitioner/therapist for:

MASSAGE A gentle massage can soothe many kinds of pain and relieve tension. Fear and tension often contribute to the level of pain.

ACUPUNCTURE Acupuncture is often used successfully to help relieve conditions such as arthritis, back pain, and chronic migraine. The principal approach is treatment of the meridians passing through the painful area.

TENS (**TRANSCUTANEOUS ELECTRICAL NERVE STIMULATION**) This can relieve back, arthritic, musculoskeletal, cancer, postoperative, labor, phantom limb, neuralgia, migraine, and sports injury pains.

ACUPRESSURE This has been known to help relieve chronic arthritis if carried out daily.

OSTEOPATHY AND CHIROPRACTIC These treatments may help particularly musculoskeletal problems such as neck and shoulder pain, backache, and sciatica.

ALEXANDER TECHNIQUE Pain that has its root in tension, or is exacerbated by tension, may be relieved by this technique. Backache, arthritis, migraine, and other problems can be successfully treated.

HYPNOTHERAPY, AUTOGENIC TRAINING, HEALING, YOGA, AND MEDITATION Any of these disciplines may also be helpful in combating pain, since they are all calming, de-stressing techniques.

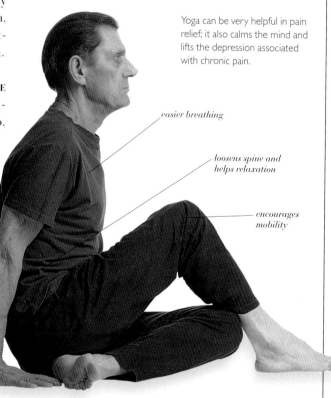

Yoga can be very helpful in pain relief; it also calms the mind and lifts the depression associated with chronic pain.

easier breathing

loosens spine and helps relaxation

encourages mobility

ACUPRESSURE *see page 94* ⮞ ACUPUNCTURE *see page 90* ⮞ ALEXANDER TECHNIQUE *see page 57* ⮞
CHIROPRACTIC *see page 39* ⮞ MASSAGE *see page 48* ⮞ OSTEOPATHY *see page 42* ⮞
TRANSCUTANEOUS ELECTRICAL NERVE STIMULATION (TENS) *see page 101*

Problems of the Nervous System

THE NERVOUS SYSTEM comprises the central nervous system (CNS), consisting of the brain and spinal cord, protected by the skull and spine, and the peripheral nervous system (PNS), made up of spinal and cranial nerves, which extend from the CNS to other parts of the body. Nerves are bundles of the long, tubelike extensions of nerve cells. Impulses traveling through them carry information throughout the body. Nerve impulses travel only in one direction. A message will, for instance, be sent to the brain from the fingertips through one nerve, and the message from the brain back to the fingers will be sent through another. Nerve cells are called neurons, and each has a cell body, branches called dendrites, and an axon. It is separated from the next nerve by a small gap called a synapse. Each neurone contacts the next in the nerve chain by releasing a chemical called a neurotransmitter from the end of the axon. This crosses the synapse and carries the message to the next neurone. The neurotransmitter found at the synapses of most peripheral nerves is called acetylcholine, although at some autonomic nerve synapses the transmitter is noradrenaline or dopamine.

WHAT NERVES DO

The action of the nerves, which is moderated by the neurotransmitters, is a sensitive process that can be increased or decreased as needed. And because the chemical structure of many of the neurotransmitters is known, they can be used as drugs to modulate some of the most important actions of the nervous system. There are also many drugs that act by simulating the action of neurotransmitters, by modifying their action or by blocking their receptor sites.

The CNS acts as a central computer to the rest of the body. It receives sensory information from the organs of the whole body, such as the ears and eyes, skin, and joints. It analyzes this information and then sends out the appropriate motor response to various muscles, such as those controlling speech or internal organs.

THE TWO SYSTEMS

There are two main divisions within the PNS: the somatic nervous system, which controls the muscles responsible for conscious or willed movement, such as speech or walking; and the autonomic nervous system, which controls involuntary body functions, such as sweating or shivering in response to cold. Organs and glands are influenced chiefly by the autonomic nervous system, which is divided into two areas: these are the sympathetic nervous system and the parasympathetic nervous system. Most of the time, these two systems are in balance, but the sympathetic system will dominate during periods of excitement or fear by stimulating functions such as the heartrate or breathing, as if preparing the body for a fight-or-flight response. In contrast, the parasympathetic system is concerned with everyday functions and dominates during sleep.

Sensory nerves carry information from the sense organs and other body receptors to the central nervous system – the brain and spinal cord – for processing. Then motor nerves carry the processed information from the central nervous system to the glands and muscles to intiate a change.

THE BRAIN

The brain controls the nervous system. The upper part of the brain is the cerebral cortex. Various parts of it are dedicated to specific processes, functions, and abilities. If the brain is damaged in any of these areas, then the skill, sense, or ability governed by that part will be affected.

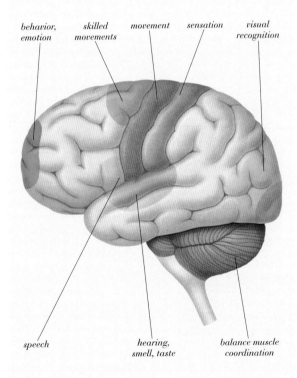

behavior, emotion   *skilled movements*   *movement*   *sensation*   *visual recognition*

speech   *hearing, smell, taste*   *balance muscle coordination*

HEAD *see page 142* ❧ NERVES *see page 189*

THE NERVES

Spinal nerves are pairs of sensory and motor nerve bundles that have their root in the spinal cord. Sensory spinal nerves send information from the sense organs and the body receptors to the central nervous system, and motor spinal nerves transmit messages to the muscles. Cranial nerves are a group of 12 pairs of sensory, motor, or mixed (having separate sensory and motor fibers) nerves that connect with the brain stem and the lower parts of the brain. Autonomic nerves are motor nerves only (part of the autonomic nervous system). They regulate a great variety of bodily functions, like the pumping action of the heart muscle, and the smooth muscles of the digestive system.

brain

spinal cord

spinal nerves of the peripheral nervous system

spine

sciatic nerve

The central nervous system comprises the brain, the spinal cord, and the set of paired nerves that lead from the spine and make a network throughout the body.

All of the CNS's responses are carried along nerves, made up of a bundle of nerve fibers (axons) of many nerve cells (neurons), which spread out from the CNS and make up the peripheral nervous system. All activity produced by the nervous system is based on transmitting impulses through this network of neurons. However, for various reasons, this activity can be disrupted.

THE RESULTS OF NERVE DAMAGE

When part of the nervous system is damaged, through disease or injury, disorders can occur. This can result in minor or temporary problems, such as pins and needles, or cause pain in certain areas (such as the face), called neuralgia, which is any pain originating in a nerve. Nerves can become trapped, as in the case of carpal tunnel syndrome, or perhaps sciatica, or they can become irritated at the spine (their root), as in the case of lumbago, neck pain, and other structural problems. But damage to the nerve may also be more severe and long term, resulting in more serious, degenerative diseases affecting the movement of the whole body, such as multiple sclerosis (MS), Alzheimer's, or Parkinson's disease, which can cause permanent disabilities. Complementary medicine has much to offer in the field of neurological disease, particularly in controlling pain and encouraging normal functioning of nerves that have become pinched or trapped (in the case of a prolapsed or "slipped disk" for instance) or damaged. Acupuncture, osteopathy, chiropractic, most of the bodywork therapies, and nutritional therapy, among others, have a useful role to play. Many modern-day neurological problems are the result of stress, which may cause muscles to spasm because of posture problems, tension, and other physical manifestations of the problem. Stress-reducing therapies, such as relaxation exercises, meditation, and yoga, often have a beneficial effect on the nervous system as a whole.

ALZHEIMER'S DISEASE *see page 194* ✧ CARPAL TUNNEL SYNDROME *see page 181* ✧
LUMBAGO *see page 174* ✧ MULTIPLE SCLEROSIS *see page 193* ✧ NEURALGIA *see pages 190-1* ✧
PARKINSON'S DISEASE *see page 194* ✧ SCIATICA *see page 191* ✧ SLIPPED DISK *see page174*

Common Problems of the Nervous System

When the nervous system is affected through irritation, damage, or disease, it can result in either partial or complete paralysis. This can be flaccid paralysis, perhaps the result of a severed nerve, which leaves the muscles floppy and without sensation, or spastic weakness of paralysis, when the muscles become rigid due to nerve damage in the brain or spinal cord, perhaps following a stroke. Paralysis can be either temporary or permanent. In diseases such as Parkinson's or MS, there may be weakness without paralysis.

NEURITIS

Numbness, tingling, pain, or muscle weakness due to the degeneration of nerve tissue, neuritis is caused by inflammation, disease, or damage. Symptoms vary according to whether it is the sensory nerve fibers or motor nerve fibers that are affected. Alcoholism may exacerbate the condition.

✌ TREATMENT

This depends on the underlying cause and severity of the damage. Specific causes include diabetes, which can be treated by rebalancing the body's sugar metabolism.

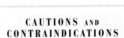

SELF-HELP

Increase your intake of foods rich in vitamins B1, B2, B12, and E, and biotin and chromium.

CAUTIONS AND CONTRAINDICATIONS

Neuralgia and neuritis should be treated as soon as symptoms set in, for the numbness and weakness they cause may lead to serious injury.

NATUROPATHY Treatment will be aimed at addressing dietary deficiencies, boosting vitamin intake and energy levels. Excessive alcohol consumption can also be treated with naturopathy to regulate diet.

DIET AND NUTRITION Restoring the body's natural chemical dehydroepiandrosterone (DHEA) may also help. Optimum levels are 750–1250ng/dL for men, 550–980ng/dL for women. Supplements of 50–100mg per day for men, and 20–75mg for women may be recommended.

HERBAL MEDICINE, AROMATHERAPY, HOMEOPATHY, AND YOGA, These all have been found helpful.

NEURALGIA

Neuralgia is pain in a particular area, and is due to nerve damage, irritation, or pressure. The pain usually lasts for only a brief period, but may be severe and is often described as a shooting sensation. It is a symptom of shingles, which is an infection of the nerves leading to areas of the skin; for instance, down one side of the trunk, neck or arm, or, more rarely, the face. Postherpetic pain, which is pain following a herpes zoster infection (the virus causing shingles, *see page 133)*, is caused by damage to the nerves, which results in repeated, strong nerve impulses being produced and sent to the brain. The pain is severe and can last for weeks or months.

✌ TREATMENT

ACUPRESSURE Trigeminal neuralgia, a spasmodic pain on one side of the face, can be self-treated by lightly pressing inward with the index fingers, just below the inner side of the brow, or from the same point, downward to the mouth. Neuralgia accompanying migraine can also be treated with light pressure or acupuncture.

BIOFEEDBACK AND HOMEOPATHY Remedies and biofeedback may be used to prevent stress, which may bring on attacks of neuralgia.

ACUPUNCTURE Particularly when used early on, this has been shown to prevent postherpetic neuralgia following shingles.

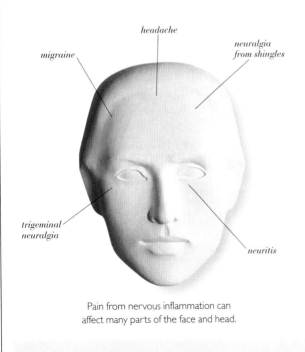

headache

migraine

neuralgia from shingles

trigeminal neuralgia

neuritis

Pain from nervous inflammation can affect many parts of the face and head.

ACUPRESSURE *see page 94* ✌ ACUPUNCTURE *see page 90* ✌ BIOFEEDBACK *see page 117* ✌
DIETARY THERAPY *see page 74* ✌ HOMEOPATHY *see page 83* ✌ NATUROPATHY *see page 24*

TENS TRANSCUTANEOUS ELECTRICAL NERVE STIMULATION This therapy uses electrodes to block these nerve impulses and stimulate the release of endorphins, the body's natural pain-relieving hormones, and is also particularly useful for pain following an attack of shingles *(see also page 133)*, and for other forms of neuralgia or face pain.

AROMATHERAPY, CHIROPRACTIC, TRADITIONAL CHINESE MEDICINE, HYPNOTHERAPY, NATUROPATHY, AND OSTEOPATHY have also proved beneficial.

SCIATICA

Pain radiating through the buttock, down the back of the thigh and lower leg, and along the length of the sciatic nerve is the result of irritation to the nerve roots at the origin of the sciatic nerve. This is commonly caused by a prolapsed intervertebral disk (slipped disk) *(see page 174)* pressing on the spinal root of a nerve or, more unusually, pressure from a clot, tumor, or even sitting awkwardly. It can be aggravated by coughing, sneezing, or bending. It is often preceded or accompanied by lumbago *(see page 174)*, and sometimes by pins and needles and numbness.

☙ TREATMENT
Bedrest on a firm mattress is advisable.

Consult a qualified practitioner/therapist for:
HYDROTHERAPY Alternating an ice or hot pack on the base of the spine helps to relieve pain.

ACUPRESSURE This can be extremely beneficial. Deep thumb pressure will be used.

ACUPUNCTURE
The acupuncture technique known as moxibustion (localized heat) may be used to relieve pain.

OSTEOPATHY, CHIROPRACTIC, MASSAGE, AND HYDROTHERAPY
The pressure applied through any of these manipulative therapies may be useful for reducing the pain of spasm.

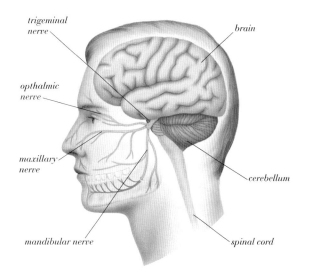

The head and face are particularly rich in nerves and therefore vulnerable to pain of many kinds when the nerves are affected.

TICS, TWITCHING, PINS AND NEEDLES
Uncontrolled repetitive contractions of a muscle cause tics and twitching, such as shrugging the shoulders, screwing up the eyes, or a "nervous" cough. These often develop in children and may be a sign of psychological disturbance or a response to situations in which the child feels tension

Pins and needles causes a prickly or tingling sensation and numbness, and is the result of a disturbance of the impulses through the nerves that carry sensation from the skin to the brain. This disturbance may be due to damage, irritation, or pressure on the nerves, and can be caused by something as simple as sleeping on an arm in an awkward way, or sitting or lying in one position for too long.

☙ TREATMENT
Although tics are often best left ignored, behavioral therapy can help discover the cause. Minor twitches and pins and needles, although irritating, need no attention.

Consult a qualified practitioner/therapist for:
TALKING TREATMENT Psychotherapy can help overcome tics caused by anxiety.

CAUTIONS AND CONTRAINDICATIONS

SCIATICA
The cause of sciatica should be diagnosed by a conventional medical practitioner before therapy is started.

SELF-HELP

SCIATICA
Local heat or ice may relieve symptoms and relax muscles that have become tense as a result of the pain. Swimming may help to release the trapped nerve if it is caused by spasm of the muscles. See your physician about preventing back problems.

ACUPRESSURE *see page 94* ☙ CHIROPRACTIC *see page 39* ☙ HYDROTHERAPY *see page 26* ☙
MASSAGE *see page 48* ☙ MOXIBUSTION *see page 31* ☙ OSTEOPATHY *see page 42*

Seizures and Epilepsy

Seizures are the tingling or twitching in small areas of the body, such as the face, or the loss of consciousness and uncontrolled jerks of the whole body. Recurrent seizures are called epilepsy. Seizures may affect only part of the brain, or be generalized, causing grand mal symptoms of headache, drowsiness, dizziness, and a feeling of discomfort or "aura," followed by unconsciousness, stiffening, or uncontrollable jerking of the body, or petit mal which usually affects children and can be difficult to detect since it may seem as if the child is just daydreaming.

Seizures are caused by sudden, uncontrolled occurrences of electrical brain activity. They can be triggered by injury, infection, or disease, or there may be no obvious reason.

Recent studies have found that infant vaccines DTP (diphtheria/tetanus/pertussis) and MMR (measles/mumps/rubella) can increase the risk of seizure. Chemicals found in aerosols, pesticides, paraffin fire fumes, diesel emissions, and solvents may also be triggers. Studies show a link between epilepsy and celiac disease, an allergy or intolerance to foods containing gluten, such as wheat, barley, rye, and oats.

Epilepsy and fits affect the brain but do not leave traces of their passage after they have gone.

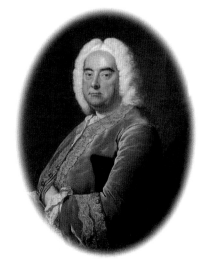

George Frideric Handel, the great German composer, suffered from epilepsy.

⊰ TREATMENT

NATUROPATHY It is believed that avoiding certain drugs, chemicals, and foods can also help prevent attacks. Naturopaths suggest a well-balanced gluten-free diet, high in vitamins D and B6, as well as zinc, calcium, and magnesium, which have anticonvulsant properties, and the amino acid taurine, to help control seizures. Avoiding caffeine and moderating your alcohol intake may also be recommended.

BACH FLOWER REMEDIES Clematis for preventing the initial feeling of vagueness and Rescue Remedy during an attack may be suggested.

OSTEOPATHY The light pressure used in cranial osteopathy has been found to help relieve symptoms.

YOGA, AROMATHERAPY, MEDITATION, AND BIOFEEDBACK Many seizures occur during times of stress and these therapies have been found to be beneficial for relaxation and body awareness.

SELF-HELP

Increase your intake of vitamin B6, magnesium, calcium, and zinc. Note: evening primrose oil is known to aggravate epilepsy and should not be taken. Carry a tag that will inform people of your condition in the event that you suffer a fit.

CAUTIONS AND CONTRAINDICATIONS

Do not reduce or stop prescribed drugs without conventional medical advice. Seek an experienced allergist or nutritionist for advice about a balanced diet.

AROMATHERAPY *see page 50* ⊰ BACH FLOWER REMEDIES *see page 86* ⊰ BIOFEEDBACK *see page 117* ⊰
MEDITATION *see page 118* ⊰ NATUROPATHY *see page 24* ⊰ YOGA *see page 61*

Multiple Sclerosis (MS)

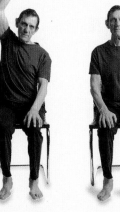

Inflammation may damage the sheath of fatty tissue, or myelin, protecting the nerve fibers in the central nervous system, causing progressively distorted messages to be sent to muscles. This causes a wide variety of symptoms, including blurred vision, and slurred speech, and motor response difficulties, including loss of coordination and paralysis. This can lead to bladder, emotional, mental, speech, and sexual problems. The causes are unknown and the symptoms are often unpredictable.

SELF-HELP

A diet low in animal fats and high in gamma linoleic acid is recommended, as is regular exercise. Ensure that your diet is rich in vitamins B6, B3, B12, C and E, and zinc and magnesium. Evening primrose oil may also be of help.

☙ TREATMENT

DIET AND NUTRITION Maintaining a low-fat (avoiding saturated fats) and low-sugar diet, with plenty of fruit and vegetables, and moderate amounts of white meat, such as fish and chicken, is advisable. Vitamin and mineral supplements have also proved helpful. A trained nutritionist or dietitian may suggest allergy-testing, since there may be a link between allergies and MS. When DHEA levels fall below 180ng/dL in men and 130ng/dL in women (optimum levels are 750–1250ng/dL in men and 550–980ng/dL in women) supplements of 50–100mg a day for men and 20–75mg for women may be taken.

MEDITATION, YOGA, AND MASSAGE These therapies can be used to prevent stressful situations from exacerbating symptoms, and the latter two are also important for maintaining muscle tone.

CAUTIONS AND CONTRAINDICATIONS

Always check that therapists are fully qualified before undergoing treatment.

CHIROPRACTIC, OSTEOPATHY, AND CRANIOSACRAL THERAPY Manipulation of the body, particularly the bones, muscles, and tissues of the spine, is helpful. Chiropractic uses this manipulation with various bone-cracking techniques to work on rebalancing. Osteopathy uses gentle manipulative techniques to improve body structure. A craniosacral therapist would lightly apply pressure to the bones of the head and spine.

ALEXANDER TECHNIQUE This can improve posture and help to realign the body to its natural position, relieving pressure, which may affect ability to function.

HERBAL MEDICINE Herbs will be prescribed to suit the condition of the individual, but they may include oats, skullcap, vervain, wood betony, damiana, lavender, mistletoe, and hyssop, among others.

HOMEOPATHY Remedies will be tailored to each individual, but specific remedies might include Phosphorus, Tarantula, Agaricus, Kali phos. and Magnesia phos.

MAGNETIC THERAPY AND HYDROTHERAPY These therapies have all been found helpful. In particular, magnetic therapy uses pulsed electromagnetic fields to promote healing.

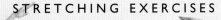

STRETCHING EXERCISES

Gentle exercises can raise the spirit and improve mobility. Seated comfortably, raise one arm above your head.

Slowly lower the arm and sit with both hands in front of you to rest. Pace yourself and do not rush.

Raise the other arm and repeat the exercise. Return to the rest position. This exercise can be repeated three times.

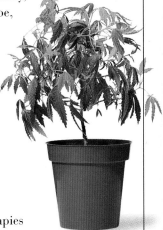

Cannabis *Cannabis indica* can be a great help to MS sufferers. At the moment, it is still illegal.

ALEXANDER TECHNIQUE *see page 57* ☙ CHIROPRACTIC *see page 39* ☙
CRANIOSACRAL THERAPY *see pages 44-5* ☙ DIETARY THERAPY *see page 74* ☙ HERBAL MEDICINE *see page 67* ☙
HOMEOPATHY *see page 83* ☙ MAGNETIC THERAPY *see page 101* ☙ OSTEOPATHY *see page 42*

The Ailments

Alzheimer's Disease

Memory loss and dementia are the key features of this progressive illness. Long-past events may be remembered, while recent events are forgotten. The patient, usually over 60, becomes disoriented, particularly at night, and possibly aggressive. The latter stages of the illness cause the sufferer to become bedridden and incontinent, and total care will be required. Alzheimer's disease occurs when the brain nerve cells degenerate and the brain shrinks. Although the cause is not known, some research suggests that the disease may be linked to levels of aluminum or toxins in the body.

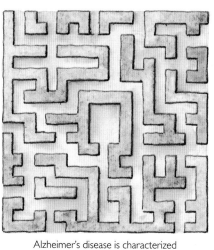

Alzheimer's disease is characterized by memory loss and confusion in once familiar surroundings.

⋘ TREATMENT

Avoid cooking with aluminum utensils and check products, such as deodorants, for content.

DIET AND NUTRITION A well-balanced diet, high in antioxidants (beta carotene, C, and E), zinc, selenium, magnesium, and folic acid can prevent harmful free radicals (in food, or caused by pollution or stress) from attacking the body, and may help minimize symptoms. When DHEA levels fall below 180ng/dL in men and 130ng/dL in women (optimum levels are 750–1250ng/dL in men and 550–980ng/dL in women), supplements of 50–100mg a day for men and 20–75 mg for women may be taken.

HERBAL MEDICINE Research shows that the herb ginko biloba may be useful. It improves the blood supply to the brain, increases nerve impulses, and may also improve memory.

HOMEOPATHY
The remedy Alumina may act as a preventive against the onset of the disease, or may help to slow its progression. For this reason it is often suggested for use in families where there is a history of Alzheimer's disease.

> **SELF-HELP**
>
> Increasing your intake of vitamins B6 and C may be beneficial.

Parkinson's Disease

Tremors in a hand or leg, along with muscular rigidity in the limbs and in the face, are the main features of this illness. This goes on to affect both sides of the body, developing into pronounced trembling, particularly when resting, and causing stiffening and an unbalanced or uncontrollable walk. Facial expressions can become fixed. Depression is common as intellect remains intact while the body degenerates.

Parkinson's is caused by the degeneration of nerve cells in the basal ganglia of the brain, which produces dopamine, a nerve transmitter. Dopamine is needed for the smooth movement of muscle control.

⋘ TREATMENT

YOGA This will help to prevent muscles from becoming stiff through disuse, and will encourage relaxation, which may reduce some symptoms. Any form of exercise will help to keep the muscles toned and flexible.

MASSAGE Gentle massage will discourage stiffening of the muscles and help to tone them.

DIET AND NUTRITION A well-balanced diet is recommended. A naturopath or dietitian will be able to advise on correct levels of vitamins and minerals. Fresh fava or broad beans contain levodopa, which the body converts into dopamine, needed for muscle control. Studies have shown some relief for patients after eating these. It is also believed that a deficiency in vitamin E early in life may leave some people vulnerable to Parkinson's in later years.

ACUPUNCTURE AND TRADITIONAL CHINESE MEDICINE Both these therapies have proved successful in the treatment of the early stages of Parkinson's disease.

> **CAUTIONS AND CONTRAINDICATIONS**
>
> Always consult your doctor if the symptoms of Alzheimer's begin to interfere with normal activities, or cause anti-social behavior. Treatment should always be carried out in conjunction with conventional medical advice.

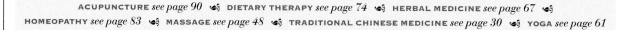

ACUPUNCTURE *see page 90* ⋙ DIETARY THERAPY *see page 74* ⋙ HERBAL MEDICINE *see page 67* ⋙
HOMEOPATHY *see page 83* ⋙ MASSAGE *see page 48* ⋙ TRADITIONAL CHINESE MEDICINE *see page 30* ⋙ YOGA *see page 61*

Motor Neurone Disease and Guillain-Barre

Motor neurone disease (MND) is characterized by weakness and wasting of muscles leading to uncontrolled muscle spasms and stiffness, usually starting in the hands and arms, then the legs, and affecting breathing and swallowing. MND is caused by the degeneration of the nerves within the central nervous system. Although the nerve degeneration cannot be controlled, some therapies can help to reduce disability. It is commonly fatal within two to four years, but some people may live much longer.

≈ **TREATMENT**
PHYSIOTHERAPY may help keep the muscles supple and working.

YOGA AND T'AI CHI
These help in heightening awareness of the body and controlling breathing patterns and pain.

MASSAGE This can help with muscle tone as well as having a general therapeutic effect.

DIET AND NUTRITION
There is also increasing evidence that antioxidants – vitamins beta carotene, C, and E – and the trace element selenium, can have positive results on MND. Foods that are high in antioxidants include red grapes, red onions, and raw or lightly cooked dark, leafy vegetables. Injections of vitamin B12 have also proved beneficial.

Supervised exercise such as yoga can help both MND and Guillain-Barre Syndrome.

SELF-HELP

MND AND GUILLAIN-BARRE
It is important to maintain mobility for as long as possible in cases of MND, and to eat plenty of proteins, which contain amino acids thought to control the condition. In Guillain-Barre, bedrest and plenty of fluids will encourage the body to gain control of an allergic reaction.

GUILLAIN-BARRE SYNDROME

Weak limbs and feelings of numbness and tingling start in the legs and spread to the arms, facial muscles, and, in the most severe cases, those controlling breathing and speech, possibly leading to paralysis. Pain is uncommon. The symptoms are the result of damage to, or inflammation of, the peripheral nerves. The cause is unknown, although we do know that it tends to develop two to three weeks after an infection and may be a reaction to this.

CAUTIONS AND CONTRAINDICATIONS

People with Guillain-Barre should be monitored carefully in hospital until it is clear that the respiratory muscles are not affected.

TREATMENT Most patients with Guillain-Barre recover fairly well with no specific intervention, but some of the following may be appropriate, depending upon the severity of the disease.

≈ **ACUPUNCTURE AND ACUPRESSURE** *Pain can be successfully reduced by releasing energy blocks.*

≈ **HYDROTHERAPY** *Joints and muscles relax in the water, which enables greater pressure to be applied.*

≈ **MASSAGE** *Gentle manipulation can also help relieve muscle tension and induce relaxation.*

≈ **FELDENKRAIS** *Considered the most effective method of rehabilitation in Switzerland, the Feldenkrais method improves posture through awareness of habitual movement patterns and through looking at new ways of moving, combined with gentle manipulation.*

≈ **YOGA AND T'AI CHI** *Muscle power and coordination can be improved, and muscle tension relieved.*

ACUPRESSURE *see page 94* ≈ ACUPUNCTURE *see page 90* ≈ DIETARY THERAPY *see page 74* ≈ FELDENKRAIS *see page 56* ≈ HYDROTHERAPY *see page 26* ≈ MASSAGE *see page 48* ≈ T'AI CHI *see page 60* ≈ YOGA *see page 61*

Problems of the Skin

SKIN FORMS a remarkable protective barrier against the outside world, helping to regulate temperature and fluid balance, keeping out harmful germs and chemicals, and offering natural protection against sunlight. It grows hair, sweats, produces oil for self-lubrication, and gives an accurate perception of touch, heat, cold, and pain, as well as the more complex sensations such as tickle, itch, and pressure.

Skin caliber varies in different body sites, from the thin, delicate tissue of the eyelid, to the thick, hard padding of the heel. Some sites have particular characteristics – luxuriant hair growth on the scalp, sweating in the armpits, highly-tuned touch discrimination in the fingertips – yet the basic structure of the skin is the same everywhere, although its actual thickness varies between different physical types. Redheads, for example, have considerably thinner skin than brunettes, and, consequently, their skin often reacts with more sensitivity.

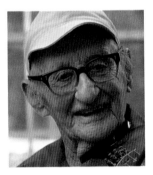

Old skin grows wrinkled through dehydration and exposure to sunlight.

The outer of the three skin layers, the epidermis, comprises the skin surface of dead "horny" cells, and underlying "prickle" cells, which move upward to replace them as they are shed (around 90 percent of household dust is dead skin cells). The epidermis also contains melanocytes, cells that secrete melanin, the pigment responsible for varying skin color. Melanin production is stimulated by sunlight: in white races this creates a tan, which offers some protection against further exposure to the sun's ultraviolet rays.

Under the epidermis is the middle layer, or dermis, a bulky fibrous and protein layer containing hair follicles, sweat, and sebaceous (oil-producing) glands, and specialized sensory receptors for conveying information about touch, temperature, and pain. Mast cells in the dermis respond to physical or chemical damage by releasing histamine, a substance leading to allergic responses.

Finally there is a layer of subcutaneous fatty tissue that gives the skin its feeling of softness and plumpness, and acts as insulation against the cold. The blood vessels supplying nourishment to the outer skin layers are carried in this layer.

STRUCTURE OF THE SKIN

The skin consists of three layers. At the bottom is a layer of subcutaneous fat that insulates the body. Above that lies the dermis, packed with blood vessels, nerves and sweat glands. On top is the epidermis, the tough, flexible, waterproof, and self-repairing outer skin. Hair follicles punctuate this layer of skin and are rooted in the dermis. Good blood circulation promotes a healthy skin on the face, and this can be helped by exercising the facial muscles regularly.

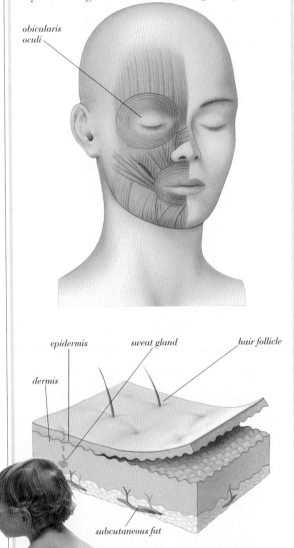

obicularis oculi

epidermis *sweat gland* *hair follicle*

dermis

subcutaneous fat

Young skin should always be protected from harmful UV rays at all times, to prevent problems later in life.

HAIR PROBLEMS *see page 197* ❧ INFECTION *see page 130*

Hair Problems

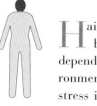

Hair reflects our inner health and becomes dry, brittle, or greasy depending on the foods we eat, the environment we live in, and the amount of stress in our lives. Natural yogurt is a wonderful natural conditioner, and rinses containing rosemary and thyme promote natural hair health.

Dry hair can indicate a deficiency of vitamins A, B12, or C; deficiency of zinc; or a lack of wholesome protein in the diet. The solution is to increase vitamin and mineral intake, avoid harsh chemical hair treatments, and massage the scalp with a few drops of olive oil. Greasy hair is caused by overactive oil glands, which can be caused by a hormonal imbalance during the teenage years or ill-health. The solution is to rinse the hair with the juice of a lemon and warm water.

Excessive hair in women can be caused by a hormonal imbalance caused by higher than usual levels of testosterone (the male sex hormone). The solution is gentle hair removal using either a sugaring or waxing process.

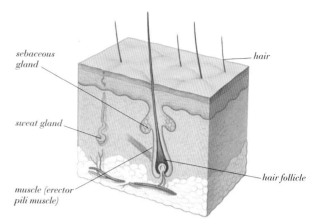

A section of skin shows how hair grows and how each individual shaft is connected to a muscle.

CAUTIONS AND CONTRAINDICATIONS

Sudden loss of hair and temporary baldness can be a sign of severe stress, which should be treated urgently.

🌿 TREATMENT

AROMATHERAPY AND HERBAL MEDICINE Promote the blood circulation in the scalp and the regrowth of hair by massaging sage, cedarwood, and rosemary oils firmly into the scalp. Rinse with an infusion of nettle.

SELF-HELP

Take dietary supplements of brewer's yeast or vitamin B complex for overall hair health.

BALDNESS

Hair loss is normal for some older men and women, but it can be caused by stress and shock. Hair loss in women can result from a dietary deficiency or hormonal imbalance (it can happen after pregnancy, during the menopause, or in a woman who also is suffering from hypothyroidism).

DANDRUFF

A dry, itchy, and flaky scalp is often the result of seborrheic eczema, and, more rarely, psoriasis or a fungal infection. Dandruff is common and usually not serious.

🌿 TREATMENT

HERBAL MEDICINE Massage vitamin E into the scalp at night. Infuse fresh or dried rosemary and sage and use it as a daily hair rinse, or make up a cedarwood rub in a lotion base and leave overnight before using it to rinse the scalp.

Natural remedies for hair problems include sage *Salvia officinalis*, fresh lemon juice, olive oil, and thyme *Thymus vulgaris*.

lemon

olive oil

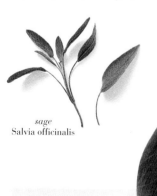

sage
Salvia officinalis

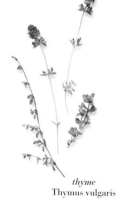

thyme
Thymus vulgaris

AROMATHERAPY
see page 50

HERBAL MEDICINE
see page 67

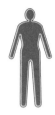

Minor Skin Problems

Although the skin is waterproof, tough, self-repairing, and self-renewing, it is still prey to minor ailments and infections. Moles, blisters, and rashes all respond to alternative therapies.

people, and those who are overweight. It may be prevented by wearing loose clothing, staying out of the sun, and taking frequent tepid (not cold) showers.

MOLES

Moles are spots of skin pigment cells (melanocytes) that can be a tiny dot or measure up to ⅓in/8mm across.

✥ TREATMENT

Most people have several moles, a few have hundreds. No treatment is needed unless they are unsightly or develop suspicious changes, which might mean they require surgical removal in case of a cancerous transformation.

Changes such as an increase in size, a wobbly edge, irregular pigmentation, a paler halo around the mole, a "daughter" mole near by, itching, crusting, or bleeding should be reported to a physician at once. Black or very dark moles should also be evaluated by a physician.

HEAT RASH (PRICKLY HEAT, MILIARIA)

A heat rash is a presentation of itchy, small red spots, especially under tight clothing or at skin creases, due to blocking of sweat ducts. It is particularly likely to occur in children, old

*echinacea
Echinacea angustifolia*

*sensitive
skin on face*

*tough skin
on knees*

*rashes
where skin
creases*

*blisters
on feet*

✥ TREATMENT

HERBAL MEDICINE Drink plenty of fluids, especially camomile, lime, or peppermint teas. Bathe the heat rash with a calendula or lavender infusion.

NATUROPATHY Lay houseleek leaves or cucumber on heat rash, to soothe.

BLISTERS

Blisters are fluid-filled bubbles that develop between two layers of skin. These painful swellings are most commonly caused by the rubbing of skin against a firm surface and by exposure to heat. Some diseases can also cause blisters but they are usually the result of ill-fitting shoes.

✥ TREATMENT

It is best not to burst a blister, but if the swelling is inconvenient, prick the blister with a sterilized, threaded needle. Remove the needle and tie a small loop in the thread along which fluid from the blister can drain.

AROMATHERAPY Apply lavender oil to the wound or use a Roman camomile antiseptic.

HOMEOPATHY Dab a mix of Hypericum and Calendula onto a punctured blister. Take Rhus tox. 6c every four hours in order to prevent blisters from getting worse.

HERBAL MEDICINE Aloe vera can be helpful. Rub the gel directly on to the affected area.

CAUTIONS AND CONTRAINDICATIONS

Moles that suddenly grow bigger or change shape should be examined by a physician.

The skin is the body's first line of defense in a hostile world, and therefore is prey to many minor ailments. Echinacea *Echinacea angustifolia* is an excellent herbal remedy for boils and the tissue salt Kali mur. (left) is useful for blisters.

✥ AROMATHERAPY *see page 50*
✥ HOMEOPATHY *see page 83*
✥ HERBAL MEDICINE *see page 67*
✥ NATUROPATHY *see page 24*

Infections and Infestation

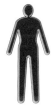

SKIN is the largest organ in the body and so offers generous space to parasites, fungi, bacteria, and viruses. Most can be easily dealt with, but contagious complaints must be treated carefully.

clean between the toes carefully to prevent infection.

RINGWORM AND ATHLETE'S FOOT

The most common fungal infections are tinea, pedis, and corporis (on the body) and capitis (on the scalp); all may be called ringworm and are due to fungal infection spread from the contaminated skin of others. Soggy, scaly, and sometimes cracked skin between the toes (athlete's foot), or round, red patches with raised scaly edges like worms (hence the term ringworm) on the body or scalp are symptoms of fungal infections.

> **CAUTIONS AND CONTRAINDICATIONS**
>
> Persistent fungal infections may indicate an immune problem or a disease such as diabetes. Check with your physician if symptoms last longer than three weeks, or recur.

Keeping the feet scrupulously clean, especially between the toes, can deter the spread of contagious fungal infections such as athlete's foot .

☙ TREATMENT

NATUROPATHY Hydrogen peroxide diluted 50/50 with water, applied twice daily, is a useful treatment. Apply Propolis ointment, vitamin C powder, or honey, and leave on the skin.

HERBAL MEDICINE Soak the affected area in cider vinegar or an infusion of golden seal root, dry with arrowroot powder, and apply tea tree essential oil.

SCABIES

The tiny scabies mite – about the size of a period – makes minute burrows under the skin. The infestation is spread by close contact. Redness and intense itching are caused, especially between the fingertips, on the wrists, and in other skin creases.

> **CAUTIONS AND CONTRAINDICATIONS**
>
> Scratching often leads to secondary bacterial infection that may require treatment. Consult a physician if pustules or boils appear in itchy areas.

☙ TREATMENT

Scabies is extremely contagious and the entire household must be treated with a special lotion from a physician.

VIRAL INFECTIONS

☙ **WARTS**
These are raised spots of rough skin, usually on the hands, face, or feet, caused by the human pappiloma virus. Verrucas on the feet (plantar warts) can make walking painful.

> **CAUTIONS AND CONTRAINDICATIONS**
>
> Check with a physician if there is any change in shape, itching, or bleeding; it could be a mole rather than a wart. Genital warts should always be seen by a physician.

TREATMENT

☙ **NATUROPATHY** *Crushed onion or garlic applied nightly can be helpful.*

☙ **HYPNOTHERAPY, AUTOSUGGESTION, AND VISUALIZATION** *Warts can sometimes be "wished" away using these techniques.*

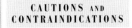

AUTOSUGGESTION *see page 114* ☙ HERBAL MEDICINE *see page 67* ☙
HYPNOTHERAPY *see page 112* ☙ NATUROPATHY *see page 24* ☙ VISUALIZATION *see page 120*

Bacterial Infections

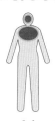

ACNE

Red spots, blackheads, and pustules, sometimes with fluid-filled swellings (cysts), appear on the face and upper trunk, resulting from blockage and infection of the oil-producing sebaceous glands.

⚘ TREATMENT

Aim to reduce stress, which can make acne worse.

HERBAL MEDICINE Blue flag root, echinacea, and burdock root are helpful.

DIET AND NUTRITION Cut down on sugar and dairy fats, and increase your intake of raw fruit and vegetables.

Consult a qualified practitioner/ therapist for:
HOMEOPATHY
Specifics include Lycopodium, especially for those self-conscious about their spots, Pulsatilla to aid skin clearance, and Graphites for suppurating pustules.

ACUPUNCTURE This therapy claims good results.

> **CAUTIONS AND CONTRAINDICATIONS**
>
> Use antiseptic preparations with caution, for they can cause sensitization reactions.

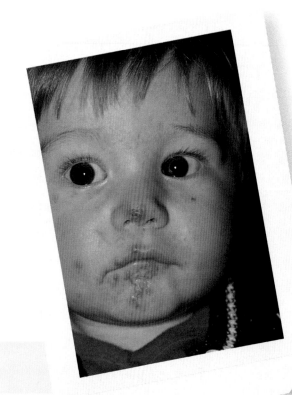

> **CAUTIONS AND CONTRAINDICATIONS**
>
> Consult a physician if red streaks develop around the boil, or if you develop a high fever.

> **SELF-HELP**
>
> The affected area can be bathed with Hypericum and Calendula solutions, made from several drops of the mother tincture in some cooled, boiled water. Avoid handling food if you have any of these conditions.

BOILS

These are sore, red, pus-filled spots, most commonly on the face, due to a staphylococcal infection. The pus needs to be drained before the boil can get better.

⚘ TREATMENT

HERBAL MEDICINE Encourage a boil to come to a head by applying a hot poultice made with comfrey, slippery elm, or burdock infusion.

DIET AND NUTRITION Garlic tablets may aid internal healing.

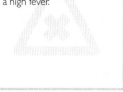

Pulsatilla (Pasque flower Pulsatilla vulgaris) helps to clear the skin.

IMPETIGO

This highly contagious skin infection is produced by the streptococcus bacterium, which possibly gains entry through minute skin breaks. It causes crusty blisters, usually in well-defined patches on the face, hands, and knees of children.

⚘ TREATMENT

Consult a qualified practitioner/therapist for:
HERBAL MEDICINE AND HOMEOPATHY Both treatments may help combat bacterial infection, and relieve symptoms, but most practitioners will probably refer you to a physician.

Impetigo, a painful and highly contagious skin complaint, usually affects children.

> **CAUTIONS AND CONTRAINDICATIONS**
>
> Because impetigo is so infectious, diagnosis and treatment by a qualified practitioner is vital. Blisters may become secondarily infected by staphylococcal bacteria, which may require antibiotic treatment. Children should be kept away from school until lesions have healed (about five days) to avoid rapid spread of the condition.

ACUPUNCTURE *see page 90* ⚘ **DIETARY THERAPY** *see page 74* ⚘ **HERBAL MEDICINE** *see page 67* ⚘ **HOMEOPATHY** *see page 83*

Psoriasis

Psoriasis is a common skin condition that is characterized by patches of well-defined plaques covered by silvery scaling. These patches occur on the knees, elbows, trunk, scalp and hairline, but do not affect the face. The patches may show pinpoint bleeding spots when scratched. Skin may be generally dry and in severe cases the nails are pitted. Severe cases may be accompanied by a form of arthritis that affects the fingers, knees, ankles, and spine, but this is rare.

Attacks of psoriasis are normally triggered by stress, illness, and damage to the skin. It is not itchy, but it can be very painful when cracks appear across the skin. Psoriasis can be very embarrassing for the sufferer because it is unsightly and still misunderstood. Psoriasis is never contagious and usually appears in the late teens and early twenties, although random cases occur in children and the elderly. It runs in families and recurs at intervals, usually throughout life.

There are four types of psoriasis: flexural, which covers the moist areas of the body; pustule psoriasis, which is characterized by small pustules, usually on the palms or soles; plaque psoriasis, which is the most common type, affecting most areas of the body and frequently the nails; and guttate psoriasis, which appears in children, usually following a throat infection.

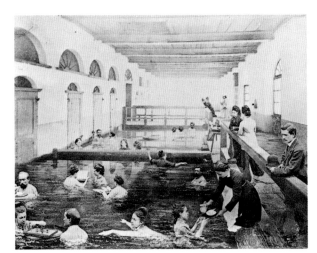

Although unsightly, psoriasis is not contagious and sufferers should try to bathe as often as possible to soothe and soften the skin.

TREATMENT

NATUROPATHY Sunlight improves psoriasis, which is usually worse during the winter months in the Northern Hemisphere.

Dandelion *Taraxacum officinale* is a blood-cleansing herb that can help psoriasis.

DIET AND NUTRITION Avoid meats, fried foods, sugar, and dairy produce; increase your intake of both fruit and vegetables. Take evening primrose oil and mineral supplements *(see pages 78–9)*.

Consult a qualified practitioner/ therapist for:
HERBAL MEDICINE A herbalist will prescribe for the individual case, but may suggest the following: dandelion and burdock to cleanse the system, nettle to improve the circulation, and echinacea as a general skin tonic.

SELF-HELP

Careful exposure to the sun will encourage healing and help to clear up an attack. Take steps to deal with stress if it exacerbates the problem. Increase your intake of zinc.

HOMEOPATHY Use Sulfur for attacks with itching, Petroleum for dryness, and Graphites for oozing plaques.

ACUPUNCTURE This claims good results in toning down symptoms, if not eliminating the problem, provided it is used in conjunction with additional suggestions, which may include dietary modification and learning techniques to deal with stress. The same applies to homeopathy.

CAUTIONS AND CONTRAINDICATIONS

About 1 in 15 people with psoriasis have associated arthritis (psoriatic arthropathy). If you suffer from psoriasis and experience any of the symptoms of arthritis (see page 178), consult a physician.

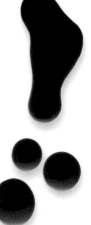

Petroleum, a homeopathic remedy particularly useful for dry, cracked, itchy skin.

ACUPUNCTURE *see page 90* • DIETARY THERAPY *see page 74* • HERBAL MEDICINE *see page 67* • HOMEOPATHY *see page 83* • NATUROPATHY *see page 24*

Allergic Reactions

THE SKIN is often the first area of the body to show an allergic reaction to a food or substance that the individual cannot tolerate. Some allergic reactions are local and temporary – heat rash, or contact dermatitis for example – and will disperse when the allergen is avoided. Others are recurring or chronic and are the result of a constitutional imbalance. Dermatitis is the general term used to describe any kind of irritating, itchy rash on the skin. Eczema usually refers to a chronic problem that appears to be linked with food intolerance of some kind, or is associated with an allergic reaction in another body system. Eczema is most commonly associated with asthma.

cosmetics, perfumes, rubber and medicated ointment. Have an allergy test *(see page 99)* if you cannot identify the cause yourself.

Consult a practitioner/therapist for:

ACUPUNCTURE AND ACUPRESSURE These can be used constitutionally. Acupressure can be used to relieve itchiness temporarily.

HERBAL MEDICINE A herbalist will prescribe according to individual need, but remedies may include the following, applied externally as ointment or lotion: purple loosestrife, chickweed, elder leaves, and aloe vera.

HOMEOPATHY Homeopaths will need to take individual cases, but acute episodes will respond well to Graphites, Petroleum, Rhus tox., and Sulfur.

Eczema and dermatitis are common allergic reactions in babies and young children.

DERMATITIS

Contact dermatitis usually attacks the skin where it is thinnest (the back of the hands, the eyelids), or only on that part exposed to the irritant. Jewelry or cosmetics can leave a very precise rash pattern showing exactly where they were in contact with the skin.

Symptoms include redness and itchiness, blistering, dry scaliness, and swelling, which can affect the parts of the body around the area with the rash.

✍ TREATMENT

Try to find out the cause of the reaction so that you can avoid it. Culprits include metal (especially nickel),

---

CAUTIONS AND CONTRAINDICATIONS

Never exclude more than one major food at a time from a child's diet, and check with a qualified practitioner before attempting nutritional changes.

SELF-HELP

Avoid any irritants that are known to cause a flareup. Use Calendula cream as a moisturiser. Take steps to deal with stress, if it exacerbates the condition. Evening primrose oil on skin may help, and extra vitamins B and C, safflower oil, and zinc should be incorporated into the diet.

ECZEMA – DIETARY TIPS

✍ *Avoid a food for at least three weeks to see if there is any effect on your eczema.*

✍ *Never cut out more than one major food group at a time without taking professional advice.*

✍ *First, try cutting out dairy products – the most common food culprit - to see if this helps.*

✍ *If dairy products are not the culprit, run through other possibilities in sequence.*

✍ *Cut down on processed and junk foods. Read the labels on every commercial food product you buy. Watch out especially for ingredients such as whey powder (a milk product) or egg.*

✍ *Eat fewer animal fats, more vegetable oils, and oily fish.*

✍ *Try supplements of evening primrose oil, fish oils (omega 3 and mega 6 fatty acids, not whole fish oils), vitamins B and E, beta carotene (25,000–200,000 units a day), zinc, selenium, and magnesium.*

ACUPRESSURE *see page 94* ✍ ACUPUNCTURE *see page 90* ✍ ECZEMA *see page 203* ✍
HERBAL MEDICINE *see page 67* ✍ HOMEOPATHY *see page 83*

ECZEMA

This infection may be due to a skin reaction to an irritant substance, to a skin allergy, or to an internal allergic reaction. Some forms of allergic eczema run in families, along with asthma and hay fever.

The symptoms of eczema are patches of dry, red, itchy skin, which may be scaly and flaky, or weeping and crusted.

✍ TREATMENT

DIET AND NUTRITION As allergies to certain foods could be part of the problem, try to figure out which ones are affecting your condition *(see box on page 202).* (Atopic eczema is less common in breastfed babies, and affected children are often allergic to cow's milk, or other foods.) Many complementary practitioners recommend nutritional modification as part of the treatment of eczema. Evening primrose oil supplements are very helpful.

HYDROTHERAPY Hot mud or sand baths, and Dead Sea bathing salts reputedly reduce long-term sensitivity. Add half a cup of sodium bicarbonate to bathwater for short-term relief from irritation.

Consult a qualified practitioner/therapist for:
HERBAL MEDICINE Drink calendula or marigold tea, and take golden seal – either by mouth (mix with honey), or as an infusion to bathe the skin. St. John's wort oil is also effective.

ACUPUNCTURE This reputedly has good success rates.

TRADITIONAL CHINESE MEDICINE Herbal teas have been proven highly effective in alleviating childhood eczema.

MASSAGE Daily local massage with essential oils such as rose, geranium, juniper, lavender, or hyssop has been found to be beneficial for some people who are suffering from eczema.

CAUTIONS AND CONTRAINDICATIONS

If there is any swelling around the mouth, or any difficulty in breathing, consult a physician immediately.

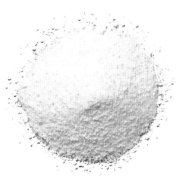

Many powdered detergents contain powerful chemicals and enzymes that can provoke allergic reaction when handled or when clothes washed in them are worn next to the skin.

URTICARIA (NETTLE RASH OR HIVES)

Urticaria is an allergic reaction to certain foods, to drugs such as antibiotics, or to direct contact (insect stings, for example). The common foods for causing urticaria are milk, wheat, corn, citrus fruit, eggs, strawberries, and shellfish. Some urticaria seems to be caused by emotional distress. No matter what the cause, stress will always exacerbate the complaint.

Urticaria is characterized by raised red patches, sometimes with pale centers, which are intensely itchy. They are normally caused by a food allergy (shellfish, strawberries, and nuts are common allergens), food additives, drugs, insect bites, extreme cases of hay fever, stress and, in people prone to this condition, heat, cold, or sunlight.

Nettle rash occurs when the skin causes the body to release histamine into the affected tissues. These raise into the characteristic weals, normally appearing on the lips, around the eyes, the limbs, trunk, and neck. Occasionally there will be swelling of the tongue and voice box (larynx), which may cause the throat to close and prevent normal breathing. In this case, urgent medical help is needed. Nettle rash can last for several days or simply a few hours.

✍ TREATMENT
NATUROPATHY
Apply vitamin E cream.

Some foods, such as avocado, can cause skin reactions.

HERBAL MEDICINE Soak infected area in an infusion of camomile or chickweed to relieve itching.

DIET AND NUTRITION Vitamin C may reduce the risk of repeated attacks.

HOMEOPATHY Take Urtica for a reaction to nettles; Apis for irritating weals; and Rhus tox. for blotchy swellings.

ACUPUNCTURE *see page 90* ✍ DIETARY THERAPY *see page 74* ✍ HERBAL MEDICINE *see page 67* ✍
HOMEOPATHY *see page 83* ✍ HYDROTHERAPY *see page 26* ✍ MASSAGE *see page 48* ✍
NATUROPATHY *see page 24* ✍ TRADITIONAL CHINESE MEDICINE *see page 30*

Problems of the Digestive and Urinary Systems

THE DIGESTIVE and urinary systems are the body's power plant and its waste-disposal mechanism. The digestive system (also called the bowel) begins at the mouth and ends at the anus. At the top, food enters the mouth where it is chewed and combined with saliva, which has enzymes to begin the breakdown of the food into useful components. It passes into the digestive tract, where more juices break the food into proteins, fats, and carbohydrates and pass it into the stomach.

Some substances (water, salts, glucose, alcohol, and certain drugs) are absorbed directly into the system from the stomach. Most food, however, is transformed by the acidic gastric juices of the stomach into a substance called chyme. Chyme passes from the stomach via the duodenum into the small intestine, where it is bathed in bile from the gall bladder and juices from the pancreas. Powerful muscular contractions (peristalsis) push the chyme along the small intestine, and as it proceeds more digestive juices and enzymes break it down into fats, carbohydrates, and proteins. These are absorbed into the bloodstream through the walls of the small intestine. From the bloodstream they pass to the liver, which is very important in the digestive process, storing sugar, fats, and proteins, and creating bile. The liver is also responsible for neutralizing toxins such as alcohol and drugs.

By the time the chyme reaches the colon (large intestine), all that is left of it is indigestible roughage and water. The water is absorbed back into the bloodstream through the intestinal walls. The main function of the the large intestine is to reclaim water from food. The bulky remains are passed into the rectum as feces, and from here they are expelled as a bowel movement.

The function of the urinary system, which is composed of the kidneys and bladder together with their connecting tubes, is to maintain the body's internal balance of water and salts. It is also responsible for filtering the blood and expelling excess waste and waste products. The kidneys also play a vital role in removing toxins and secreting important hormones. The kidneys

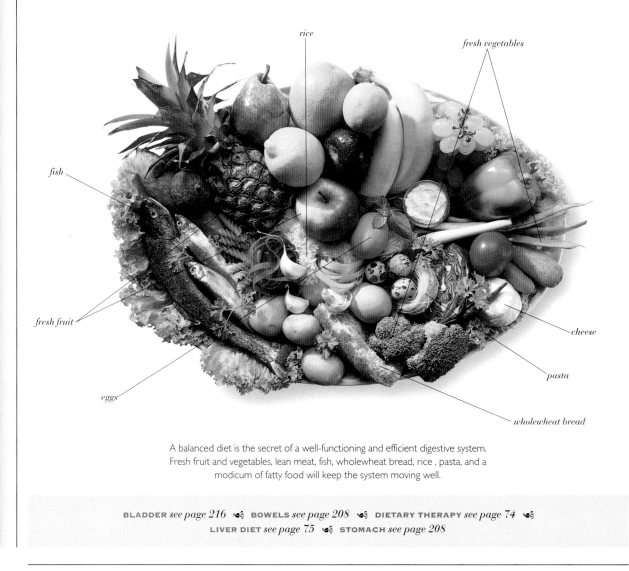

rice

fresh vegetables

fish

fresh fruit

cheese

pasta

eggs

wholewheat bread

A balanced diet is the secret of a well-functioning and efficient digestive system.
Fresh fruit and vegetables, lean meat, fish, wholewheat bread, rice , pasta, and a
modicum of fatty food will keep the system moving well.

BLADDER *see page 216* ❧ BOWELS *see page 208* ❧ DIETARY THERAPY *see page 74* ❧
LIVER DIET *see page 75* ❧ STOMACH *see page 208*

are made up of nephrons, which are responsible for filtering out the smaller molecules from the blood, including water, glucose, and waste products. The kidneys have an impressive blood supply – more than 300pt/150l of blood passes through them each day to form the 2pt/1l of urine that the body produces daily. Urine formed in the kidneys passes down the ureters and is stored in the bladder until it is convenient to empty it. The bladder drains through the urethra. In the female, the urethra is about 1½in/4cm long but it is 10in/25cm long in males. The bladder is a fibrous organ that stretches as it fills with urine. When it reaches its capacity it sends a message to the brain, which acknowledges that water should be passed.

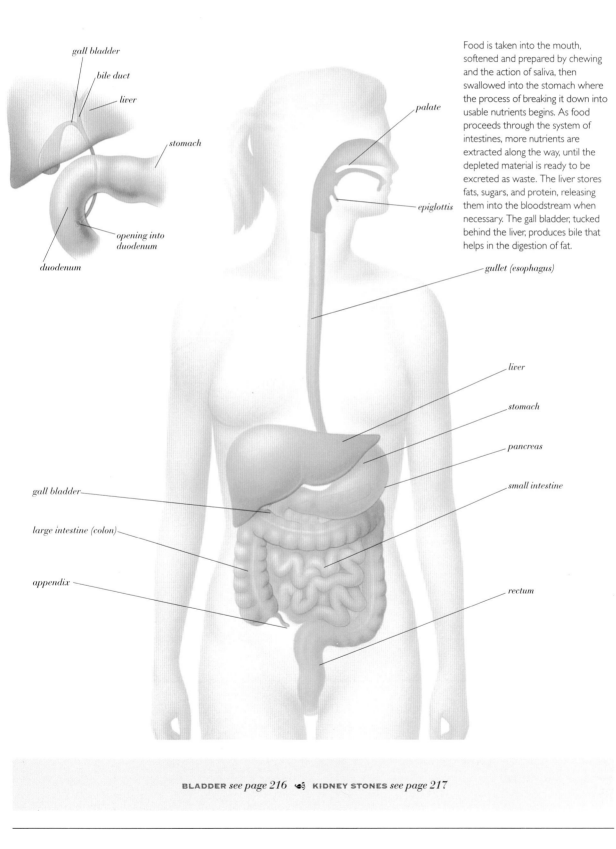

gall bladder

bile duct

liver

stomach

opening into
duodenum

duodenum

palate

epiglottis

Food is taken into the mouth, softened and prepared by chewing and the action of saliva, then swallowed into the stomach where the process of breaking it down into usable nutrients begins. As food proceeds through the system of intestines, more nutrients are extracted along the way, until the depleted material is ready to be excreted as waste. The liver stores fats, sugars, and protein, releasing them into the bloodstream when necessary. The gall bladder, tucked behind the liver, produces bile that helps in the digestion of fat.

gullet (esophagus)

liver

stomach

pancreas

small intestine

gall bladder

large intestine (colon)

appendix

rectum

BLADDER *see page 216* **KIDNEY STONES** *see page 217*

Nausea and Gastroenteritis

Nausea and vomiting can be due to food-poisoning, which results from eating toxic foodstuffs, including shell-fish or moldy meat, and can lead to bacterial infections such as gastroenteritis. An allergic reaction to certain foods may also cause nausea and vomiting *(see page 99)*, as may a disturbance in the balancing mechanism of the ear (in motion sickness, for example). Morning sickness in early pregnancy is also common, but usually stops after the twelfth week. Migraine is often associated with nausea and vomiting.

They may be prevented by avoiding foods that are old, past their sell-by date, or in any way dubious; eating fresh vegetables and fruit, and ensuring they are thoroughly washed; drinking bottled water where tap water may be impure.

TREATMENT

HERBAL MEDICINE An infusion of ginger, Roman camomile, or black hore-hound (not to be taken in pregnancy) helps reduce nausea and vomiting.

HOMEOPATHY Pulsatilla 6c, Ipecacuanha 6c, and Arsenicum alb. 6c.

ACUPRESSURE This may be beneficial.

DIET AND NUTRITION Avoid dairy products, maintain fluid intake, and gradually introduce a light diet.

SELF-HELP

Drink plenty of fluids to discourage dehydration, and avoid solid foods for 24 to 48 hours. Ensure you have adequate zinc and vitamin B6 in your diet, which may discourage further bouts.

CAUTIONS AND CONTRAINDICATIONS

Any nausea and vomiting that persist for more than 24 hours should have medical attention. If they are accompanied by severe abdominal pain, or follow a head injury, or if there is blood in the vomit, seek emergency medical attention.

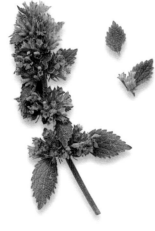

Black horehound *Ballota nigra* is excellent for nausea or vomiting caused by nervousness or motion sickness.

HANGOVER PREVENTION

HERBAL MEDICINE Extract of milk thistle can reduce the likelihood of experiencing that unpleasant "morning after" feeling.

TREATMENT
Drink plenty of clean water (not sparkling water).

HOMEOPATHY Take Nux vomica 6c.

DIET AND NUTRITION Vitamin C (1g effervescent tablets in a glass of water are best).

NATUROPATHY Take Spirulina extract.

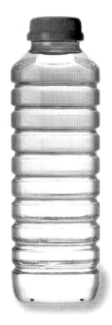

Drinking still mineral water can help the system recover after bouts of nausea.

GASTROENTERITIS

Gastroenteritis is usually caused by bacteria or toxins in contaminated food or water. The symptoms of the illness include nausea, vomiting and diarrhea, stomach pain, and cramp.

TREATMENT
DIET AND NUTRITION Drink plenty of fluids (but not ice-cold fluids, milk and milk-based products, or citrus fruit juice). Water mixed with a little salt and honey or sugar should help prevent dehydration. Do not eat until symptoms have eased, and then stick to plain whole-grain foods and fresh vegetables for several days. Eat plenty of live, natural yogurt to restore the protective bacteria of the digestive system.

HERBAL MEDICINE An infusion of ginger and Roman camomile or black horehound (not to be taken if pregnant) or meadow-sweet, can be helpful.

HOMEOPATHY Arsenicum alb. 6c, Pulsatilla 6c, and Ipecacuanha 6c can all be helpful.

CAUTIONS AND CONTRAINDICATIONS

In the case of infants and the elderly, a physician should be consulted immediately, and for anybody else, after 48 hours.

ACUPRESSURE *see page 94*   DIETARY THERAPY *see page 74*
HERBAL MEDICINE *see page 67*   HOMEOPATHY *see page 83*   NATUROPATHY *see page 24*

Celiac Disease

Celiac disease is an intolerance to gluten, normally hereditary but occasionally the result of a bout of gastroenteritis in childhood. The term is derived from the Greek word *koiliakos*, which means "suffering in the bowels." As far as is known, there is an inability of the cells lining the upper part of the small intestine to break down gluten, which is a protein found in wheat, oats, barley, and rye. The disease reduces the intestines' ability to absorb nutritive substances from the diet and so is a cause of malabsorption. It is a condition that presents itself in small children, but is only diagnosed by a biopsy, which means removing a small sample of tissue from the colon in order to analyze it. Tests for celiac disease using blood and urine are currently being developed.

Celiac disease is less prevalent in children who are breastfed or introduced late to foods containing gluten. Many complementary practitioners believe that restoring the balance of beneficial bacteria in the bowel and improving the efficiency of the immune system will provide a cure. Constitutional treatment by a homeopath may also work to make the sufferer less sensitive to gluten – to the point that a gluten-free diet may be finally unnecessary.

Signs of possible celiac disease include an inability to gain weight, constipation, or, alternatively, bulky, smelly, frequent bowel movements, decreased muscle tone, protruding stomach, and general lethargy. The only effective treatment is to remove gluten from the diet, permanently or temporarily, but this must be done under the supervision of a physician or practitioner.

Some sufferers outgrow their intolerance and can eventually return to eating a normal diet.

Nontropical sprue is a disease that occurs in adults. It is very like celiac disease and is treated in the same way, by excluding all gluten from the diet.

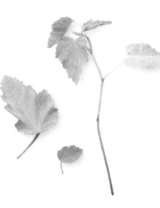

The root of marshmallow *Althea officinalis* is used to soothe irritation in the digestive tract.

Symptoms of celiac disease often mimic other problems such as lactose intolerance (a sensitivity to the sugar in milk), as well as allergies, cystic fibrosis, immune deficiencies, or emotional problems. It is important that these are ruled out first, before removing gluten from the diet.

❧ TREATMENT

DIET AND NUTRITION Breastfeed babies if possible: research indicates a possible link between celiac disease and formula-feeding. Avoid foods containing gluten for the first year of the child's life, including bread, cookies, cakes, and gravy thickened with flour. Switch to rice crackers and corn products. Avoid commercially prepared foods that often contain flour. Read all ingredient labels carefully. An allergy to milk may be involved in this condition: avoid cows' milk where possible. Eat fresh fish, vegetables, fruits, and nuts.

Consult a qualified practitioner/therapist for:

HERBAL MEDICINE
A herbalist may prescribe slippery elm, marshmallow, camomile, or papain. Research indicates that papain – an extract of papaya, which is available as a supplement – may break down the gluten so that it does no harm.

Bread and wheat or oat products of all kinds are intolerable to celiacs since they contain gluten. Rice or soybean flour may be used as an alternative.

DIETARY THERAPY *see page 74* ❧ HERBAL MEDICINE *see page 67*

The Ailments

Stomach and Bowels

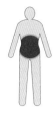

STOMACHACHE

Various specific problems can be the cause of a stomachache *(see Indigestion, Constipation, Ulcer)*, but it is often simply a symptom of tension.

TREATMENT

Lie down with a hot-water bottle on the stomach.

HERBAL MEDICINE Camomile, peppermint, slippery elm, and lemon balm teas can soothe muscular spasm and aid relaxation.

HOMEOPATHY Arsenicum alb. 6c and Bryonia 6c are especially effective.

> **CAUTIONS AND CONTRAINDICATIONS**
>
> Consult a physician if other symptoms include vomiting blood, dizziness, sweating, and pallor, or if a stomachache lasts for more than six hours.

DIET AND NUTRITION Follow a wholefood diet. Eat a little and often. Cut down on caffeine and alcohol intake.

ACUPRESSURE This can relieve pain.

RELAXATION TECHNIQUES Yoga and biofeedback are good ways of learning to cope with stress.

INDIGESTION/HEARTBURN

Indigestion is often caused by eating too quickly, eating too much, or eating rich or highly spiced food. Stress can also play a role. The symptoms of this condition are discomfort after eating, including pain in the stomach – and in the lower part of the esophagus (gullet) in the case of heartburn – nausea, and gas.

> **CAUTIONS AND CONTRAINDICATIONS**
>
> Acute stomach pain, particularly if accompanied by fever, vomiting, or nausea, may indicate serious illness and should be considered a medical emergency.

> **SELF-HELP**
>
> Indigestion may be avoided by eating smaller meals, at regular times; following a wholefood diet; cutting down on sugar and avoiding junk foods; avoiding rich or highly spiced foods; eating slowly and, if possible, in a relaxed environment.

TREATMENT

HERBAL MEDICINE A meadowsweet infusion, and coriander (eaten raw or drunk as a tea) reduce the effects of indigestion and heartburn.

AROMATHERAPY AND REFLEXOLOGY Both of these therapies help in treating indigestion.

HOMEOPATHY Arsenicum alb. 6c and Argentum nit. 6c can reduce pain and excess gas.

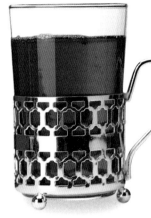

A glass of peppermint tea is a pleasant remedy to soothe general stomachache and discomfort.

FLATULENCE

Flatulence is a buildup of gas that can be uncomfortable and embarrassing, but is not usually a symptom of disease. It is often caused by swallowing excessive amounts of air, and by certain foods. Symptoms of flatulence include feelings of bloatedness and an excessive release of gas, either from the mouth (belching) or the anus (farting).

Flatulence may be prevented by practicing regular breathing using the diaphragm rather than the muscles of the chest; talking slowly; chewing food slowly and sitting upright when eating; not drinking with meals; avoiding beans, pulses, and fizzy drinks; eating garlic as often as possible (or taking garlic pearls twice a day); chewing caraway seeds or cloves; using the herbs sage, thyme, and marjoram in cooking.

TREATMENT

DIET AND NUTRITION *Ginger root capsules and charcoal tablets or capsules can be beneficial. For some sufferers, digestive enzymes may be helpful.*

HERBAL MEDICINE *Sip a cup of peppermint or camomile tea between meals.*

REFLEXOLOGY *This can help relieve gas.*

ACUPRESSURE *see page 94* • AROMATHERAPY *see page 50* • DIETARY THERAPY *see page 74* • HERBAL MEDICINE *see page 67* • HOMEOPATHY *see page 83* • REFLEXOLOGY *see page 52* • RELAXATION *see page 116*

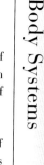

Constipation and Diarrhea

CONSTIPATION

This is usually caused by insufficient fiber in the diet. However, lack of fluid, too little exercise, and too much stress can also contribute. Symptoms of the condition include difficult, irregular, and infrequent movements of the bowel. Consult a physician if constipation persists, or immediately if it is associated with vomiting, fever, or abdominal pain

✌ TREATMENT
HERBAL MEDICINE
Camomile, hops, fennel, and a natural laxative such as linseed, will ease constipation. Drink herbal teas rather than coffee.

REFLEXOLOGY AND MASSAGE Both can be helpful.

Consult a qualified practitioner/therapist for:
ACUPUNCTURE This can help to relieve stress.

DIARRHEA
Intolerance of certain foods, a virus, or bacteria can be responsible for diarrhea. It can also be caused by anxiety and a change of diet.

✌ TREATMENT
DIET AND NUTRITION Drink lots of water and peppermint tea to replace lost fluid. If symptoms persist, replace lost salts by regularly drinking a mixture of 1 pt/500mlt water to 1 tablespoonful of sugar and 1 teaspoonful of salt. The water strained off boiled

---

> **SELF-HELP**
>
> Constipation may be prevented by: eating wholewheat bread, fresh vegetables, and fruit; drinking more water; and taking regular exercise.

---

rice is also helpful. Eat plenty of live yogurt or take half a teaspoonful of *Lactobacillus acidophilus* with a teaspoonful of *Lactobacillus bulgaricus* in a glass of water three times a day. Avoid solid food.

HERBAL MEDICINE Golden seal, and an infusion of agrimony, plantain, or geranium are helpful, as is peppermint tea.

HOMEOPATHY Arsenicum alb. 6c and Pulsatilla 6c.

TRADITIONAL CHINESE MEDICINE Dandelion, golden thread and skullcap root are all recommended.

ACUPRESSURE This can help.

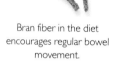

Bran fiber in the diet encourages regular bowel movement.

FECAL INCONTINENCE
A temporary loss of bowel control can occur as a result of diarrhea. Regular lack of control may result from an injury to the anal muscles (during childbirth or surgery), or from paralysis or dementia. It can also result from fecal impaction, a condition in which feces become stuck in the bowel. This can cause inflammation and lead to the uncontrolled release of small pieces of feces from the rectum.

✌ TREATMENT
DIET AND NUTRITION Follow a high-fiber, wholefood diet, and drink plenty of water (at least six large glasses a day).

ACUPRESSURE AND YOGA Both of these treatments are helpful, especially the practice of abdominal breathing techniques.

HOMEOPATHY Causticum 6c is often recommended.

Regular exercise eases and prevents constipation.

> **CAUTIONS AND CONTRAINDICATIONS**
>
> Consult a physician if diarrhea lasts more than 48 hours (or 24 hours for children), or if it is accompanied by vomiting, slimy mucus or blood in the motions.

> **SELF-HELP**
>
> **CONSTIPATION**
> For constipation rest in bed with a hot-water bottle on the stomach.

ACUPUNCTURE *see page 90* ✌ DIETARY THERAPY *see page 74*
HERBAL MEDICINE *see page 67* ✌ HOMEOPATHY *see page 83*
TRADITIONAL CHINESE MEDICINE *see page 30* ✌ YOGA *see page 61*

Hemorrhoids and Varicose Veins

Hemorrhoids (piles) and varicose veins are common conditions caused by blood collecting in veins and not returning properly to the heart for recycling – usually as a result of a weakness in the valves in the veins but also because of an obstruction. Constipation (causing piles) and pregnancy (causing varicose veins) are the usual culprits, though obesity, inactivity, the habitual use of laxatives and long periods of standing have also been blamed. Veins become "lumpy" and visible as well as painful and itchy. Piles also bleed frequently.

An estimated 50 percent of adults are affected by hemorrhoids at some time in their lives. They often occur during pregnancy (but usually disappear after childbirth), and as a result of constipation. Symptoms of the condition are swollen veins in and around the anus, itching, and pain, and sometimes bleeding when motions are passed. The veins can remain inside the anus or protrude from it.

Daily supplements of vitamin C (500mg), E (400iu), rutin, and lecithin can help both piles and varicose veins. Increased fiber (bran, oats, cereals, whole-wheat bread, linseed/flaxseed, peas, and beans), fluid intake, and exercise can also help prevent constipation and relieve piles. Raw beets are said to help varicose veins and also fruit such as apricots, cherries, rosehips, blackberries, and buckwheat.

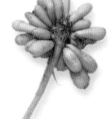

Pilewort *Ranunculus ficaria*, as its name suggests, is a traditional herbal remedy for hemorrhoids, or piles.

HERBAL MEDICINE For piles apply ointments of pilewort, comfrey, horse chestnut, and witch hazel. Witch hazel is best for bleeding piles. An infusion of yarrow herb may be beneficial for its astringency and its influence on blood vessels. It is also good applied as a compress.

Consult a qualified practitioner/therapist for:

AROMATHERAPY
Essential oils such as cypress, juniper, peppermint, or camomile, either applied directly or mixed into a warm bath, ease discomfort.

HOMEOPATHY A homeopath will prescribe according to the individual case, but Ratanhia 6c, Hamamelis 6c, Sepia 6c, and Sulfur 6c might be recommended. Hamamelis, or peony ointment, or suppositories are often used for acute cases. Hamamelis is particularly good for a bruised feeling with bleeding. Aloes, Nux vomica, Aesculus, and Pulsatilla are other possible forms of remedy.

YOGA Positions such as "the inverted corpse" (lie with the legs at 45 degrees to a wall for three minutes every day) can help, and so can yoga breathing exercises.

MASSAGE For varicose veins, gentle massage on the legs, toward the heart, can help. Massage can also help to improve circulation.

CAUTIONS AND CONTRAINDICATIONS

Consult a physician for a proper diagnosis before starting any of the therapies given here.

SELF-HELP

Apply peony ointment to external hemorrhoids, and peony suppositories for internal hemorrhoids. Warm salt baths may be soothing, and ensuring that your feet are kept up for a few hours every day will help. Avoid tea, coffee, eggs, gelatine, refined carbohydrates, and milk until symptoms disappear.

TREATMENT
Hot baths and compresses applied to the anus will help ease pain. Keep the anal area clean by washing with hot water after bowel movements.

NATUROPATHY "Sitz" baths – or hot and cold bathing *(see Chilblains, page 165)* – is recommended and ice packs can help relieve discomfort. Sitting in the water for five to ten minutes is recommended for piles.

DIET AND NUTRITION Follow a wholefood diet to reduce constipation and ease bowel movements. Drink plenty of water. Take a large spoonful of linseed seeds with water once a day (not at mealtimes).

CAUTIONS AND CONTRAINDICATIONS

Any bleeding of the anus should be brought to the attention of your physician, for it can indicate more serious illness. Seek emergency treatment if pain or bleeding lasts for more than 12 hours.

AROMATHERAPY *see page 50* • DIETARY THERAPY *see page 74* • HERBAL MEDICINE *see page 67* • HOMEOPATHY *see page 83* • SITZ BATHS *see page 26* • YOGA *see page 61*

Irritable Bowel Syndrome (IBS)

Irritable Bowel Syndrome, or IBS, is also known as irritable or spastic colon, and there is no real understanding of why it exists, although it seems to occur when the muscles that line the walls of the intestines and the colon, go into spasm. The muscles contract for no apparent reason, causing pain and diarrhea alternating with constipation. Other symptoms include a cramping pain in the abdomen, swelling, general malaise and lethargy, back pain, and often, excessive wind. Symptoms can subside and even disappear for long periods of time, but many sufferers continue to experience symptoms recurrently throughout their lives. It is a chronic, irritating, and uncomfortable condition, but it is not life-threatening and the symptoms can be reduced in many cases by proper treatment.

It is estimated that about 30 percent of people in the West has suffered from IBS at some stage, and 13 percent of those do so regularly.

IBS appears to be brought on and exacerbated by anxiety, stress, and nervous problems. Symptoms often appear worse during menstruation. Other causal factors include food intolerance.

Orthodox medical treatment has been largely unsuccessful in the treatment of IBS. Antispasmodic drugs are often recommended but in many cases they are ineffective. The best way of controlling the condition is by reducing and learning to cope with stress, and by eating a diet that does not exacerbate the condition.

✺ TREATMENT

DIET AND NUTRITION Research shows that eating more fiber, in the form of oats, dried beans, peas, fresh fruit and vegetables, can greatly reduce the symptoms of IBS, but improvement may take months rather than weeks. Also, bear in mind that wheat bran, often prescribed as the standard treatment for IBS, can actually make the condition worse for some sufferers. Eat plenty of natural, unsweetened live yogurt or take daily supplements of *Lactobacillus acidophilus* to boost the levels of healthy bacteria in the digestive system.

Different food combinations can cause IBS symptoms in different individuals: keep a detailed record of everything you eat and drink, and of all bowel movements and their consistency.

Consult a qualified practitioner/ therapist for:
COUNSELING AND HYPNOTHERAPY Both have been shown to be very effective in reducing the symptoms. Hypnotherapy has a particularly good record.

MASSAGE, RELAXATION TECHNIQUES (INCLUDING YOGA, MEDITATION, AND BIOFEEDBACK) All these therapies are beneficial.

HERBAL MEDICINE A soothing tea of camomile, peppermint, and fennel is recommended. Herbalists may prescribe cramp bark, golden seal, wild yam, and licorice.

AROMATHERAPY Essential oils of peppermint or sassafras help relaxation and reduce painful spasms.

ACUPUNCTURE This can be beneficial in helping to relieve IBS.

SELF-HELP

Try eliminating foods from your diet to pinpoint a potential allergy that may be causing the condition. Increase your intake of fiber, and take steps to deal with any stress that may be exacerbating the condition.

CAUTIONS AND CONTRAINDICATIONS

It is important to visit a physician for a checkup to exclude other more serious conditions before trying any of the therapies given here.

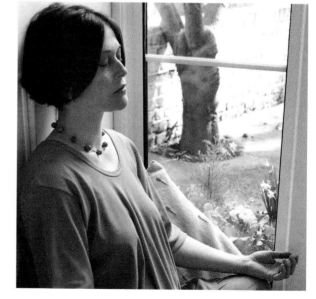

Relaxation techniques can help calm and soothe the symptoms of irritable bowel syndrome.

ACUPUNCTURE *see page 90* ✺ AROMATHERAPY *see page 50* ✺ DIETARY THERAPY *see page 74* ✺
COUNSELING *see page 103* ✺ HERBAL MEDICINE *see page 67* ✺ HYPNOTHERAPY *see page 112*

Diverticulitis, Ulcers, and Appendicitis

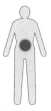

DIVERTICULITIS

This condition is often triggered by constipation and irregular bowel movements. Little "pouches" form in the walls of the large intestine and can get clogged with fecal material and become infected. Symptoms include pain in the lower abdomen and bloating.

✑ TREATMENT

DIET AND NUTRITION Follow a wholefood diet, high in fiber, and drink plenty of water. Avoid coffee and alcohol. Eat at least three cloves of raw garlic a day.

HERBAL MEDICINE Slippery elm can soothe the inflamed lining of the intestine.

MASSAGE, ACUPUNCTURE, AND REFLEXOLOGY All these can help ease constipation.

CAUTIONS AND CONTRAINDICATIONS

If there is blood in the feces, or severe pain and fever, seek emergency medical treatment.

SELF-HELP

Take regular exercise. Make sure you have enough fiber in your diet.

APPENDICITIS

The appendix is a small tube-like part of the bowel, branching off from the large intestine. It can become inflamed and cause problems. Symptoms include loss of appetite, pain around the navel area moving to become a sharp pain in the lower right side of the stomach, fever, nausea, sometimes constipation or diarrhea.

TREATMENT

Immediate medical attention is required. In severe cases, surgery to remove the inflamed appendix is necessary.

Before surgery:

✑ BACH FLOWER REMEDIES *Choose a Bach flower remedy that can reduce anxiety.*

After surgery:

✑ HOMEOPATHY *This can relieve pain and aid healing. A solution of Hypericum and Calendula cleans the wound and prevents infection. Arnica 6c relieves pain. Phosphorus 6c can ease the nausea and/or vomiting that are common after effects of an anesthetic.*

ULCERS

A layer of mucus normally protects the inner walls of the digestive system from the acid used to break down food. If this protective layer becomes too thin, or breaks down, an ulcer can develop at the site. Symptoms can vary according to the type of ulcer: a gastric (stomach) ulcer involves acute pain in the top part of the abdomen soon after eating, sometimes accompanied by nausea and vomiting and, in severe cases, by blood, either vomited or in the feces, which appear black and tarry; a duodenal ulcer causes less acute pain, slightly lower down, usually on the left side of the body, up to two hours after eating.

CAUTIONS AND CONTRAINDICATIONS

Always consult a physician; recent research shows that *Helicobacter pilori*, a bacterium often found in the stomach, can prevent an ulcer from healing, and a physician can advise on ways to deal with this.

✑ TREATMENT

DIET AND NUTRITION Cut down on foods known to cause ulcers – alcohol, coffee, and tea, for example. Avoid aspirin and products containing aspirin: they can irritate the stomach lining. Eat regularly and slowly and avoid hot, spicy foods. Small, frequent meals are best. Avoid smoking, or give it up entirely if you can.

SELF-HELP

Smoking, stress, anxiety, and overwork all increase the risk of an ulcer, so learning a relaxation technique is helpful.

HERBAL MEDICINE Marshmallow, coriander, camomile, lemon balm, and celery juice are recommended.

Consult a qualified practitioner/therapist for:
HOMEOPATHY Arsenicum alb. and Nux vomica can provide relief.

ACUPUNCTURE *see page 90* ✑ BACH FLOWER REMEDIES *see page 86* ✑ DIETARY THERAPY *see page 74* ✑ HERBAL MEDICINE *see page 67* ✑ HOMEOPATHY *see page 83* ✑ MASSAGE *see page 48* ✑ REFLEXOLOGY *see page 52*

Inflammatory Bowel Disease (IBD)

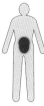

Inflammatory Bowel Disease covers a number of bowel disorders. It can describe colitis, which affects the colon, or regional enteritis (known as Crohn's disease), which affects the small intestine.

Body Systems

COLITIS

The cause of colitis, an inflammation of the large intestine, is not properly understood, although a lack of fiber in the diet is thought to be partly to blame. Symptoms of this illness include abdominal pain, diarrhea, and sometimes blood or mucus in the motions.

HOMEOPATHY Podophyllum 6c and Arsenicum alb. 6c are particularly helpful.

ACUPRESSURE AND ACUPUNCTURE Both of these can be effective.

CROHN'S DISEASE

Crohn's disease is caused by recurrent inflammation of the small intestine. The digestive system can also become damaged, reducing its ability to absorb nutrients from food. Symptoms of the disease include pain, fever, diarrhea, and weight loss.

SELF-HELP

Cut down on milk and dairy products. Try to avoid refined and processed food.

CAUTIONS AND CONTRAINDICATIONS

Specialist medical care is always necessary. However, many sufferers find that the therapies mentioned below can reduce the severity of their symptoms.

CAUTIONS AND CONTRAINDICATIONS

Always see your physician for a medical diagnosis. It is important to exclude more serious conditions with similar symptoms.

SELF-HELP

Avoid sugar and other refined carbohydrates, and increase your intake of vitamins A, B, and D, and zinc. Avoid milk if there is any possibility of an intolerance or allergy.

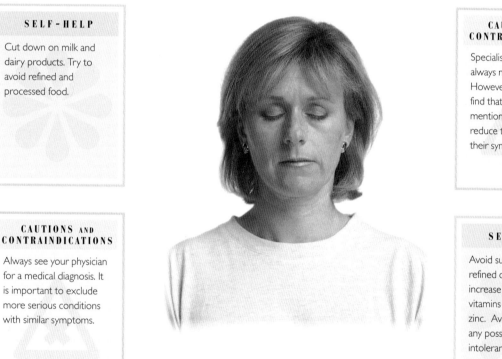

Stress is always a factor in diseases of the digestive system, and relaxation techniques have proved very helpful, both in their own right and as a support therapy to conventional medicine.

❧ TREATMENT

DIET AND NUTRITION Follow a wholefood diet with plenty of brown rice, fruit (stewed apples especially), and vegetables. As colitis can sometimes be caused by allergies to certain common foods – milk products and cereals such as wheat or oats, for example – cut them out of your diet for at least two weeks to see if there is any improvement. Eat plenty of garlic or, if you do not like it, take garlic capsules.

Consult a qualified practitioner/therapist for:
HERBAL MEDICINE Slippery elm to reduce inflammation is often prescribed.

❧ TREATMENT

RELAXATION TECHNIQUES Yoga, meditation, and biofeedback can reduce stress, which often plays a major role in this disease.

AROMATHERAPY Essential oil of lavender is particularly beneficial.

MASSAGE This, together with regular exercise, is very beneficial.

HERBAL MEDICINE Slippery elm is recommended, alternated with astringent teas such as agrimony.

AROMATHERAPY *see page 50* ❧ DIETARY THERAPY *see page 74* ❧ HERBAL MEDICINE *see page 67* ❧ MASSAGE *see page 48* ❧ RELAXATION *see page 116*

Obesity, Edema, and Gallstones

OBESITY

People who are at least 20 percent overweight are generally considered to be obese. Occasionally obesity may be caused by a physical disorder, such as a hormonal imbalance, but the vast majority of those who are overweight are that way because they eat too much of the wrong food, and exercise too little.

❧ PREVENTION/TREATMENT

DIET AND NUTRITION Do not "crash diet." This seldom has lasting benefits and can lead to nutritional deficiencies and unhealthy eating habits. Permanent weight loss is best achieved gradually through a change in lifestyle. Switch to a wholefood diet with plenty of fresh vegetables and fruit. (*For more information about eating disorders, see pages 224–5.*)

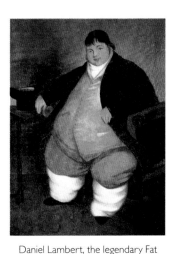

Daniel Lambert, the legendary Fat Man of Lincolnshire, England, weighed over 700lb/312kg when he died.

EDEMA

Fluid retention, known medically as edema, can be caused by various disorders, including heart failure, kidney problems, and varicose veins, or too much salt in the diet. It can also be a side effect of some medicines, and can occur naturally in pregnancy and as part of premenstrual syndrome (PMS). Sometimes, however, there is no apparent cause. Symptoms of the condition include increased weight, especially noticeable at the ankles and in the lower limbs, which become swollen and uncomfortable. Edema may be generalized (all over the body), or localized.

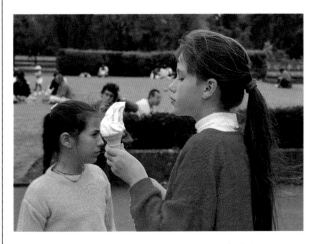

Malnutrition occurs in rich nations when sugar-loaded food that is empty of calories predominates in the daily diet.

❧ TREATMENT

HERBAL MEDICINE Parsley, taken either as an infusion or eaten raw (but not if pregnant), or dandelion leaves, either drunk as a "coffee" or eaten in salad, are both recommended. Cut down on salt, eat lots of vegetables, salads, and fruit, and drink fruit juices.

AROMATHERAPY Lavender is particularly helpful.

MASSAGE AND ACUPRESSURE Both of these can be beneficial. Effleurage is the most effective massage technique.

GALLSTONES

These pebblelike lumps, made up of calcium, cholesterol, and other chemicals, can develop in the gall bladder, a pear-shaped organ near the liver. The gall bladder stores bile, a substance made by the liver, and supplies it to the digestive system, where it helps break down food.

Gallstones occur in up to 10 percent of the population of the Western world and are linked to a low-fiber, high-fat diet. They are more common in pregnancy, in people who are obese, and in those suffering from diabetes. The condition is often hereditary. Gallstones do not cause problems unless they block the flow of bile. If this happens surgery or ultrasound treatment may be needed to remove the stone.

Symptoms include pain, often at the right shoulder or at the hip, indigestion, jaundice (yellowing of the skin, whites of the eyes, and urine), and fever.

❧ TREATMENT

DIET AND NUTRITION Follow a low-fat, wholefood diet with lots of fresh fruit and vegetables. Avoid dairy products and animal fats. Switch to olive oil. Drink plenty of water and take a vitamin C supplement daily.

Consult a qualified practitioner/therapist for:
HERBAL MEDICINE Rosemary, dandelion, and balmony may be prescribed. (Pregnant women should seek medical advice before taking any herbal medicines.)

AROMATHERAPY Essential oil of Scots pine helps to ease the pain.

ACUPUNCTURE This can also be helpful.

ACUPRESSURE *see page* 94 ❧ ACUPUNCTURE *see page* 90 ❧ AROMATHERAPY *see page* 50 ❧
DIETARY THERAPY *see page* 74 ❧ HERBAL MEDICINE *see page* 67 ❧ MASSAGE *see page* 48

Malnutrition

In the Western world, good, clean food is in ready supply, and there is no real reason why any one of us should suffer from malnutrition – which is the result of inadequate nutritional intake. However, failure to understand the changing needs of our bodies, for instance, in pregnancy, illness, and as we grow older, and the dismaying lack of nutrition available in our food due to environmental factors, means that cases of malnutrition are on the increase in richer countries. The great Western diet has come up short for many people. The links between diet and disease are not fully understood as yet, but we do know that malnutrition can cause pathological illness affecting all parts of the body. Some of the most common effects of malnutrition are

❋ heart disease and circulatory problems as a result of obesity

❋ normal headaches or migraine

❋ night blindness, from a vitamin A deficiency

❋ bleeding gums, loose teeth and general fatigue resulting from a lack of vitamin C (the body does not store vitamin C and daily requirements vary from person to person)

❋ anemia from insufficient iron

❋ lack of motor function in the legs, painful feet, numbness, lesions in the spinal cord, and neurological disease, may all be the result of vitamin B deficiency

❋ digestive disorders, including diarrhea, nausea, cramps, IBS, pain, and piles, may be a result of inadequate diet

❋ rashes, itching, allergies, sensitivities and other skin problems may be the result of vitamin deficiencies

❋ loss of hair, or dry, dull hair reflects deficiency in some area of the diet

❋ insufficient fluid causes stones to form in the kidneys; excess fat causes them to form in the gall-bladder (gallstones)

❋ enlargement of the thyroid may be the result of an iodine deficiency

❋ defective bone growth in children due to lack of vitamin D, a component of fish, milk, and eggs

❋ softening of the bones and early osteoporosis may be a result of a calcium and vitamin D deficiency, becoming increasingly common in the West where they are in adequate supply.

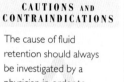

CAUTIONS AND CONTRAINDICATIONS

The cause of fluid retention should always be investigated by a physician in order to exclude any serious underlying disorder.

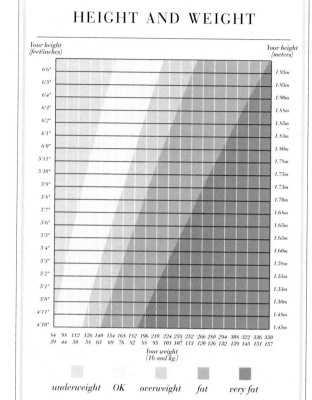

HEIGHT AND WEIGHT

underweight   OK   overweight   fat   very fat

The chart above offers an at-a-glance guide to the ideal height to weight ratios. If you find yourself in one of the danger zones (underweight, fat or very fat) you should consult a physician before embarking on any kind of diet. Very obese persons may need hospital treatment to lose weight safely.

If you think that you need to lose weight, choose a diet that you can comfortably live with, and aim at slow but steady weight loss – 1lb/500g a week is enough. That way, your body can get used to your lower calorie requirements (as you lose weight, you need less fuel to keep you going). It is thought that the diet and binge pattern, where weight is lost then quickly regained, places more strain on the body system than remaining steadily at the same slightly too heavy weight.

Diet alone is a very slow way to lose weight. If you exercise at the same time, you will burn up more calories. Walk or cycle wherever possible rather than traveling by car or public transportation. Take up a form of regular, pleasant exercise, such as swimming, or dancing and aim at three sessions a week.

BONE PROBLEMS *see page 172* ✺ CIRCULATION *see page 164* ✺ HEADACHES *see page 144* ✺ HEART DISEASE *see pages 168-9* ✺ OSTEOPOROSIS *see page 177* ✺ VITAMIN C *see page 76*

Bladder Problems

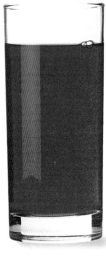

The Ailments

CYSTITIS and urinary tract infection are both caused by an inflammation of the lining of the bladder and the urinary tract. This is usually the result of a bacterial infection spread from the anus either through poor hygiene or through sexual intercourse.

CYSTITIS

Both men and women can suffer from cystitis, but women are usually more susceptible due to their shorter urinary tract. Bacteria can reach the bladder more quickly. Symptoms include painful urination, cloudy urine, with fever and backache in severe cases.

Cystitis can also be caused by vaginal infections such as thrush, sexually transmitted diseases, and vaginal deodorants. Bruising (as a result of sexual intercourse or childbirth) can also trigger the condition.

Cranberry juice is a very effective naturopathic cure and preventive for cystitis.

✑ TREATMENT

DIET AND NUTRITION Drink lots of water, camomile tea and cranberry juice. Cut out alcohol, coffee, and all acidic fruit juices. Apply live yogurt to the vagina to help "recolonize" it with healthy bacteria.

HERBAL MEDICINE An infusion of yarrow, couch grass, and buchu are recommended.

HOMEOPATHY Cantharis 6c and Staphysagria 6c are beneficial.

AROMATHERAPY Sandalwood, juniper, lavender, or bergamot – used for a stomach massage, or in the bath – will help to ease pain and discomfort.

ACUPRESSURE This can also relieve pain.

SELF-HELP

This condition may be prevented by: maintaining a high standard of hygiene after going to the lavatory; always going to the lavatory as soon as you need to pass urine; emptying the bladder before and after sexual intercourse; washing or showering before intercourse (both partners); ensuring there is sufficient lubrication during intercourse (use a lubricating jelly if necessary); avoiding tight underwear and pantyhose; and not using douches or vaginal deodorants.

URINARY TRACT INFECTION

All parts of the urinary tract may develop infections. The infection causes inflammation of the affected part, and the clinical syndrome associated with inflammation of that part tends to be characteristic.

Inflammation of the urethra (urethritis) causes pain when water is passed. If there is infection present, pus or blood may also be evident in the opening of the urethra.

Urethritis in women is commonly caused by bruising during intercourse rather than infection.

Urethritis in men is more often caused by sexually transmitted infections such as gonorrhea or chlamydia *(see page 237)*. Such infections do not usually manifest any symptoms in women, but it is important that both partners are adequately treated to prevent long-term complications such as infertility. Urethritis usually lasts for two or three days.

✑ TREATMENT

Follow the advice about complementary therapies suitable for the treatment of cystitis.

Massage and acupressure to the lower abdomen can soothe the symptoms of cystitis.

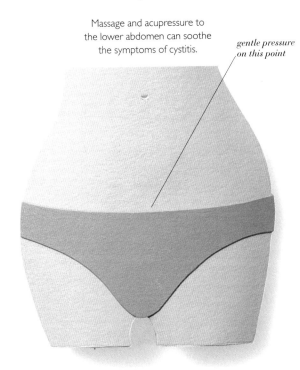

gentle pressure on this point

ACUPRESSURE *see page 94* ✑ AROMATHERAPY *see page 50* ✑
DIETARY THERAPY *see page 74* ✑ HERBAL MEDICINE *see page 67* ✑ HOMEOPATHY *see page 83*

Kidney Stones and Urinary Incontinence

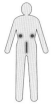

KIDNEY STONES

These are hard deposits of chemical salts. They can be caused by inadequate fluid intake and by too much calcium and animal protein in the diet. In the United States it is believed that a deficiency of magnesium and vitamin B6 can contribute considerably to calcium oxalate kidney stones. Mild pain in the lower back on one side indicates stones in the kidney. Severe pain indicates stones that have got stuck in the ureter, one of the two tubes that carry urine from the kidneys to the bladder.

✧ TREATMENT

DIET AND NUTRITION Drink several pints of water daily. Reduce your intake of calcium-rich foods such as dairy products. Avoid foods containing calcium oxalate – chocolate, strawberries, rhubarb, grapes, spinach, blueberries, and beets. Use a water filter to remove calcium in hard water areas. A tablespoon of apple cider vinegar, mixed with a bit of honey in a little warm water and taken every day, can also help.

> **CAUTIONS AND CONTRAINDICATIONS**
>
> Conventional medical treatment is needed if the stones are large, or stuck in the ureter. Mild cases can be helped by the various therapies mentioned below.

Consult a qualified practitioner/therapist for:
HERBAL MEDICINE Remedies include gravel root, stone root, and parsley piert.

HOMEOPATHY Remedies to relieve pain caused by kidney stones blocking the ureter include Berberis, Magnesia Phos., and Calcarea.

ACUPUNCTURE This can help reduce pain and infection.

URINARY INCONTINENCE

This condition can be caused by a weakness of the muscles controlling the bladder, injury (sometimes during childbirth), or disease. Drugs prescribed for some medical conditions – high blood pressure, for example – can also affect bladder control.

The symptom of this condition is inability to control urination. An early sign is involuntary micturation, a leakage of urine when laughing, coughing, or lifting. In men this can also be a symptom of prostate problems *(see page 234)*.

> **SELF-HELP**
>
> Do exercises to strengthen the pelvic floor muscles.

✧ TREATMENT

DIET AND NUTRITION Lose weight if necessary – being overweight can strain the muscles controlling the bladder. Follow a wholefood diet rich in fresh fruit and vegetables, and drink plenty of water: strained bowel movements due to constipation put pressure on the bladder muscles.

HOMEOPATHY Pulsatilla 6c and Causticum 6c are often prescribed.

TRADITIONAL CHINESE MEDICINE Golden lock tea is recommended.

ACUPRESSURE This can also be helpful.

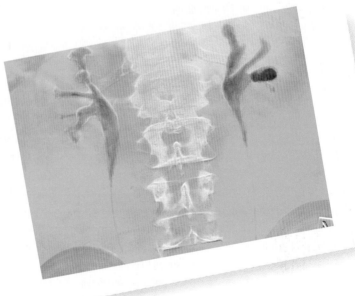

A body scan shows small stones forming in both of the kidneys.

ACUPRESSURE *see page 94* ✧ ACUPUNCTURE *see page 90* ✧ DIETARY THERAPY *see page 74* ✧
HERBAL MEDICINE *see page 67* ✧ HOMEOPATHY *see page 83* ✧ TRADITIONAL CHINESE MEDICINE *see page 30*

Diabetes

DIABETES is caused by a deficiency of insulin, a hormone produced by the pancreas and necessary for converting glucose to energy. There are two types of diabetes – Type I and Type II.

Diabetes is largely considered a disease of affluence, a product of the Western diet. Genetic factors are also important. Type II diabetes, for instance, is usually associated with obesity and can often be cured simply by medically supervized dieting and weight loss.

Type I diabetes is the more serious form. It is an autoimmune disease triggered when insulin-producing cells in the pancreas are attacked and destroyed. The only treatment is daily injections of insulin, but people with diabetes must also pay attention to their diet, following a pattern of healthy eating and regular exercise. Uncontrolled and untreated Type I diabetes can result in a life-threatening coma. It is essential to seek specialist advice.

Diabetics can regulate their own lives by using an insulin kit with which they can test their own insulin levels and administer the required dose when necessary.

With Type II diabetes a certain amount of insulin is produced, but the body is unable to use it properly, making it less effective.

Diabetes tends to run in families, although not all members who carry the gene will go on to acquire the disease. It is more common to develop Type II than Type I. In addition to hereditary factors, damage to the pancreas may cause diabetes, particularly by viruses (such as mumps or rubella).

Other factors that may cause the disease in susceptible people are
❋ pregnancy – this is called gestational diabetes and is more common if previous babies have weighed upward of 9lb/4kg at birth; urine tests during prenatal checks will show high levels of glucose, and you will be given a glucose tolerance test; positive cases will require dietary changes under medical supervision, or in the more severe instances, insulin treatment
❋ other illnesses, including diseases of the pancreas, thyrotoxicosis and hyperthyroidism
❋ treatment of existing conditions with corticosteroids.

Symptoms of diabetes include:
❋ frequent urination and thirst
❋ lethargy and apathy
❋ weight loss
❋ lowered resistance to infection (particularly urinary tract infections)
❋ cramps
❋ blurred vision
❋ menstrual problems.
Longer-term complications include:
❋ scarring of the retina
❋ damage to the peripheral nerves
❋ chronic kidney failure
❋ atherosclerosis
❋ associated disorders of the thyroid.

SPECIAL NOTE ON COMA

It is important in diabetes to distinguish between diabetic coma and hypoglycemic coma.
❋ Hypoglycemic (low blood sugar) coma occurs as a result of taking too much insulin, or of not following insulin with enough sugar or carbohydrate. As the food and insulin levels become quickly out of balance, sweating, erratic and often violent behavior very quickly results, followed by coma – usually within 15 to 30 minutes. This reaction is known as "a hypo" and can be corrected just as quickly by taking in sugar, preferably as glucose, in food or drinks.
❋ Diabetic coma is much more serious, and requires immediate medical help. The causes of this kind of coma are a buildup of acids (ketones), and metabolic poisoning as a result of having too little insulin in the body for too long. The condition causes rapid breathing and dehydration, followed by life-threatening coma if not checked.

Insulin pens supply the precise premeasured dosage and can be refilled when necessary.

DIETARY THERAPY *see page 74* ❧ OBESITY *see page 214* ❧ PREGNANCY *see page 246*

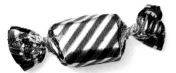

Diabetics must be careful
not to eat too many candies.

❧ TREATMENT

The key to successful treatment of both types of diabetes is in maintaining the correct balance between food and insulin. There is no cure, either conventional or alternative, but research in the United States has shown that careful control of blood sugar levels can reduce the risk of diabetic complications by as much as 60 percent.

Research shows that the blood sugar levels of diabetics can best be controlled by a high-fiber, high-carbohydrate, low-fat diet. In the past, carbohydrate content comprised about 40 percent of the energy intake, but this has now been altered so that at least 50 percent of total energy intake is drawn from carbohydrates. Evidence has also shown that blood sugar levels do not rise as rapidly when a high-fiber diet is eaten. Because high-fiber foods take longer to digest, the increase in blood sugar is slower and more monotonous and the diabetic does not have to contend with a sudden increase such as that supplied by refined sugars in fizzy drinks, for instance, or candies.

❧ TYPE I DIABETES

The only treatment is daily injections of insulin, but people with diabetes must also pay attention to their diet, following a pattern of healthy eating and regular exercise. Several alternative therapies can help, but you always should consult a qualified practitioner.

❧ TYPE II DIABETES

DIET AND NUTRITION Undertake a weight-loss diet; this encourages the body to take up insulin. Change your diet by introducing high-fiber foods and cutting down on sugar and fat. Replace saturated fats with monosaturated oils such as olive oil.

Scientists are in the process of creating "functional foods" specifically for diabetic control. These contain natural, therapeutic ingredients that can help to lower swings in blood glucose levels after meals. Guar gum, oat bran, and different Nigerian beans are being studied, as well as plants such as "karela" which is used in India.

Some everyday foods – for example onions, cabbage, potatoes, garlic, and fenugreek seeds – contain natural plant chemicals that play a part in lowering blood glucose levels. The problem is that very large amounts of these foods must be consumed in order to provide this benefit. Research has shown that supplements of evening primrose oil can be an effective treatment for diabetic neuropathy and retinopathy, and that vitamin E supplements can produce small improvements in metabolic control.

LIVING WITH DIABETES The recommendations for a diabetic diet are much the same as those for the rest of the population, but there are a few extra rules that should be observed. Eat a high-fiber diet. Reduce intake of sugar. Eat little but regularly. Maintain your ideal body weight. Reduce fat intake.

RELAXATION THERAPIES Meditation, autogenic training, biofeedback, and hypnotherapy can all help sufferers to regain a sense of control and promote well-being. (Diabetes can be aggravated, or triggered, by stress.)

AROMATHERAPY Massage with essential oils can be useful for healing wounds such as leg or foot ulcers. Oils for managing the complications of diabetes include sage (circulation), orange blossom (stress), lemon (circulation and high blood pressure), frankincense (skin problems and stress), and lavender (to soothe). A bath oil containing camphor, eucalyptus, geranium, juniper, lemon, and rosemary can help balance secretions from the pancreas.

Consult a qualified practitioner/therapist for:
HOMEOPATHY Homeopaths will prescribe to suit the individual case. Although remedies can be prescribed to boost overall health and treat diabetic complications, nothing can restore insulin-producing cells.

YOGA Sessions of yoga have a positive impact on blood glucose levels, blood pressure, and weight. Specific abdominal exercises and yoga breathing are useful – consult your medical practitioner first and then seek advice from a qualified Hatha yoga teacher.

CAUTIONS AND CONTRAINDICATIONS

Always seek conventional medical attention. There is no cure for diabetes; never be tempted to give up insulin or prescribed tablets without specialist advice.

SELF-HELP

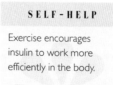

Exercise encourages insulin to work more efficiently in the body.

AROMATHERAPY *see page 50* ❧ DIETARY THERAPY *see page 74* ❧
HOMEOPATHY *see page 83* ❧ RELAXATION *see page 116* ❧ YOGA *see page 61*

PROBLEMS OF THE MIND
Emotional and Mental Health Disorders

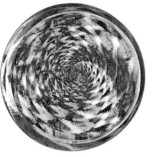

THERE are very few conditions or illnesses that are entirely psychological or physical, and mental or emotional illnesses do become inextricably entangled with physical symptoms, which even the best therapist or doctor would find difficult to separate. Most mental problems are either pathological (caused by disease) or they are caused by problems in childhood and growing up, or stressful events of life. Stresses and problems affect every individual differently, and each person will adapt – or fail to do so – according to his or her physical and psychological makeup. Depressions are very common after illness because resistance is low emotionally, spiritually, and physically. Illness is common after depression for much the same reason.

The patterns of mental and emotional life are different for each individual.

Very few people suffer from problems that require hospitalization, and conditions can differ in severity from person to person. Common emotional or mental problems include addictions, agoraphobia, amnesia, anger, anxiety, bereavement, confusion, delirium, depression, eating disorders, fears, fright, grief, hallucinations, hypochondria, hysteria, insecurity, manic depression, memory loss, obsessions, panic attacks, paranoia, schizophrenia, sexual problems, sleep problems, stress, and unusual behavior.

Mental health problems are very common. Most of us experience depression or stress at some point in our lives, and literally millions of people in the Western world are diagnosed as mentally ill each year. Often fear of being out of control or of experiencing painful emotions means that we neglect our mental health, ignoring the warning signs of stress.

Alternative therapies and medicines can be helpful in preventing mental health problems by reducing stress, aiding relaxation, and reminding us that physical and mental health go together. For people who have already had mental health problems, alternative medicine can help reduce the chances of a relapse. It can also counteract the side effects of prescribed drugs.

Drugs can control symptoms and give short-term relief, but they do not get to the root of the problem. Alternative medicine's holistic approach – which looks at the underlying causes of symptoms in the context of the person's life and emotions – makes it ideally suitable for the treatment of many mental health problems.

An alternative practitioner should treat you as an individual, giving you attention and time to discuss your problems.

The so-called talking treatments of psychotherapy and counseling may seem the obvious treatment choice for people in mental distress, but there are many other alternative therapy options. For example, aromatherapy or acupuncture can aid relaxation, and ease pain, anxiety, and depression. Buying herbs, remedies, or oils for your own use is an option, but for a full assessment and individually tailored treatment, a professional should be consulted.

It is vital that you feel comfortable with your chosen practitioner. A good one will tell you if they do not think they can help you, and suggest another form of treatment, or another practitioner. They may also advise you to see a physician if they feel it is appropriate.

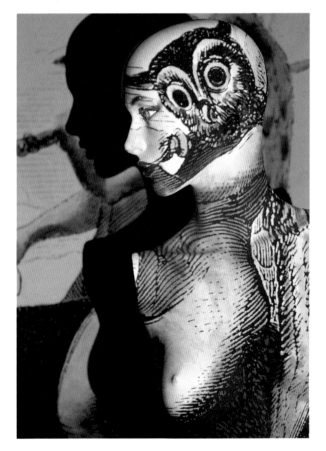

When there is an imbalance or problem in emotional or mental health, there may be confusion about the self in the world; we may project the wrong ideas or not see others as they really are.

ACUPUNCTURE *see page 90* • AROMATHERAPY *see page 50* • COUNSELING *see page 103* • DEPRESSION *see page 228* • HERBAL MEDICINE *see page 67* • STRESS *see page 223*

Anxiety and Insomnia

Anxiety and worry are facts of life. Most people will feel worried if they are about to take an exam, start a new job, or have an operation. The anxiety normally goes away after the stressful event, especially if all has gone well. But sometimes anxious feelings feed on themselves and start to interfere with everyday life. Anxiety can often lead to other symptoms, such as insomnia or panic *(see page 222)*.

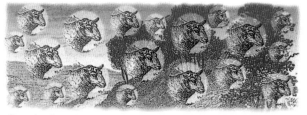

Counting sheep jumping over a fence is a traditional method of self-hypnosis, combining visualization of a soothing scene and the mantra-like repetition of numbers.

ANXIETY

Symptoms of anxiety include difficulty in concentrating, irritability, tense muscles, aches and pains, nausea, dizziness, breathlessness, sleep problems, dry mouth, decreased or increased appetite.

❧ TREATMENT

DIET AND NUTRITION Caffeine, alcohol, and smoking can all contribute to anxiety states and so are best avoided. Magnesium supplements may be helpful.

AROMATHERAPY Lavender and camomile oils are relaxing and calming. Use them in a relaxing bath or in a burner to scent a room.

VISUALIZATION Practice imagining situations where you feel peaceful and relaxed and "go there" when you start to feel anxious. Relaxation tapes and classes can help you learn how to do this.

BACH FLOWER REMEDIES Agrimony, Rock Rose, and Red Chestnut are possible choices.

Consult a qualified practitioner/therapist for:
COUNSELING AND TALKING TREATMENTS Behavioral psychotherapy aims to help you unlearn problem behavior. Cognitive therapy can help you recognize and change patterns of thinking that reinforce your anxiety.

HOMEOPATHY A homeopath will tailor remedies to the individual case, but Aconite and Argentum nit. are recommended for the physical effects of anxiety.

HERBAL MEDICINE A herbalist may prescribe sedatives such as passiflora, camomile, or valerian as infusions.

AROMATHERAPY *see page 50*
BACH FLOWER REMEDIES *see page 86*
COUNSELING *see page 103*

INSOMNIA

Insomnia (sleeplessness) is a common symptom of anxiety and stress. If the underlying problems are dealt with, the insomnia usually clears up.

❧ TREATMENT

AROMATHERAPY A bath with a few drops of essential oil of meadowsweet and orange blossom will soothe.

RELAXATION THERAPIES Yoga and meditation can help you to relax and free your mind from worry and stress.

HERBAL MEDICINE Infusions of lime blossom, hops, or Californian poppy all have a sedative effect.

Consult a practitioner/therapist for:
HOMEOPATHY Depending on the case, a homeopath may choose from Aconite for insomnia caused by fear, Arnica for the overtired, Coffea for the racing mind, Phosphorus for nightmares that wake you, Ignatia for the fear that you will never sleep again, and Nux vomica for insomnia caused by heavy drinking.

SELF-HELP

Any exercise is good for anxiety, stress, and depression, but aerobic exercise, such as swimming, cycling, and walking, is particularly good. Tension is released, breathing improves, and the body's natural antidepressants, known as endorphins, are released. Exercise can also help you sleep more soundly.

Calm, steady breathing into a brown paper bag is a simple but effective cure for anxiety-induced hyperventilation.

HOMEOPATHY *see page 83*
RELAXATION *see page 116*
VISUALIZATION *see page 120*

Panic and Stammering

Generalized anxiety and stress can sometimes crystallize into a specific event such as a panic attack or palpitations. If this happens often, sufferers begin to worry about having a panic attack, which makes matters worse.

PANIC ATTACK

A rapid buildup of anxiety produces a panic attack where the body suddenly overreacts, producing powerful physical effects. Panic symptoms include a pounding heart, sweating, chest pains, rapid breathing or a feeling of being unable to breathe, and dizziness.

TREATMENT

BACH FLOWER REMEDIES Designed specifically for self-help, Rescue Remedy calms you after a sudden shock.

RELAXATION TECHNIQUES When panic sets in, the sufferer takes rapid, shallow breaths (hyperventilation), using the upper nose only. This makes the panic worse. Slow, rhythmic breathing, using the whole ribcage and diaphragm, will aid relaxation.

HOMEOPATHY Aconite is used for an acute panic attack. Causticum and Ignatia may also be useful.

SELF-HELP

STAMMERING
There is some evidence that copper can exacerbate the problem, so it is sensible to remove it from the diet and environment. Take steps to deal with stress if it exacerbates the problem.

CAUTIONS AND CONTRAINDICATIONS

Stammering in children may be a sign of stress, insecurity and lack of confidence, which should be addressed before they manifest themselves as other health and behavior problems.

PALPITATIONS

This is the conscious registering of the heartbeat, usually because it is going faster than normal. Palpitations may be a response to a genuine emergency, or they can result from too much coffee, tea, alcohol, nicotine, or some medical drugs.

TREATMENT

Avoid stimulants such as tea or coffee and cut down on nicotine.

RELAXATION TECHNIQUES Biofeedback *(see page 117)*, where the person learns to monitor and control their own bodily reactions, is the best help.

STAMMERING

Stammering is a complex problem affecting the flow of speech. Although it is not caused by anxiety – stammerers are no more anxious than other people – sufferers often worry about the stammer and feel tense in particular situations. Feelings and thoughts about the stammer can become part of the problem and make the stammer worse.

The cause of stammering is unknown and there is no known cure. It usually starts in early childhood, and a combination of physical, emotional, and social factors (particularly family and school) seems to be involved.

TREATMENT

RELAXATION TECHNIQUES *Learning relaxation techniques, using tapes or at classes, and developing self-confidence and assertiveness can help control a stammer.*

Consult a qualified practitioner/therapist for:

ALEXANDER TECHNIQUE *This can help reduce physical tension.*

HYPNOTHERAPY *This may be helpful if it teaches you how to relax.*

PSYCHOTHERAPY AND COUNSELING *These can help in understanding and dealing with stammer.*

BACH FLOWER REMEDIES Rescue Remedy.

HOMEOPATHY Aconite can help as a first aid measure.

HERBAL MEDICINE Hawthorn or valerian will help.

Consult a qualified practitioner/ therapist for:
ACUPUNCTURE An acupuncturist would treat the Heart meridian.

HYPNOTHERAPY This helps if palpitations are caused by an emotional issue.

ACUPUNCTURE *see page 90* • ALEXANDER TECHNIQUE *see page 57* •
BACH FLOWER REMEDIES *see page 86* • COUNSELING *see page 103* • HERBAL MEDICINE *see page 67* •
HOMEOPATHY *see page 83* • HYPNOTHERAPY *see page 112* • RELAXATION *see page 116*

Stress

Stress is sometimes described as the "fight or flight" response: the body prepares for running or fighting, and the muscles, lungs, heart, and brain gear up for action. Breathing is quicker, heartbeat gets faster, and blood pressure goes up. The cause of stress need not be a physical threat, but our bodies have this physical reaction to any pressure around us. Stress is a normal part of life. It may be caused by work, relationships, surroundings (such as noise, bad housing, or traffic), or any number of other factors.

A little stress can give you energy and keep your mind alert. It keeps you "alive." But there is no such thing as the right level for everyone. We all differ, so the right amount of stress for one person could be too much for another. Too much stress for too long can lead to mental and physical exhaustion and illness. Panic attacks are a common response to long-term stress *(see page 222)*.

Symptoms of stress may include aching and tense muscles, diarrhea, constipation, asthma, migraines, skin problems, tiredness, insomnia, frequent colds, anxiety, fear, depression, anger, irritability, hostility, impatience, mood swings, and tearfulness. Difficulty in concentrating, smoking and drinking more, and never finishing anything are all signs of too much stress having gone on too long.

Everyday life takes its stressful toll on all of us.

TREATMENT

Take positive steps to reduce the stress in your life. Try to avoid several major life changes at one time. Be good to yourself, eat well, have breaks, and do things you enjoy. Don't set yourself unrealistic targets. All the treatments listed under anxiety are all relevant for stress too, and aerobic exercise for 20 to 30 minutes two or three times a week in particular is also a powerful antidote to stress.

RELAXATION TECHNIQUES The best stress treatments are those that help you to manage your stress levels yourself. Examples are yoga, meditation, and autogenic training where you learn specific relaxation exercises.

BIOFEEDBACK Stress-related conditions can be helped by recognizing how your body responds to stress. Treatment involves using a biofeedback machine and is normally given by a psychologist.

TALKING TREATMENTS Talking about your feelings to friends and family when under stress is important. However, if you want to understand your work and family situation better or get to the root of recurring problems, a qualified counselor or psychotherapist should be consulted.

SELF-HELP

Knowing the signs and taking action to counteract stress is the key to keeping it under control.

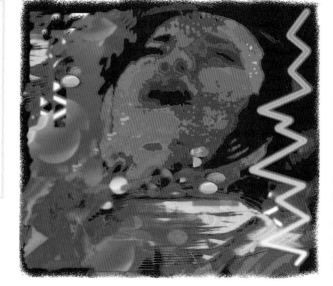

CAUTIONS AND CONTRAINDICATIONS

Untreated stress can lead to serious health problems affecting the body, mind, and spirit, self-destructive behavior, and an unusual tendency to accidents.

When stress overwhelms us, problems loom out of all proportion; even simple tasks become impossible.

BIOFEEDBACK *see page 117* ❧ COUNSELING *see page 103* ❧ RELAXATION *see page 116*

Eating Disorders

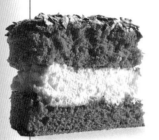

EATING DISORDERS are an outward expression of emotional turmoil or deep unhappiness. Sufferers concentrate on food and eating as a way to avoid looking at their problems and to exert control over their own body, when they may otherwise feel powerless in the world.

Although anorexia nervosa and bulimia nervosa are probably the best-known expressions of this condition, there are many kinds of eating disorders, some more extreme than others. Compulsive eating, compulsive dieting, binge eating, comfort eating, laxative abuse, and faddy eating are all forms of eating disorder.

People with eating disorders do not like food; for them it is an addiction. Anorexics regard it as an enemy to be avoided at all costs. Bulimics choose food that will be easy to regurgitate; binge eaters will eat whatever is in the refrigerator or cupboards, however unappetizing it may be; comfort eaters choose indulgent, easy-to-eat foods – cookies, cakes, candies, white bread, all of which produce short-term contentment by releasing serotonins in the brain.

Such distorted views of food and eating are different in every individual case and often have their roots in family history. Anorexia nervosa, for example, is characteristically associated with adolescent girls who suffer from low self-esteem and who may feel powerless in their relationship with the rest of the family. There are other factors that affect young people with this disorder; it is argued, with some success, that outside pressures have a great effect especially on adolescents who feel under pressure to conform to the current popular notion that "thin is beautiful."

However, other eating disorders will also respond to an examination of this area; staying fat in a world where thin is considered beautiful may allow you to step out of the arena of courtship, which may be a goal for people who are uncomfortable with sexual relationships. Deciding to be fat may be a form of revenge, especially in a mother-daughter relationship where the mother has been too dominant. Counseling and psychotherapy from a trained practitioner can help these cases, once the reason why the decision to either eat yourself to obesity or to starve yourself into a nonperson have been addressed.

Very few cases have a physical origin, although naturopaths and nutritionists may make a careful analysis of thyroid activity to see if any minor imbalance in the production of thyroxine may be causing excess weight gain or loss. People who eat for comfort may respond to a course of enjoyable exercise to produce serotonin. Once they have done that, a sensible eating regime can be established, and they can address the problem of why they are unhappy from a more rational standpoint.

However, once recovery is underway, a naturopath or nutritionist should be consulted to help establish a healthy, enjoyable, and nutritious diet and to prescribe supplements to support recovery and maintain the new status.

Chocolate cake, an occasional treat for most people, or an addictive substance to comfort eaters.

Anorexics suffer from distorted body image; they consistently believe themselves to be fatter than they are, even when presented with evidence to the contrary in the mirror.

SELF-HELP

Zinc is recommended for sufferers from eating disorders.

COUNSELING *see page 103* ◦§ DIETARY THERAPY *see page 74*
NATUROPATHY *see page 24* ◦§ THYROID DISORDERS *see page 143*

Anorexia and Bulimia Nervosa

Anorexia nervosa affects mostly adolescent girls. Anorexics practice self-starvation, and say they are looking and feeling better as a result. The symptoms are severe weight loss, fear of becoming fat, distorted self-image, excessive exercising, loss of menstrual periods, constipation, poor circulation, sleep problems, isolation, anxiety and irritability. Many anorexics develop bulimia and the two conditions often coexist. Most reported cases (90 percent) are girls or women.

Bulimia nervosa is an advanced form of compulsive eating; bulimics binge on large quantities of food and then purge themselves by vomiting and using laxatives to keep their weight down. Symptoms of bulimia include binge eating, secretive behavior, menstrual disturbance, dehydration, poor skin condition, sore throat, dental problems, and lethargy.

CAUTIONS AND CONTRAINDICATIONS

In cases of severe weight loss, hospitalization may be necessary.

TREATMENT

As anorexia and bulimia are aspects of the same disorder, treatment is the same for both. Sufferers of anorexia and bulimia have very low self-esteem and little confidence, so any therapy or activity that helps them to relax and feel good about themselves can be helpful (see pages 221–3). For recovery, the underlying emotional problems must be fully dealt with. Research suggests various causes for anorexia and bulimia. Some experts believe they result from disturbed family relationships in which the adolescent uses food intake as a means of control.

➤ **AROMATHERAPY OR REFLEXOLOGY** *A massage or using essential oils at home can improve mood and sense of well-being.*

➤ **TALKING TREATMENTS** *Supportive counseling where you are not judged, and family therapy can be helpful.*

➤ **SELF-HELP GROUPS** *It can be helpful to talk to others with similar problems.*

➤ **EXPRESSION THERAPIES** *Art, drama, music, or dance therapy can help express buried feelings.*

➤ **ASSERTIVENESS TRAINING** *Learning to express what you really feel can help.*

Consult a qualified practitioner/therapist for:

➤ **COUNSELING, PSYCHOTHERAPY, AND GROUP THERAPY** *As eating disorders are normally the result of deep-rooted problems, these are the treatments that generally work best. (Any therapy that increases self-esteem is beneficial.)*

➤ **ART THERAPY AND DANCE THERAPY** *Many sufferers find these two therapies particularly helpful ways of exploring emotional difficulties.*

➤ **MASSAGE** *This can put sufferers "back in touch" with their bodies.*

➤ **ACUPUNCTURE** *This helps to restore the body's energy balance and increase self-confidence.*

➤ **TRADITIONAL CHINESE MEDICINE** *Practitioners concentrate on strengthening the digestive system, which can become weakened by long periods of starvation.*

ACUPUNCTURE *see page 90* ➤ AROMATHERAPY *see page 50* ➤ ART THERAPY *see page 111* ➤ COUNSELING *see page 103* ➤ DANCE THERAPY *see page 110* ➤ MASSAGE *see page 48* ➤ REFLEXOLOGY *see page 52* ➤ TRADITIONAL CHINESE MEDICINE *see page 30*

Obsessions, Addictions, and Phobias

OBSESSIONS are recurring thoughts or ideas that are distressing and frightening. Like phobias, obsessions are irrational and uncontrollable and are rooted in anxiety. Compulsions or rituals often follow, when sufferers cannot stop themselves from taking particular actions or following particular routines to ward off the imagined danger.

Most people experience mild obsessions – for example, the urge to check or count things – but an obsessive person might not be able to leave the house without going back countless times to check the door was locked. Someone with an obsession about cleanliness might be compelled to wash his or her hands hundreds of times a day.

Doctors sometimes call this type of behavior "Obsessive Compulsive Disorder." Performing a ritual means the sufferer feels better for a while but the anxiety soon starts again and the ritual has to be repeated. Obsessions and rituals interfere with daily life as they are very time consuming.

TREATMENT
Anything that helps reduce anxiety and tension can help *(see pages 221–3)*. Relaxation techniques are useful for calming the body and mind. Some people find that sharing experiences and information with other sufferers can help.

ADDICTIONS
A person is addicted when they are compelled to do any activity repeatedly and to depend on it. Smoking, drinking, and taking drugs are well-known addictions, but people can also be addicted to activities such as gambling, eating, or sexual intercourse.

Addictions are normally classified as psychological dependence or physical dependence. Psychological dependence involves powerful cravings for the activity, while physical dependence induces physical symptoms when the object of the addiction is withdrawn.

TREATMENT
PSYCHOTHERAPY, COUNSELING, AND SELF-HELP GROUPS For some treatments sufferers have to agree to stop the addiction before therapy begins, while others concentrate on reducing the harm being done to them. One of the best-known self-help groups for alcohol addiction is Alcoholics Anonymous (AA).

Consult a qualified practitioner/therapist for:
ACUPUNCTURE It is claimed that acupuncture can reduce a number of cravings, alleviate pain, and help sufferers to relax.

AROMATHERAPY, MASSAGE, MEDITATION, YOGA, AND HYPNOTHERAPY These can all help people cope with physical withdrawal symptoms by aiding relaxation and improving general well-being. In all cases, strong willpower is essential. It is also vital to take care not to replace one source of addiction with another.

SELF-HELP

Various self-help groups exist for dealing with all kinds of obsessions, addictions, and phobias.

CAUTIONS AND CONTRAINDICATIONS

Severe obsessive behavior may lead to depression and depression-related illness and should be treated by your physician as soon as symptoms arise. Unchecked, it will cause disruption to work, family, and social life.

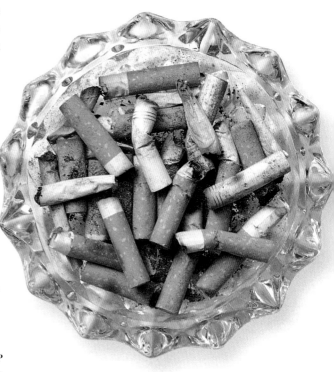

Addiction to the nicotine in tobacco is one of the hardest to throw off, despite the known health risks of smoking.

ACUPUNCTURE *see page 90* • AROMATHERAPY *see page 50* • COUNSELING *see page 103* • HYPNOTHERAPY *see page 112* • MASSAGE *see page 48* • MEDITATION *see page 118* • PSYCHOLOGICAL THERAPIES *see page 102* • YOGA *see page 61*

Phobias

A phobia is an uncontrollable and irrational fear of an object or a situation, such as a fear of flying, or heights, or insects, a social phobia (fear of meeting people, of going to school), claustrophobia (fear of enclosed spaces), or agoraphobia (fear of going outside, of being away from the security of the home, or of being alone).

Most people have some phobia (it is estimated that about 10 percent of the population suffer from one or more phobias) but manage to keep it controlled either by avoiding the stimulus or by suppressing their fears. Phobias are only serious when fear becomes disabling and begins to affect lifestyle to the extent that it has to be altered or normal situations avoided.

The causes of a phobia may be unknown or the result of an experience that has left a long-lasting impression. It can, however, be copied or adopted from parents, teachers, or carers, or very occasionally be the result of some organic disease, such as epilepsy or brain injury. Panic and anxiety are also the result of low blood sugar, and can be more common in people with borderline diabetes or a sensitivity to sugar. Phobias can also be the result of prolonged stress (which in itself can cause blood sugar levels to drop), anxiety, or panic. Anxious, nervy, or easily stressed people are more vulnerable than others to phobias.

Symptoms of a phobia include overt fear and feeling overwhelmed when confronted with the object of that fear. Physical symptoms include breathlessness, palpitations, sweating, nausea, giddiness, and trembling. A sufferer may go to extreme lengths to avoid a confrontation with the object of their fear.

LEARNING TO COPE
There is some evidence that sufferers can help themselves, usually through graduated exposure. In the case of a serious phobia, people are unable even to think about it. The first step is being able to do so, and then taking it one step further by drawing pictures of the object of a phobia, looking at pictures in a magazine, perhaps watching them on television, and so on.

In the case of a situation phobia, like flying, it may be suggested that you go to the airport and watch airplanes taking off and landing. Then, on the next visit, you might go as far as the departure lounge (many airlines offer sessions for phobics and do not consider this unusual). On the third visit you might sit on an airplane, or try an electronically simulated flight. You will gradually learn to control your phobia.

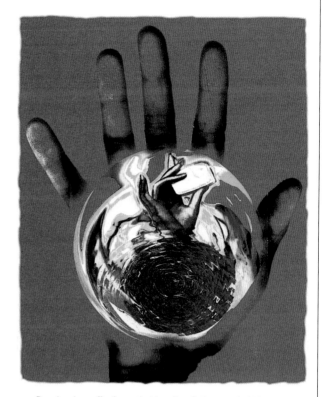

People who suffer from phobias often feel trapped within their fears and need a helping hand to control what seems to others to be an irrational response to the world.

Take one step at a time. Draw lists, keep diaries that provide a record of your progress. Even when you find you are progressing at a very slow rate – some sufferers complain of taking two steps back for every one step forward – there are changes in your situation and your acceptance of it, and a diary makes them obvious. The key to overcoming a phobia is harnessing the panic, and with practice it is possible to do so. Panic can be overwhelming, and it may appear uncontrollable, but in time you can learn to distance yourself from the feelings and learn how to turn them off. Many exposures to panic may be necessary to do so, but eventually it becomes clear that panic attacks do end and go away and that it is possible to master feelings about a phobic situation or object.

TREATMENT
PSYCHOTHERAPY Treatment may involve relaxation techniques and desensitization.

HOMEOPATHY Treatment would be constitutional but specific remedies include: Borax and Sulfur for fear of heights; Lycopodium, Gelsemium, and Anarcardium for stagefright and fear of performing in public.

HOMEOPATHY *see page 83* • PANIC *see page 222* • PSYCHOLOGICAL THERAPIES *see page 102*

Problems of the Mind

Depression

MOST PEOPLE experience depression at some point in their lives. It can be a normal part of grieving for somebody who has died, for example, or at the end of a relationship, or when your life changes in some way.

Many people have times when they feel bad about themselves or dissatisfied with some aspect of their lives. Mild depression need not affect normal day-to-day life, but things seem more of a struggle and less worthwhile. In the case of severe depression, sufferers may feel in total despair or suicidal.

In such cases a physician should be consulted. Alternatively, you can contact appropriate telephone helpline services.

Symptoms of depression may include waking in the very early hours or sleeping for longer than usual, over- or undereating, increased use of tobacco, alcohol, or drugs, social withdrawal, "negative" thinking, difficulty concentrating or making decisions, irritability, impatience, and loss of sex drive.

Women are more ready to admit to depression and ask for help than men.

✎ TREATMENT
Anything that improves self-image or helps sufferers to understand and cope with their feelings is acceptable.

AROMATHERAPY Jasmine and bergamot oils are uplifting and refreshing, while lavender is calming and relaxing. Use a few drops in the bath, on a handkerchief, with water in a burner, or mixed in almond oil for performing a massage.

MASSAGE Whether performed by a friend or qualified practitioner this can help you feel better.

BACH FLOWER REMEDIES Use Gorse for despair and hopelessness, Elm for a feeling of being unable to cope, and Larch for lack of confidence. Remedies should be diluted with water.

Consult a qualified practitioner/therapist for:

COLOR THERAPY Color affects our mood and behavior. Many people already know their color "preferences". A color therapist can help identify colors that may work therapeutically for you.

EXPRESSION THERAPIES Art, drama, or music therapy can help you express feelings that may have become buried by using your creative talents.

CRANIAL ELECTRICAL STIMULATION This therapy can in many cases bring sufferers out of their depression within two weeks.

TALKING TREATMENTS Counseling can help you find solutions to your current problems, while psychotherapy can help you come to terms with past events. Cognitive therapy can help depressed people overcome negative thinking and lack of motivation. *(See page 109 for further information.)*

CAUTIONS AND CONTRAINDICATIONS

If you, a friend, or relative feels suicidal as a result of depression, seek medical attention immediately. Depression is a serious threat to health and should be treated as such.

SELF-HELP

Take steps to relieve any stress that may be exacerbating the condition, and ensure that you get adequate exercise and nutrition. Exercise is particularly helpful in depression because it stimulates circulation, and releases serotonins in the brain, the hormones that encourage contentment and cheerfulness.

HAPPY EATING

Depression may be the result of inadequate nourishment. If the brain is not receiving sufficient fuel, it will not function properly. Vitamin B deficiency is often a physical cause of depression. To combat depression:

- ✎ *eat more wholefoods*
- ✎ *give up sugar, tea, coffee and alcohol*
- ✎ *increase your intake of vitamin B complex, vitamin C, folic acid, calcium, potassium, and magnesium.*

AROMATHERAPY *see page 50* ✎ BACH FLOWER REMEDIES *see page 86* ✎ COLOR THERAPY *see page 126* ✎ COUNSELING *see page 103* ✎ MASSAGE *see page 48*

SEASONAL AFFECTIVE DISORDER

Seasonal Affective Disorder (or SAD) is a severe form of "winter blues." Most people slow down a little in the winter and experience some form of winter blues, but full-blown SAD can be extremely disabling. Many sufferers are unable to function in winter without continuous treatment.

It happens when insufficient light passes into the light-sensitive pineal gland – the part of the brain controlling appetite, sleep, mood, and sex drive – and this increases levels of a hormone called melatonin. This in turn causes many bodily functions to slow down or stop, and the higher its levels the slower we become, which is why most people want to sleep at night.

It is not known why some people (those between 18 and 30) are more likely to get it than others and why it seems to affect women more than men. The only permanent cure is to live within 30 degrees of the equator!

Symptoms of SAD include depression, lethargy, feeling sleepy in the daytime, oversleeping, overeating, anxiety, irritability, withdrawing from people, and loss of sex drive. Symptoms occur regularly each winter (you will not normally be diagnosed as having SAD until after three or more winters of symptoms).

TREATMENT

PHOTOTHERAPY OR LIGHT TREATMENT *Spending between one and four hours a day in winter exposed to very bright "full spectrum" lighting (ten times the power of domestic lights) has proved successful in 85 percent of diagnosed SAD cases. Full spectrum lighting is also known as "natural lighting." Light treatment suppresses the over-production of melatonin, which makes us sleep in the dark. Light boxes can be bought from specialist retailers or through a national charity organization. Getting outdoors in bright daylight as much as possible and sitting near windows in light-colored rooms can also help.*

TALKING TREATMENTS *(See page 228.)*

RELAXATION *Any therapy that helps you relax.*

POSTNATAL DEPRESSION

After the birth of a baby it is common for some mothers to suffer a period of mild depression, sometimes called the "baby blues." This can last from a few hours to a few days. Postnatal depression begins later and lasts longer than a few days. It affects around one in six new mothers and seems to be caused by the extensive changes in hormone levels after childbirth.

Symptoms of postnatal depression include tearfulness and hopelessness, inability to cope, guilt, anxiety, panic, inability to concentrate, hostility to partner, sleep problems, loss of sex drive. The most severe form of postnatal depression – puerperal psychosis – is rare, affecting one in 500 women. Sufferers can become manic or deluded and out of touch with reality. If this happens a physician should be contacted as soon as possible.

TREATMENT

Adequate rest is important, but is difficult with a small baby. It is important to take some time out, even if it is only ten minutes with your feet up. Support from friends and family, and contact with other mothers can help in practical and emotional ways.

DIET AND NUTRITION Eating regularly is important. Vitamin B6 and a good multivitamin and mineral supplement may help.

Men's cultural bias against talking about feelings can make depression worse.

COUNSELING Supportive counseling can help you explore your feelings and look at coping strategies.

MASSAGE, AROMATHERAPY, AND BACH FLOWER REMEDIES *(See listings on page 228.)*

CAUTIONS AND CONTRAINDICATIONS

Never look directly into bright light, especially the sun.

AROMATHERAPY *see page 50* ◦ BACH FLOWER REMEDIES *see page 86* ◦ COUNSELING *see page 103* ◦ DIETARY THERAPY *see page 74* ◦ LIGHT THERAPY *see page 126* ◦ MASSAGE *see page 48*

Psychotic Disorders • Autism

CHILDREN and adults with autism are unable to relate to others in a meaningful way. They have difficulty developing relationships or understanding other people's feelings and often develop strange obsessions or odd behavior patterns. Autism is believed to be a brain development disorder, and while there is no cure there is hope.

Autism is rare, affecting every two to four children in 10,000, and nearly three times more boys are affected than girls. It is also more common in higher social classes. Most cases present themselves before the age of two and a half or earlier. Although the cause is unknown, it has been linked to epilepsy (10 to 15 percent of sufferers develop epilepsy) and later schizophrenia (there is some indication that autism may be a form of schizophrenia, although it does not, as yet, respond to the same medication).

Most sufferers remain educationally subnormal, although some have an isolated special ability, for instance, with numbers or music.

✍ TREATMENT
There are a vast range of approaches that can help people with autism develop, communicate, and become more independent.

DIET AND NUTRITION High doses of vitamin B6 and magnesium *(see Megavitamin therapy, page 80)* have been found to be helpful in improving sleeping habits and attention span, decreasing hyperactivity, irritability, and aggression in autistic people.

Consult a qualified practitioner/therapist for:
MASSAGE Hand and foot massage (with or without essential oils) can help autistic people learn to enjoy positive touch and be calm. Carers can be taught how to massage.

MUSIC THERAPY Trained therapists have had good results using music to communicate with autistic children and help them express themselves.

"HOLDING" THERAPY When combined with other treatments, holding – where the parent insists on comforting an unwilling child – has been found to be effective in improving the behavior patterns of autistic children. Families will find that they need support and advice from experienced therapists when attempting to use this form of therapy.

RELAXATION TECHNIQUES Learning relaxation techniques can help avoid violent outbursts.

OSTEOPATHY Autistic children can benefit from gentle manipulation by specialized osteopaths.

TALKING TREATMENTS These can help the family deal with an autistic child. Behavior therapy may help reduce difficult behavior and teach new skills.

CAUTIONS AND CONTRAINDICATIONS	SELF-HELP
Symptoms of autism can be detected early in life. If you suspect that your child has autism, consult your practitioner.	Increase your intake of foods which contain vitamins B3, B5, B6, and C, zinc and magnesium. Avoid copper.

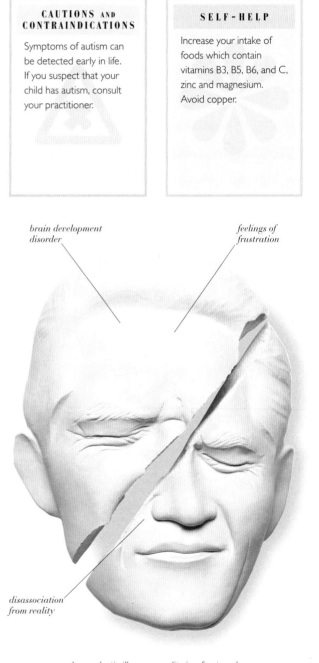

brain development disorder

feelings of frustration

disassociation from reality

In psychotic illnesses, reality is a fractured, unreliable experience for the sufferer.

BEHAVIORAL THERAPY *see page 109* ✍ DIETARY THERAPY *see page 74* ✍ MASSAGE *see page 48* ✍
MUSIC THERAPY *see page 111* ✍ OSTEOPATHY *see page 42* ✍ RELAXATION *see page 116*

Schizophrenia and Manic Depression

Mental health problems are severe when the person becomes out of touch with reality. They may develop false beliefs about who they are or what is happening, feel persecuted by external forces, or believe they have been given special powers. They may hear voices, discussing their thoughts or behavior, or telling them what to do, or they may see things that are not there (hallucinations).

When someone is out of touch with reality in this way, they are called psychotic. Some people have only one episode of psychotic illness in their life, others have several with remission in between, and others have them most of the time. Alternative therapies can be useful for all these people but may not be appropriate in a crisis. Conventional drug medication can usually prevent psychotic episodes, but people who are very distressed or dangerous to themselves or others may need the shelter and protection of a hospital or specialized care unit.

SCHIZOPHRENIA

Each sufferer's experience of schizophrenia is unique. Thoughts and feelings are dramatically disturbed and the world is experienced very differently. The person's behavior may appear bizarre to others. Schizophrenia does not mean "split personality" as is widely believed, but is a word used to describe a wide range of symptoms and conditions.

It is not known what causes schizophrenia: one theory is that a person's genetic makeup makes him or her vulnerable, and that it is triggered off by stressful events. People diagnosed as schizophrenic are rarely violent, but they are often very frightened and isolated because of their distressing symptoms.

Symptoms of schizophrenia include jumbled, disordered thinking, paranoia, false beliefs, hearing voices, apathy, lack of concentration, and depression.

MANIC DEPRESSION

Manic depression involves mood swings: periods of deep depression and over-excited or manic behavior. There may be periods of varying stability in between these extreme highs and lows.

During mania, sufferers are euphoric, feel self-important, excited, and extremely talkative. They may go on spending sprees, be unable to sleep, be irritable, or angry. They have no awareness of changed behavior. During the depressive periods (usually longer) they feel despair, guilt, and worthlessness.

Music, which can access mood states without recourse to language, may be a helpful therapeutic tool in the treatment of psychotic illness.

❧ TREATMENT

It is important to avoid stressful situations, and finding the right therapy and therapist is vital.

RELAXATION TECHNIQUES

Meditation, visualization and relaxation exercises can all help. In particular, *see Anxiety, pages 221–3, and Depression, pages 228–9,* for ways of dealing with symptoms of the illness and the side effects of medication.

> **SELF-HELP**
>
> People diagnosed schizophrenic or manic depressive can find it helpful to meet, and to share experiences and ways of coping.

Consult a qualified practitioner/therapist for:

TALKING TREATMENTS Taking part in supportive psychotherapy and counseling can help reduce the risk of a relapse by helping sufferers to understand the condition and cope better with problems and stresses. Group or family therapy can help with the communication process. It is thought, however, that psychotherapy, which probes into the past, can be too stressful for people with manic depression or schizophrenia, but some sufferers do find it helpful. Some sufferers may prefer cocounseling.

> **CAUTIONS AND CONTRAINDICATIONS**
>
> Psychotic illnesses are very serious and a qualified practitioner should be consulted if the condition is suspected. Schizophrenics and manic depressives should not abandon drug treatment without medical advice.

❧ TREATMENT

Conventional drug treatment can help control some of the symptoms of schizophrenia (such as hallucinations) but may also create many new symptoms. Alternative therapies can be used alongside conventional treatment for these problems.

COUNSELING *see page 103* ❧ PSYCHOLOGICAL THERAPIES *see page 102* ❧ RELAXATION *see page 116*

SEXUAL AND REPRODUCTIVE PROBLEMS

A MAN'S reproductive organs are responsible for producing the male sex hormone testosterone, and for the manufacture and storage of sperm. The organs are mostly outside the body and consist of the penis and the testes or testicles.

The penis is largely made up of three groups of spongy tissue, with a network of blood vessels and nerves. When a man is sexually stimulated the spongy tissue fills with blood and the penis becomes erect. The average length of an erect penis is 6in/15cm, although its size bears no relation to sexual potency. A cylinder running along the underside of the penis holds a muscular dual-purpose tube called the urethra, which carries urine from the bladder or semen from the testes to the tip of the penis.

The testicles are egg shaped glands supported by the scrotum, a loose sac of skin. Inside each testicle are hundreds of tubules, and it is in these that the manufacture of sperm takes place. Hundreds of millions of sperm are produced every day. The testicles also contain cells which manufacture testosterone, the hormone responsible for male characteristics such as body hair and deep voice, and for male pattern fat distribution.

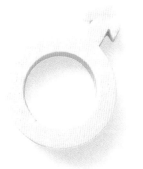

The biological symbol for the masculine principle. It is the same as the sign used in astronomy to indicate the planet Mars.

Attached to the back of each testicle is the epididymis, a comma-shaped structure 1in/2.5cm long, consisting of a cluster of tiny tubules that collect sperm from the testicles. The sperm mature within the epididymis over two to three weeks, and are stored there until they are ready to be ejaculated. Just before ejaculation, sperm are transported from the epididymis through a long duct called the vas deferens, toward the base of the bladder. The prostate, a small chestnut-shaped gland that is situated at the base of the bladder and surrounds the urethra, produces secretions that mix with seminal fluid.

Erections are controlled by nerve centers in the brain that react to erotic stimulation. What is sexually stimulating differs from man to man. Expectations and confidence also play a large part: in a highly competitive society, many men have unrealistic sexual expectations and equate sexual performance and penis size with success. Stress and anxiety about performance are common reasons for impotence.

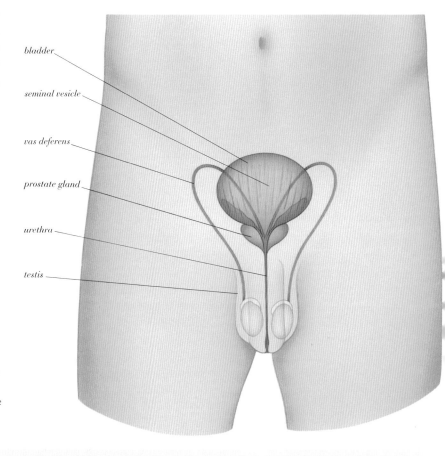

bladder

seminal vesicle

vas deferens

prostate gland

urethra

testis

Most of the male sexual organs are situated on the outside of the body. This is because sperm manufacture, which takes place in the testes, needs a slightly cooler temperature than that which is normal inside the body.

ANXIETY *see page 221* • STRESS *see page 223*

Men's Problems

ALTHOUGH individual men may suffer from low sperm counts or poor quality sperm making it difficult for them to father children *(see Infertility, page 234)*, a more worrying statistic has recently come to light. This is the fact, discovered by scientists from the University of Copenhagen in 1990, that the sperm count in 20 of the world's countries has fallen by 50 percent over the last 50 years. In 1940, men produced around 113 million sperms per milliliter of seminal fluid; today only 66 million are produced, and by the year 2000, this figure is predicted to fall to 50 million. In theory, a lower sperm count does not equal infertility, but some scientists believe that the count will be down to zero in 70 or 80 years, unless something is done.

The reason for this catastrophic decline is still in debate, although it is considered by many authorities to be the result of artificial substances, such as plastics and pesticides leaching hormone-disrupting chemicals into the soil, water, and food chain. These chemicals can mimic the female hormone estrogen, disrupt the production of the male hormone testosterone, or disturb the functioning of the endocrine system, which regulates the production of the body's hormones. Evidence indicates that birds and animals are also suffering from hormonal disruption. The fear is that these chemicals

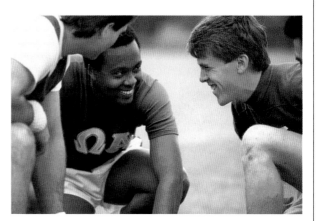

Competition with the peer group is the hallmark of male bonding patterns. Many biologists believe that competition between males is imperative for the spread of successful genes.

may also be linked to breast, testicle, and prostate cancer, endometriosis, and general damage to the immune system.

Some countries have reacted by banning PVC and other plastics for food packaging, but the chemical industry as a whole is awaiting the results of more research before it takes any action. There seems to be little that an individual can do since these chemicals are now ubiquitous, although taking steps to strengthen the immune system *(see page 135)* may help.

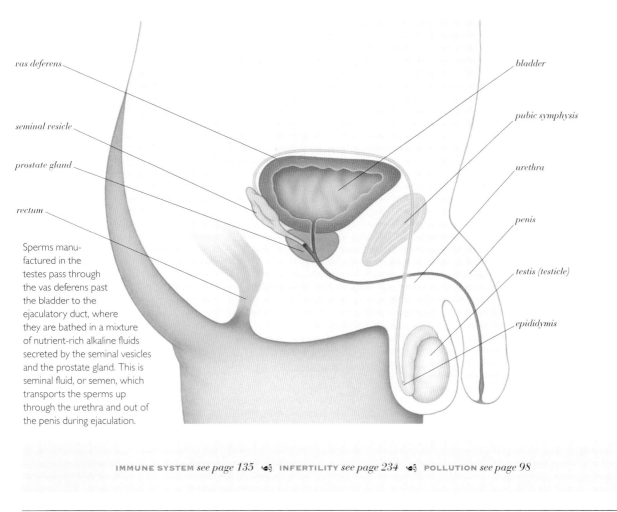

vas deferens

seminal vesicle

prostate gland

rectum

Sperms manufactured in the testes pass through the vas deferens past the bladder to the ejaculatory duct, where they are bathed in a mixture of nutrient-rich alkaline fluids secreted by the seminal vesicles and the prostate gland. This is seminal fluid, or semen, which transports the sperms up through the urethra and out of the penis during ejaculation.

bladder

pubic symphysis

urethra

penis

testis (testicle)

epididymis

IMMUNE SYSTEM *see page 135* • INFERTILITY *see page 234* • POLLUTION *see page 98*

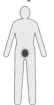

The Ailments

Physical Problems

HERNIA

A hernia is the protrusion of an organ, or part of an organ, through the wall of its containing cavity. This usually occurs as a result of straining (for example, to empty the bowels, or when lifting heavy objects), but it may be an inborn weakness. Symptoms include a swelling in the groin or abdomen, and general debility.

❧ TREATMENT

Hernias can be controlled by wearing a truss – a padded belt that acts as a support. Surgery is the only other option.

> **CAUTIONS AND CONTRAINDICATIONS**
>
> Consult a physician at once if a hernia is suspected. There is a danger that it may become strangulated.

PROSTATIS

Inflammation of the prostate gland is usually caused by an infection. Symptoms include a burning sensation or pain between the legs when urine is passed, pain in the genital area, back, lower abdomen, or inner thighs, and fever.

❧ TREATMENT

DIET AND NUTRITION Cernilton (pollen extract marketed under the name of Prostabrit) has an anti-inflammatory effect on prostatic tissue.

HERBAL MEDICINE Dandelion tea can help.

PROSTATE ENLARGEMENT

Enlargement of the prostate gland is common in men over 50, although young men can also suffer. As the prostate enlarges, it puts pressure on the bladder and the urethra. This causes symptoms such as passing urine more frequently than usual, having to get up often during the night, weak, dribbling urine stream, and difficulty or delay in passing water.

> **CAUTIONS AND CONTRAINDICATIONS**
>
> Consult a physician if you have any of the symptoms listed, before attempting to t.eat yourself.

❧ TREATMENT

DIET AND NUTRITION A trained nutritionist might recommend zinc, antiglan, protat, and cernilton (Prostabrit). Drink plenty of fluids; cut out coffee, tea, and alcohol.

HERBAL MEDICINE Use saw palmetto, fygeum, horsetail, and couch grass. The first two taken together are particularly effective.

Consult a qualified practitioner/therapist for:
ACUPUNCTURE Particular attention is paid to pressure points on the Bladder, Large Intestine, Spleen, and Kidney meridians.

INFERTILITY

The usual reason for infertility is a low sperm count, or a complete absence of sperm, resulting in failure of your partner to become pregnant after six months.

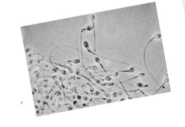

A low sperm count (measured in sperms per milliliter of seminal fluid) means that fertilization may be difficult or impossible.

❧ TREATMENT

Excessive heat can reduce sperm production. Wear loose boxer shorts rather than close-fitting underwear; avoid saunas and long soaks in hot baths. Splashing the testicles with cold water regularly each morning can raise the sperm count significantly.

DIET AND NUTRITION High-potency multivitamins and minerals might be recommended; vitamin E can improve potency and fertility; zinc may assist growth and development of the sexual organs.

> **CAUTIONS AND CONTRAINDICATIONS**
>
> If none of the measures given here help, check with your physician. There may be a physical or genetic reason for a low sperm count.

Consult a qualified practitioner/therapist for:
AUTOGENIC TRAINING This can help if the problem of infertility is stress related in origin.

ACUPUNCTURE *see page 90* ❧ AUTOGENIC TRAINING *see page 117* ❧
DIETARY THERAPY *see page 74* ❧ HERBAL MEDICINE *see page 67*

Psychological Problems

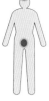

ERECTION PROBLEMS

Psychological impotence often arises after an erection failure (which all men experience at some time) because it can cause a man to lose confidence. Subsequently the anxiety felt when he next has sexual intercourse makes it likely that he will fail again.

In some cases, the problem is physical in origin, so you should always have a thorough medical checkup before embarking on any psychotherapeutic regimes.

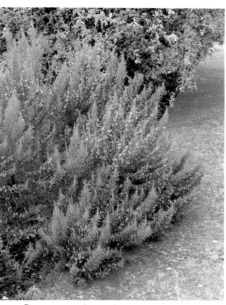

Rosemary can be used to treat a wide range of complaints, and oil of rosemary is particularly effective in reducing psychological tension.

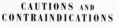
TREATMENT
Treatment is aimed at reducing anxiety and the fear of having to perform sexually. Agree with your partner not to attempt intercourse for a while, to remove pressure. Instead, concentrate on nongenital touching, using stroking and massage, and focus on your feelings. Only progress to genital touching when you feel completely at ease and have learned about your own and your partner's sexual responses. Do not attempt intercourse again until you feel absolutely ready to undertake it.

AROMATHERAPY Massage scalp with oil of rosemary.

HYDROTHERAPY Take a daily bath in cold water, sitz baths, or cold water frictions.

HERBAL MEDICINE Saw palmetto tea is thought to be an aphrodisiac. Fygeum is also helpful.

CAUTIONS AND CONTRAINDICATIONS
If the problem persists, consult a physician to check that there is no physical cause. If the problem is deep rooted, a psychosexual counselor or therapist may be needed.

Impotence and unsatisfactory sexual performance can be caused by outside factors, such as work. However, once it has gained hold, men can fall into a spiral of decline, in which the problem assumes paramount importance and contributes more stress to the situation. The only way out is to break the circle, relax, and address the difficulty from a different angle.

PREMATURE EJACULATION

Anxiety and stress are common causes of premature ejaculation, particularly anxiety about sexual performance. The symptom of the condition is ejaculation almost immediately after, or sometimes before, penetration. It is important to make love in relaxed and comfortable surroundings, without fear of being disturbed: furtive sexual encounters with one eye on the clock can also lead to the development of this distressing condition.

TREATMENT
The stop-start method can work well. Your partner stimulates you manually until you are on the point of orgasm, and just as you are about to ejaculate she squeezes the tip of your penis. Repeat four times a session: this will stop the orgasm and should eventually reestablish control after a few weeks.

Consult a qualified practitioner/therapist for:
AUTOGENIC TRAINING This can induce a feeling of deep relaxation.

EASTERN TRADITIONS Tantric Buddhism regards male orgasm and ejaculation as separate and has evolved methods of controlling ejaculation that may be helpful. Read tantric literature for more information.

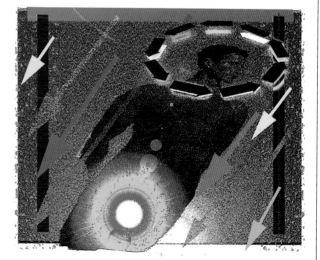

AROMATHERAPY *see page 50* ● AUTOGENIC TRAINING *see page 117* ●
HERBAL MEDICINE *see page 67* ● HYDROTHERAPY *see page 26*

Sexual and Reproductive Problems

The Ailments

Sexually Transmitted Diseases (STD)

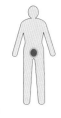

STDs ARE infections passed from one partner to the other during sexual intercourse (vaginal, oral, or anal sex). Many sexually transmitted diseases share the same symptoms. Because the more serious ones can cause infertility, and even death if left untreated, it is vital to be properly diagnosed by a specialist hospital clinic or physician. In all cases the use of barrier contraceptive methods, such as diaphragm or sheath, can limit the spread of infection.

GENITAL HERPES

These genital sores are caused by the herpes simplex 2 virus *(see page 133)*. Nothing can actually cure herpes, although there are a number of ways of relieving an attack. Symptoms of genital herpes are a crop of small painful sores on the penis or vagina. These turn into blisters, which eventually burst and dry up.

❧ TREATMENT

NATUROPATHY Bathe the affected area in a salt solution (1 teaspoonful salt to 1pt/500ml of warm water).

HERBAL MEDICINE Tea tree oil can be applied directly to the blisters, and witch hazel helps dry out the sores.

AROMATHERAPY Three drops each of eucalyptus, thyme, and geranium in a carrier oil put into a bath can soothe irritation.

GENITAL WARTS

The symptoms of this condition are painless, but often itchy, lumps of skin in the vagina, or on the vulva or penis, which can grow uncomfortably large.

❧ TREATMENT

Have genital warts dealt with by a specialist as soon as they are detected, as there may be a link between genital warts and cervical cancer.

Consult a qualified practitioner/therapist for:
HERBAL MEDICINE Thuja ointment or tincture.

NONSPECIFIC URETHRITIS

This condition, also known as NSU, is often the result of unprotected sexual contact while one partner has cystitis or a urinary tract infection *(see page 216)*, or thrush *(see page 240)*. The symptoms include soreness, painful intercourse, and a discharge that smells unpleasant. Orthodox treatment is antibiotics.

❧ TREATMENT

Scrupulous hygiene to prevent infection in the first place. You can also follow the advice about complementary therapies suitable for the treatment of cystitis *(see page 216)*.

penis

vagina

The nature of intercourse means that any disease or infection is very easily transferred between partners. If you have more than one sexual partner, it is doubly important that you protect yourself and them from the spread of infection.

AROMATHERAPY *see page 50* ❧ HERBAL MEDICINE *see page 67* ❧ NATUROPATHY *see page 24*

HUMAN IMMUNODEFICIENCY VIRUS (HIV), which can lead to Aids, is dealt with under Infections *(see pages 136–7).*

SYPHILIS

A painless raw ulcer (chancre) at the site of infection that heals in a few weeks, even though the disease is still spreading characterizes this disease. It is caused by the syphilis spirochete, a kind of bacterium. There may be glandular swelling, fever, and skin rashes.

✌ TREATMENT
It is essential to seek medical help when the chancre first appears. The only effective treatment is penicillin, or a similar drug.

Consult a qualified practitioner/therapist for:
HOMEOPATHY Syphilis and its after effects can be treated constitutionally by a homeopath.

CHLAMYDIA

Chlamydia is caused by a bacterial parasite called chlamydia trachomatis and is thought to be the most common sexually transmitted disease in the world. It can be present for years without any symptoms being experienced, but when they are, they include a discharge and a feeling of urgently needing to pass water. The cervix is tender, and will bleed with contact. Untreated, chlamydia spreads throughout the reproductive system causing pain, PID (pelvic inflammatory disease), chronic illness, and infertility. Orthodox treatment is by antibiotics, taken two to four times per day for several weeks. The health and hygiene habits of yourself and your partner will need to be addressed in order to discourage the spread of symptoms.

✌ TREATMENT
NATUROPATHY Colonic irrigation with Lactobacillus implant will flush out the parasitic bacteria and provide an environment in which the chlamydia cannot exist.

Consult a qualified practitioner/therapist for:
HERBALISM AND HOMEOPATHY Remedies will be individually tailored to symptoms.

PUBIC LICE OR CRABS
The pubic louse is a minute insect, *Pthirus pubis.* Although it is described as a crab, it looks like a tiny grayish, flattened spider. Symptoms of the condition are itching around the genital area, and sometimes tiny white specks can be seen in the pubic hair if the infestation has spread.

✌ TREATMENT
The insects can be removed with a metal nit comb, although the simplest remedy is to shave the pubic area, and wash thoroughly.

GONORRHEA
Gonorrhea is caused by bacteria that infect the opening of the urethra. It manifests in sores around the genitals, a green creamy discharge from the penis or vagina, abdominal pain, and pain on passing urine.

✌ TREATMENT
Seek medical help from a physician immediately. Gonorrhea can only be treated successfully with a course of antibiotics.

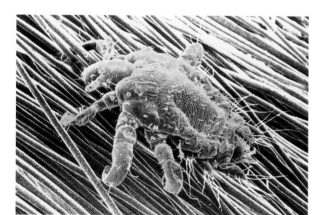

Pubic lice pass easily between partners, so both should be treated at once to prevent reinfestation.

COLONIC IRRIGATION *see page 27* ✌ HERBAL MEDICINE *see page 67* ✌
HOMEOPATHY *see page 83* ✌ NATUROPATHY *see page 24*

Women's Problems

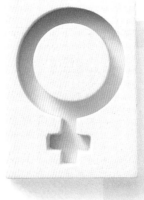

The biological symbol for the feminine principle. It is the same as the sign used in astronomy to indicate the planet Venus.

THE FEMALE reproductive system consists of the uterus (womb), a muscular pear-shaped expandable organ about 3in/7.5cm long and 2in/5cm wide, two ovaries (connected to the uterus by the Fallopian tubes), and the cervix, which joins the lower end of the uterus to the top end of the vagina.

The system is activated by hormones in the bloodstream. These are produced by the pituitary, a tiny gland at the base of the brain. Their output is controlled by a different part of the brain, the hypothalamus. During a woman's menstrual cycle the ovaries produce the sex hormones estrogen and progesterone in varying amounts, and small amounts of testosterone and other male hormones. These hormones do not work in isolation: estrogen, for example, works with testosterone to give a woman her sex drive. Estrogen and progesterone are responsible for the regulation of the menstrual cycle during a woman's reproductive life, her female characteristics, and her sex drive and fertility. If she becomes pregnant, these hormones enable the womb to support the growing baby by making the endometrium (lining of the womb) thick and rich with tiny blood vessels.

CONTRACEPTION

Natural contraception, or birth control, is becoming increasingly popular as it becomes clear that the artificial methods carry unknown risks and side effects. Alternative therapies encourage us to get to know our bodies, and it is a natural progression to use that knowledge for contraceptive purposes. Natural birth control methods include

- *calendar method, which involves recording the dates of periods on a calendar and then calculating "unsafe" dates*
- *temperature method, which requires diligent temperature taking to ascertain when ovulation will occur*
- *cervical mucus method, which involves noting the changes in the mucus produced by the cervix*
- *withdrawal, also called coitus interruptus, meaning interrupted intercourse, before ejaculation can occur*
- *breastfeeding, which is temporary and often ineffective.*

See your local family planning center or physician for details of how to apply these methods successfully.

Hormones enable the ovaries to release an egg each month for possible fertilization. If sperm are present, the egg is fertilized in the Fallopian tube and passes down into the uterus, where it attaches itself to the endometrium and grows. If the egg is not fertilized, the levels of estrogen and progesterone fall, the endometrium shrinks because there are no hormones to support it, and the uterus expels this and the unfertilized egg as a menstrual period. The whole cycle then starts up all over again.

Most women have around 400 menstrual periods throughout their lives. Although the level of hormones fluctuates throughout each cycle, it is essential that the balance is correct, for even the smallest imbalance can cause menstrual disorders, or even infertility. Many problems associated with the menopause are due to the diminishing levels of hormones.

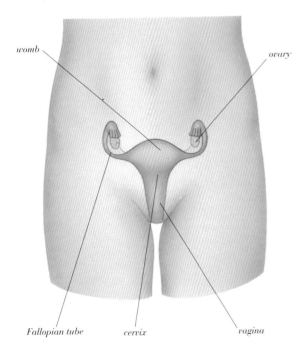

womb

ovary

Fallopian tube　　*cervix*　　*vagina*

The female reproductive organs are contained entirely within the body. They consist of the vagina, cervix, womb, and ovaries.

BRAIN *see page 188* • **MENSTRUATION** *see page 244*

Female Infertility

CAUSES AND TREATMENT

Hormonal problems, failure to ovulate, and blocked Fallopian tubes are the most common causes of a woman's infertility, resulting in failure to conceive after attempting to do so for six months.

TREATMENT

Ensure you make love during the fertile period (days 9–16 of the menstrual cycle) as often as possible.

LIFESTYLE *Cut down on alcohol and give up smoking: both can affect fertility. Stress can sometimes cause spasms in the Fallopian tubes and often make it impossible to establish a relaxed mood for successful lovemaking; learning a relaxation technique can be beneficial.*

DIET AND NUTRITION *Eat plenty of sesame and pumpkin seeds, nuts, avocado, dried apricots, carrots, olives, soybeans, and oily fish.*

> **CAUTIONS AND CONTRAINDICATIONS**
>
> It is important that the cause is properly diagnosed by a physician. Sometimes surgical treatment is the only option.

Consult a qualified practitioner/therapist for:

ACUPUNCTURE *If the problem is based on a hormonal disorder, this can stimulate the body's natural hormonal production.*

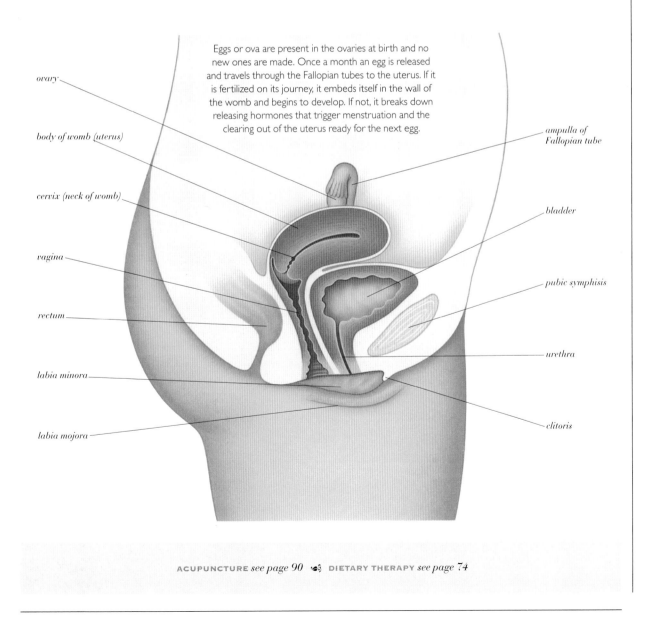

Eggs or ova are present in the ovaries at birth and no new ones are made. Once a month an egg is released and travels through the Fallopian tubes to the uterus. If it is fertilized on its journey, it embeds itself in the wall of the womb and begins to develop. If not, it breaks down releasing hormones that trigger menstruation and the clearing out of the uterus ready for the next egg.

ovary

body of womb (uterus)

cervix (neck of womb)

vagina

rectum

labia minora

labia mojora

ampulla of Fallopian tube

bladder

pubic symphisis

urethra

clitoris

ACUPUNCTURE *see page 90* • **DIETARY THERAPY** *see page 74*

Genital Problems

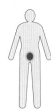

BACTERIAL VAGINOSIS (BV)
This mild, noninflammatory condition is thought to be linked to a high pH level (low acid balance) in the vagina. It causes symptoms that include a gray-white discharge with a strong, fishy smell.

➳ TREATMENT
NATUROPATHY Dip a tampon in live, natural yogurt and leave in the vagina for an hour.

DIET AND NUTRITION A tub of live, natural yogurt daily will help prevent further attacks. Take two capsules of *Lactobacillus acidophilus* daily.

HOMEOPATHY Sepia and Kreosotum are both helpful remedies.

> **CAUTIONS AND CONTRAINDICATIONS**
> Although BV is relatively harmless there is an association with premature labor: consult a physician if you experience symptoms during pregnancy.

THRUSH
Thrush is a fungal overgrowth caused by the *Candida albicans* organism, which occupies the gut and vagina along with a host of other bacteria. Normally it is kept under control by "friendly" vaginal bacteria and does not cause any problems. If anything upsets that delicate bacterial balance (for example, antibiotics, stress, illness, poor nutrition) the yeast can start to grow out of control and eventually manifests itself as a fungal infection. Symptoms of the infection are a thick white curdy or watery discharge that resembles cottage cheese, together with itching around the vulva or the vagina. Sexual intercourse and passing urine may be painful.

➳ TREATMENT
NATUROPATHY Itching can be eased by dipping a tampon in live, natural yogurt and leaving it in the vagina for an hour.

DIET AND NUTRITION Eat two or three tubs of live yogurt daily during an attack. Two capsules of Lactobacillus acidophilus daily will replenish vaginal bacteria and guard against future attacks. Cut out food that the yeast feeds on: sugar, refined carbohydrates, bread, mushrooms. Eat salads, fruit, and wholegrain cereals, and try to incorporate more garlic into your daily diet.

AROMATHERAPY Add drops of rose, lavender, and bergamot to 2pt/1l of warm water and use as a douche.

HERBAL MEDICINE Tea tree oil applied topically acts as an antifungal. Make a compress from golden seal, myrrh, or camomile to relieve symptoms.

HOMEOPATHY Helonias or Borax veneta may be helpful. If the problem recurs, consult a qualified practitioner.

> **CAUTIONS AND CONTRAINDICATIONS**
> **THRUSH**
> Avoid intercourse during an attack; spores can be passed on to your partner who can in turn reinfect you.

> **SELF-HELP**
> **VAGINITIS**
> Avoid disinfectants and perfumes in the bath, soap and strong laundry detergents. Antibiotics should be avoided, if possible. Douche the vagina with Hypericum and Calendula solution (about 5 drops of the mother tincture in about 10fl oz/300ml cooled, boiled water). A cold water compress on the lower abdomen may help. Increase your intake of vitamins C and B, as well as evening primrose oil.

VAGINITIS
An irritation or abrasion of the vagina, often brought about by insufficient lubrication during intercourse, is the main cause of vaginitis, particularly after the menopause. The symptoms of vaginitis are vaginal itching, soreness, and dryness, and occasionally a blood-stained discharge.

➳ TREATMENT
NATUROPATHY Bathe the vagina in a salt solution (1 teaspoonful salt to 1pt/500ml of warm water) to soothe inflammation.

AROMATHERAPY Lavender sitz baths can soothe itching, and jojoba oil is a good lubricant. As for the menopause, tea tree oil, diluted in a concentration of 1 to 3 percent essential oil to base, can help to eliminate vaginal dryness.

Consult a qualified practitioner/therapist for:
HOMEOPATHY Treatment will be tailored to individual cases but may include Natrum Mur., Sepia, or Argentum nit.

AROMATHERAPY *see page 50* ➳ DIETARY THERAPY *see page 74* ➳
HERBAL MEDICINE *see page 67* ➳ HOMEOPATHY *see page 83* ➳ NATUROPATHY *see page 24*

Cervical Cancer

Cervical cancer is cancer of the cervix, which is the neck of the womb. This type of cancer is more common in women in their forties and fifties, but the proportion of women under the age of 35 is growing all the time. It is second only to cancer of the breast as the greatest cause of death by cancer in women. In the United States about 13,500 new cases of invasive cervical cancer occur every year and about 40 percent of these eventually die from the disease. Cancer of the cervix is preceded for many years by a recognizable and easily diagnosable preinvasive condition, known as carcinoma in situ (CIN). About 55,000 cases of CIN occur each year in the United States. There is some evidence that barrier methods of contraception have a protective effect against cervical cancer, but risk factors include

❋ having sexual intercourse at an early age, particularly before the age of 20

❋ having many different sexual partners

❋ smoking and exposure to others' smoke

❋ two viruses: human papilloma (wart) virus and the herpes simplex virus.

There are no obvious symptoms of cervical cancer and when they do present, the condition is usually at an incurable stage. Therefore, it is vital that women look after their own health and keep up their screening program. Cervical smear screening is crucial for detecting the condition in an early, precancerous stage. Early treatment can offer a complete cure, since this is one cancer that can be stopped in its tracks.

> **CAUTIONS AND CONTRAINDICATIONS**
>
> Consult a physician if there is a blood-stained discharge. Itching (pruritis vulvae) can also be a symptom of diabetes.

∾ TREATMENT

HOMEOPATHY A homeopath believes that cancer represents a profound breakdown of health on every level and will prescribe constitutional treatment.

HERBAL MEDICINE Treatment to boost the immune system and to help ease any harmful side effects of orthodox treatment may be offered. Useful remedies include echinacea to promote healing, sweet violet, cleavers, red clover, and burdock to cleanse the system and improve immune response. Some remedies such as clematis or echinacea may encourage the body's immune system to function at optimum levels.

AROMATHERAPY This can be very useful at all stages of the disease. Consult an aromatherapist to help you select suitable oils. Early stage sufferers should avoid massage, which may speed up the spread of the condition, but oils used in warm baths or vaporizers will deliver the aromatherapeutic benefits. Terminal sufferers may find massage very relaxing and useful in encouraging a sense of well-being.

> **SELF-HELP**
>
> Make sure that you have the smear test every two to three years, and more often if abnormalities are uncovered.

ACUPUNCTURE Treatment will encourage recovery and help the body to deal with the toxic side effects of chemotherapy and radiotherapy. Energy levels will also be improved, and pain may be controlled through regular sessions.

Women have a cultural bias toward sharing feelings, talking, and cooperating. Support groups of fellow sufferers can help with diseases such as cervical cancer.

ACUPUNCTURE *see page 90* ∾ AROMATHERAPY *see page 50* ∾
CANCER *see page 140* ∾ HERBAL MEDICINE *see page 67* ∾ HOMEOPATHY *see page 83*

Serious Problems

The female reproductive system is complicated, and many things can go wrong. It is particularly vulnerable to infection, and any pain or symptoms in the area should be discussed with a practitioner or therapist as soon as possible.

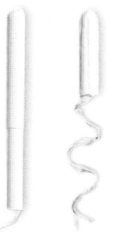

Internal tampons are convenient but should be removed with care and changed regularly. A condition known as toxic shock, a form of blood poisoning, can occur if a tampon is left in place for too long or is forgotten.

PELVIC INFLAMMATORY DISEASE (PID)

PID is a collective term for inflammation or infections of the Fallopian tubes, ovaries, cervix, or uterus. It can be caused by an intrauterine device (IUD), endometriosis, pelvic surgery, sexually transmitted diseases (*see pages 236-7*), or if an infection develops after an abortion. It may be acute or chronic. Symptoms can include sharp abdominal pain, backache, high fever (acute); abdominal pain and tenderness, tiredness, vaginal discharge, general feeling of unwellness (chronic).

❧ TREATMENT
DIET AND NUTRITION Prevent recurrent attacks by eating well.

CAUTIONS AND CONTRAINDICATIONS

Acute PID should always be diagnosed and treated by a physician in the first instance: any delay could lead to the development of abscesses on the Fallopian tubes or womb. As a result, scar tissue could form, causing infertility or an ectopic pregnancy. Failure to treat PID properly can lead to peritonitis, which is life-threatening.

SELF-HELP

Getting sufficient sleep is important. Learn to manage stress levels. Talk to a physician about alternative forms of contraception if you use an IUD.

The cuttlefish is the source of the homeopathic remedy Sepia, a specific in treating menstrual disorders.

Consult a qualified practitioner/therapist for:
ACUPUNCTURE Helpful for pain control and to promote bodily healing.

UTERINE PROLAPSE

A prolapse is the falling or sagging of the uterus due to slack muscle tone. The pelvic organs are supported by a sling of muscles and ligaments, and if strain is put on these muscles during pregnancy, or because of obesity, or because the muscles have lost their elasticity due to the menopause, the pelvic organs start to sag. Symptoms of this condition are a dragging sensation, or heaviness in the back or lower abdomen, incontinence, a frequent desire to urinate even when the bladder is empty, constipation, and a feeling of looseness in the pelvis.

SELF-HELP

Lose weight if you need to. Exercising the muscles of the pelvic floor by contracting them as though you were trying to prevent a bowel movement, or prevent the passing of urine, can improve muscle tone.

❧ TREATMENT
DIET AND NUTRITION
Eat a diet rich in fiber.

Consult a qualified practitioner/therapist for:
HOMEOPATHY
Treatment will be constitutional, and will probably include Sepia and Helonias. The tissue salt Calc. fluor. can help.

CAUTIONS AND CONTRAINDICATIONS

If prolapse persists, consult a gynecologist. A pelvic floor repair operation may be necessary.

HERBAL MEDICINE
Uterine tonics include black cohosh, raspberry leaf, and chaste tree.

Psychosexual Problems

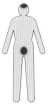

LOSS OF SEXUAL DESIRE (FRIGIDITY)

A woman's sex drive fluctuates and is related to her menstrual cycle, but various factors – problems with a relationship, illness, tiredness, stress, depression, bad sexual experiences, and some antidepressant drugs and tranquilizers – can affect sexual responsiveness. Pelvic pain caused by underlying disease can also cause loss of sexual desire, and sometimes the problem can be as simple as inadequate stimulation during intercourse.

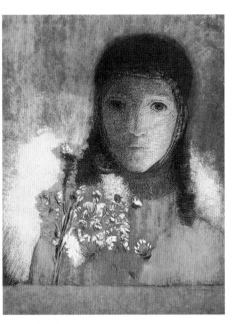

Frigidity or lack of desire may result if a woman feels insecure or anxious.

☙ TREATMENT

Try to discover the root cause. Consider masturbation, when you are alone, relaxed, and comfortable. If you can arouse yourself, you should feel more relaxed about letting your partner know how you like to be stimulated.

AROMATHERAPY Many essential oils act as aphrodisiacs, including jasmine, sandalwood, patchouli, and ylang ylang (but avoid using them on the genital area). A mixture of five drops jasmine, five drops rose, ten drops sandalwood, and five drops bergamot in two cups/500ml of base oil – used in the bath or as a sensual massage oil for you and your partner – should help you to get to know each other's sexual responses and reawaken sexual desire.

Consult a qualified practitioner/therapist for:
ROLFING If the problem is psychological, this body-mind therapy can release physical tensions and enable you to deal with emotional problems more easily.

COUNSELING If the problem persists, seek help from a psychosexual counselor or therapist.

CAUTIONS AND CONTRAINDICATIONS

Before you embark on any psychological treatment, consult a physician to check that there is nothing wrong with you physically.

VAGINISMUS

Vaginismus (involuntary contractions of the vagina) often makes intercourse impossible because the muscles around the entrance of the vagina go into spasm as soon as penetration is attempted. The spasm is a reflex action, and the vaginal muscles are so powerful that it becomes impossible to penetrate them. The muscles may remain contracted for some time, an effect that is increasingly painful and causes considerable anxiety. In fact, anxiety – in particular a subconscious fear of intercourse – is often the main cause of vaginismus. It can happen after a bad or painful sexual experience, or even after painful childbirth.

☙ TREATMENT

Learn a relaxation technique. On your own, when you are feeling relaxed and comfortable, try inserting your little finger into your vagina. When you can do that comfortably, try two fingers. Carry on until you feel relaxed enough to let your partner try.

AROMATHERAPY

Sensual mutual massage with your partner (*see Loss of Sexual Desire, above*) will help you to relax. Use oils such as jasmine, ylang ylang, rose, or sandalwood in a carrier oil. Avoid rubbing into the genital area.

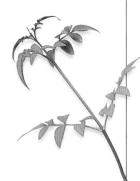

Essential oil of jasmine Jasminum officinale *is ideal for a sensual massage to help reawaken sexual desire.*

Consult a qualified practitioner/therapist for:
COUNSELING Psychosexual counseling and therapy, combined with learning a relaxation technique, can help over a period of time.

HOMEOPATHY Treatment will be tailored to individual cases, but may include Causticum, Natrum. Mur., Argentum Nit., or Sepia.

AROMATHERAPY *see page 50* ☙ COUNSELING *see page 103* ☙ HOMEOPATHY *see page 83* ☙ ROLFING *see page 46*

Menstruation

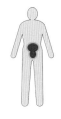

Problems with menstruation are very common and are usually caused by hormone imbalance. Periods may be too heavy, too scant, too frequent, too rare, annoyingly irregular, or very painful.

DYSMENORRHEA (PAINFUL MENSTRUAL PERIODS)

When menstruation starts, the muscles of the uterus contract to expel the lining. These contractions are caused by hormonelike substances known as prostaglandins. If the body produces too much, the contractions are stronger and more painful, causing a dull ache or cramplike pain in the lower abdomen or back, and sometimes sickness and diarrhea.

✥ TREATMENT

YOGA Classic positions such as the Bow, Cobra, and Cat Hump postures are all helpful.

DIET AND NUTRITION Take evening primrose oil (100g), plus vitamin E (400iu daily).

SHIATSU This can be applied to pressure points on the legs, feet, abdomen, and beside the lumbar vertebrae.

HERBAL MEDICINE A raspberry leaf tea or ginger decoction can be beneficial.

AROMATHERAPY Use caraway oil in the bath.

HOMEOPATHY Chamomilla is a helpful remedy.

> **CAUTIONS AND CONTRAINDICATIONS**
>
> Consult a physician if you suddenly experience pain after years of trouble-free periods. It could be a symptom of an underlying disease such as endometriosis, in which patches of endometrial tissue start to grow in the pelvic cavity and respond to the hormones that regulate the menstrual cycle.

> **CAUTIONS AND CONTRAINDICATIONS**
>
> Consult a physician if your menstrual periods suddenly become heavy. It could indicate some sort of infection, or problems with the lining of the uterus, or a hormonal imbalance. Always seek medical advice if you experience bleeding between periods.

MENORRHAGIA (HEAVY BLEEDING)

Menorrhagia is usually caused by fibroids, benign solid growths of muscle and fibrous tissue on the uterus. It is estimated that 20 percent of women over 30 have fibroids, and many are unaware of them until a physician feels them during an internal examination. Although they can cause excessive menstrual bleeding, they often cause no further problems, and it is very rare for them to turn cancerous. The growth of fibroids is stimulated by estrogen, the production of which is influenced by the amount of fat consumed in the diet. The symptom of this condition is blood loss during menstruation so heavy that normal sanitary protection cannot cope with it.

Grapes are a healthy source of vitamin C, which can strengthen blood vessels.

✥ TREATMENT

DIET AND NUTRITION A low-fat diet made up largely of vegetables, fruits, and starches can lower estrogen levels significantly. Foods rich in bioflavonoids with vitamin C, such as citrus fruits, grapes, apricots, tomatoes, broccoli, peppers, cherries, and rosehips, can strengthen blood vessels.

Consult a qualified practitioner/therapist for:
ACUPUNCTURE This can regulate the body's natural hormone production.

The yoga pose known as the Cobra is very helpful during painful periods.

ACUPUNCTURE *see page 90* ✥ AROMATHERAPY *see page 50* ✥ DIETARY THERAPY *see page 74* ✥
HERBAL MEDICINE *see page 67* ✥ HOMEOPATHY *see page 83* ✥ SHIATSU *see page 96* ✥ YOGA *see page 61*

Premenstrual Syndrome and Menopause

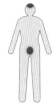

PREMENSTRUAL SYNDROME

This is a collective term for a variety of symptoms that occur each month before the start of a period. Some may be caused by changes in hormone levels. Symptoms can include bloatedness, water retention, breast tenderness or soreness, depression, tension, headaches, irritability, sugar craving, and mood swings.

✍ TREATMENT

DIET AND NUTRITION
Cut down on cola drinks, caffeine, sugar, and salt, all of which can aggravate symptoms. Eat plenty of green vegetables and salads. A trained nutritionist might recommend supplements: optivite, vitamin B6 or B complex, especially folic acid, and evening primrose oil.

AROMATHERAPY
A lemongrass bath can be emotionally calming.

Consult a qualified practitioner/therapist for:
HOMEOPATHY Take Lycopodium, for depression; Sepia for tender breasts, pain, tiredness or mood swings; and Pulsatilla for tearfulness.

MENOPAUSE

As the body's reproductive system gradually winds down, the ovaries shrivel and generate less and less estrogen, although they carry on producing small quantities of hormones for some years after the menopause. The most common symptoms of the menopause are hot flushes and night sweats, vaginal dryness, incontinence (*see page 217*), depression, forgetfulness, confusion, feelings of unreality rather like a panic attack, poor memory, inability to concentrate, a general feeling of unwellness, tiredness, and lack of energy.

> ### SELF-HELP
>
> Avoid salt, fatty food, tea, and coffee. Limit your consumption of dairy produce and refined carbohydrates. Eat raw fruits and vegetables, and include the following supplements in your diet:
> * vitamins C, E, and B6
> * magnesium
> * evening primrose oil
> * pancreatic enzymes
> * zinc
> * iron.
> Take steps to deal with stress, which may be exacerbating the condition. Try to include some exercise in your daily routine.

✍ TREATMENT

Hot flushes can be helped by wearing natural fibers next to the skin, and not using nylon sheets.

DIET AND NUTRITION A trained nutritionist might recommend evening primrose oil, vitamin B6, and calcium. Avoid spicy foods, smoking, and drinking alcohol or coffee late at night: these all affect the blood vessels. Eat plenty of calcium-rich foods including yogurt, skimmed milk, spinach, oranges, apples, and cottage cheese to minimize the risk of osteoporosis (brittle bone disease).

HERBAL MEDICINE Vaginal dryness can be helped by applying jojoba oil just before intercourse.

AROMATHERAPY Rose oil is calming for psychological problems; geranium oil mixed with ylang ylang can improve muscle tone when rubbed into the breasts; tea tree oil, diluted in a concentration 1 to 3 percent essential oil to base, can help vaginal dryness, or add ten drops of oil to a bath.

Consult a qualified practitioner/therapist for:

HOMEOPATHY A homeopath will take a detailed history and prescribe remedies for the mental as well as the physical state. They may include: Lachesis, Sepia, and Pulsatilla (for mood changes); Belladonna (for hot flushes); Graphites (for loss of libido and emotional instability); Cimicifuga (depression, irritability, restlessness); Caulophyllum (nervous tension, anxiety, emotional instability, joint pains); and Arnica (backache, tiredness, aching muscles).

ACUPUNCTURE Can help psychological symptoms such as anxiety, depression, and irritability, and alleviate hot flushes and back pain.

Keeping a PMS diary will help you monitor mood swings and changes in behavior or appetite.

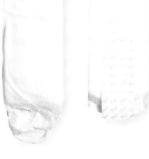
During the menopause, vaginal dryness makes sanitary towels more comfortable than tampons.

ACUPUNCTURE *see page 90* ✍ AROMATHERAPY *see page 50* ✍
DIETARY THERAPY *see page 74* ✍ HERBAL MEDICINE *see page 67* ✍ HOMEOPATHY *see page 83*

The Ailments

Pregnancy and Childbirth

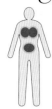

IT IS NORMAL to experience some minor discomforts during pregnancy, but it is best to avoid taking drugs, unless they have been prescribed by a physician. Alternative remedies can be helpful, but some can be harmful during pregnancy. Always consult a qualified practitioner before undertaking any treatment.

MORNING SICKNESS

Morning sickness is a feeling of nausea, or actual vomiting, usually in the morning, although it can happen at any time of day. It is thought to be caused by an increase in hormone levels in early pregnancy.

✍ TREATMENT
DIET AND NUTRITION
Eat small frequent meals that are high in carbohydrates; avoid fatty, rich, or spicy foods. Drink plenty of fluids. A trained nutritionist might recommend supplements: 500mg of magnesium and 100mg of vitamin B6 per day.

HERBAL MEDICINE
Try camomile or peppermint tea or an infusion of fresh ginger.

HOMEOPATHY
Nux vomica, Pulsatilla, and Ipecacuanha are useful remedies.

AROMATHERAPY
Place one or two drops of lemon oil in a burner placed in the room where you sleep.

SORE BREASTS
One of the first signs of pregnancy is sore breasts, as they begin to increase in size in preparation for feeding the baby.

✍ TREATMENT
Wear a well-fitting bra throughout pregnancy to give the breasts support.

HOMEOPATHY Conium and Bryonia can ease soreness. Cracked nipples respond to Castor equi.

AROMATHERAPY Add two drops of lavender oil or geranium oil to a warm bath. Allow the water to cover your breasts, or hold a soaked facecloth over them.

HEARTBURN
This problem is caused by acid from the stomach and is often experienced during the last months of pregnancy. It creates a strong burning sensation in the chest.

✍ TREATMENT
DIET AND NUTRITION Eat small, regular meals based on wholefoods, with moderate amounts of protein. Cut out fatty and spicy foods and avoid tea, coffee, and alcohol. A milky drink at bedtime can also help.

HERBAL MEDICINE
Meadowsweet tea and marshmallow infusion will help soothe the lining of the stomach.

AROMATHERAPY
Add 2 drops of sandalwood to 2.5 teaspoonfuls of carrier oil and massage into the solar plexus.

> **CAUTIONS AND CONTRAINDICATIONS**
> If you have symptoms that you are concerned about, discuss them with your midwife or physician. Always check that any remedies are suitable for use during pregnancy.

A serene newborn baby is the result of a healthy pregnancy and a labor that has proceeded with as little intervention as necessary.

> **CAUTIONS AND CONTRAINDICATIONS**
> **MORNING SICKNESS**
> If frequent vomiting occurs, consult your physician.

AROMATHERAPY *see page 50* ✍ DIETARY THERAPY *see page 74* ✍
HERBAL MEDICINE *see page 67* ✍ HOMEOPATHY *see page 83*

Ways to Ease Labor and Childbirth

Many women feel that natural childbirth is less traumatic for the baby and gives them more control over the birth. Start preparation for this early in pregnancy by taking regular gentle exercise, such as swimming and walking, which tones the muscles and improves overall fitness. Eat a sensible diet and take supplements or folic acid in recommended amounts. Draw up a birth plan which sets out how you want the birth to be managed. If it is your first baby, join a natural childbirth class to learn breathing techniques.

RELAXATION AND BREATHING Concentrating on breathing can have a soothing effect and help you relax.

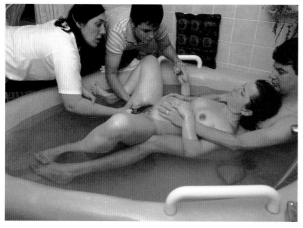

Properly supervised, water births allow the mother to relax and deal calmly with her contractions. The baby makes a gentle transition through the warm water from the amniotic fluid of the womb to the dry, bright air of the world.

WATER BIRTH Immersion in a pool filled with warm water helps relieve the pain of contractions, and some women go on to give birth in the water. Find out if your hospital provides a birth pool, or if you can hire one.

HERBAL MEDICINE Raspberry leaf tea drunk over the last three months of pregnancy helps tone the womb.

AROMATHERAPY Rosemary oil, lavender, and camomile, rubbed on your wrists, forehead, and neck, relieves pain during labor.

MASSAGE Gentle downward strokes can ease pain, especially in the lower back.

Consult a qualified practitioner/therapist for:
ACUPUNCTURE Permission from the hospital where you are giving birth will be needed if you intend to use this form of pain relief.

TENS (TRANSCUTANEOUS ELECTRICAL NERVE STIMULATION) This is a version of acupuncture. It works by sending electrical impulses to the brain. These block the pain messages and stimulate the release of endorphines, the body's natural painkillers.

HYPNOSIS To help ease tension it is important to practice the necessary techniques from early on in pregnancy. Permission from the hospital where you are giving birth will be needed if you want a hypnotist to attend you at the delivery.

TORN PERINEUM

The perineum is the skin between the vagina and the anus. It is stretched during childbirth and may sometimes tear. In some cases, stitches will be needed to repair the damage.

PREVENTION

Massage the area regularly before your estimated date of delivery so that it becomes more supple.

AROMATHERAPY Rub half a teaspoonful of jojoba oil into the area daily for eight weeks before your expected delivery date.

TREATMENT

If you had stitches after delivery, apply a cold compress to the area (try a bag of frozen peas wrapped in a face cloth), then dry the area thoroughly. The warm air from a hairdryer works well.

AROMATHERAPY Add two drops of lavender and two drops of cypress oil to a warm bath and soak the area for 10 to 15 minutes.

STRETCH MARKS

These are pink or reddish streaks on the skin which eventually fade to silver. They are caused by overstretching the skin.

TREATMENT/PREVENTION

MASSAGE Essential oils of frankincense, lavender, or rosewood should be rubbed into the abdomen and upper legs during pregnancy.

HOMEOPATHY Biochemic tissue salts Calc. fluor.

DIET AND NUTRITION Increase intake of vitamin E, or alternatively rub vitamin E oil into the skin.

ACUPUNCTURE *see page 90* • AROMATHERAPY *see page 50* • DIETARY THERAPY *see page 74* •
HERBAL MEDICINE *see page 67* • HOMEOPATHY *see page 83* • HYPNOSIS *see page 112* • MASSAGE *see page 48*

The Ailments

CHILDREN'S AILMENTS • Babies' Problems

MANY childhood ailments and diseases can be successfully treated with alternative medicines, used on their own, or alongside conventional medicines. However, when administering them to a baby or toddler you should always seek professional advice. If a child does not respond to a treatment or you are concerned about his or her health, consult a physician immediately.

baby's stomach in a clockwise direction with one drop of fennel in half a teaspoonful of carrier oil (such as wheatgerm or almond oil).

HOMEOPATHY Depending on the other symptoms, Chamamilla, Colocynthis, Dioscorea, or Magnesia phos. may be prescribed. Consult a homeopath for a remedy suited to your baby.

BABIES' COLIC
Colic is a distressing pattern of excessive crying during the first few months after birth. The cause of colic is unknown.

TREATMENT
DIET AND NUTRITION If you are breast-feeding, consider your own diet: many different foods can affect a baby through the mother's milk. A special counselor can offer advice. Some formula-fed babies are allergic to cows' milk, and a change to a soybean alternative may be required. Always seek professional advice before changing your baby's formula.

HERBAL MEDICINE Half a teaspoonful of peppermint, catnip, and fennel tea every half-hour may be helpful. If you are nursing, take an infusion yourself.

AROMATHERAPY Offer a gripe water containing the essential oil of fennel. Externally gently massage the

CRADLE CAP
Flaky patches of white or yellow scales on the top of the scalp caused by the glands in the hair follicles overproducing oil.

TREATMENT
NATUROPATHY Rub almond or olive oil into the hair at night and comb gently the next morning to remove the scales.

HERBAL MEDICINE Add 2 drops of tea tree oil to a mild shampoo.

> **CAUTIONS AND CONTRAINDICATIONS**
>
> Some treatments are unsuitable for babies and very young children: buy specially formulated remedies and consult a qualified practitioner.

Gentle alternative therapies are suitable for children, whose young systems allow them to respond to remedies very quickly.

Barrier cream (below left) can help prevent any soreness caused by bedwetting.

BEDWETTING

There are two types of bedwetters – a child who has never been dry, and one who was dry and then starts wetting the bed again after bladder control has been established. These conditions are known as primary and secondary enuresis. Most primary enuresis is caused by slow development of bladder control. Anxiety is usually the cause of secondary enuresis, which may start when the child begins school or a sibling is born. Other causes include urinary infections *(see page 216)*.

TREATMENT

HERBAL MEDICINE *St. John's wort or horsetail tea are helpful.*

HOMEOPATHY *Belladonna, Causticum, Pulsatilla, and Silica may all be helpful.*

Consult a qualified practitioner/therapist for:

COUNSELING *Both child and parents should be involved, and the child is usually given a positive role where dryness is rewarded with praise and prizes.*

AROMATHERAPY *see page 50* • DIETARY THERAPY *see page 74* •
HERBAL MEDICINE *see page 67* • HOMEOPATHY *see page 83* • NATUROPATHY *see page 24*

Skin Rashes and Teething

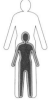

Problems during a baby's first six months are usually skin rashes or teething. Diaper rash afflicts nearly all babies and can easily become very painful unless dealt with. Eczema is usually caused by an allergy. The discomfort of teething can be soothed with various gentle herbal or homeopathic remedies.

DIAPER RASH

This is usually caused by prolonged skin contact with urine or feces. Symptoms are red, spotty, and sore skin. The diaper may smell of ammonia.

TREATMENT

Change the diaper frequently. Wash and rinse baby's bottom with plain water, and dry the area thoroughly. Leave the diaper off for as long as possible every day so that the skin is exposed to fresh air.

🌿 HOMEOPATHY *Infant remedies include Sulfur and Rhus tox.*

🌿 NATUROPATHY *Use almond or olive oil after every change.*

🌿 HERBAL MEDICINE *Apply comfrey ointment.*

Diaper rash is very uncomfortable; if possible, leave the baby's skin exposed to the air whenever you can.

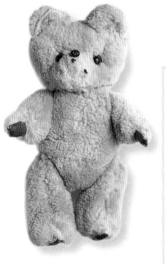

The comfortable presence of a familiar cuddly toy is an essential part of the healing process in young children.

ECZEMA

If a baby shows signs of eczema before starting solids it is likely to be caused by an allergy to cows' milk – even breast-fed babies can suffer if the mother has a cows' milk allergy. Allergies play an important part in eczema: foods such as eggs, wheat, cows' milk, oranges, and apples can be the cause of eczema, or even make it worse. For more about Eczema *see pages 202–3.*

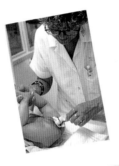

CAUTIONS AND CONTRAINDICATIONS

Diet and allergies have to be taken into consideration. It is therefore advisable to consult a qualified practitioner before starting any treatment.

🌿 **TREATMENT**
Try to identify any allergies. Avoid petroleum-based products, baby oils, and scented talcum powder. Never wash the affected areas with soap of any kind. Avoid detergent washing powders and fabric softeners.

HOMEOPATHY Apis, Graphites, Pulsatilla, Rhus tox., and Sulfur may be helpful.

HERBAL MEDICINE Marigold tea, calendula ointment, or aloe vera gel are all helpful.

AROMATHERAPY Add 12 drops of fennel, geranium, or sandalwood to 2fl oz/60ml of carrier oil.

TEETHING

Most babies begin cutting their teeth at around six months of age. It is a painful process and causes irritability, dribbling, and chewing, and sometimes a flushed cheek.

🌿 **TREATMENT**
Offer your baby something hard to chew on, or massage the gums with a clean finger.

HOMEOPATHY Infant remedies such as Chamomilla or Pulsatilla can be purchased as powders.

AROMATHERAPY Add 1 to 2 drops of camomile or lavender oil to a vaporizer and place in baby's room.

CAUTIONS AND CONTRAINDICATIONS

If the diaper rash persists it may be caused by a thrush infection, and medical advice should be sought.

AROMATHERAPY *see page 50* 🌿 HERBAL MEDICINE *see page 67* 🌿
HOMEOPATHY *see page 83* 🌿 NATUROPATHY *see page 24*

The Ailments

Childhood Diseases

OST BABIES are born with at least temporary immunity to any infectious diseases that their mothers have had. The colostrum in breast milk adds to this protection so that breast-fed babies are protected until their own immune system develops and they are better able to cope with an illness. This is why most common childhood diseases tend to affect children as they get older. Many children get through them without any form of medical intervention. If treatment is required it is necessary to assess which one is most suited to the child's symptoms. If concern about the child's health persists, seek professional advice.

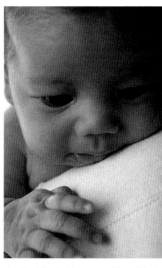

Avoid giving babies powerful antibiotics for minor ailments; save them for serious bacterial infection.

GLUE EAR

A discharge of thick yellow mucus from the ear and some loss or impairment of hearing, usually after ear or viral infections, are symptoms of this condition. Cases of glue ear have increased over the last decade or so, and some alternative therapists believe that the condition is a side effect of immunization.

❧ TREATMENT

Conventional medical treatment may include an operation to insert small drainage tubes called grommets in the affected ear. If this becomes necessary, alternative therapies such as homeopathy can help support the child before and after the operation.

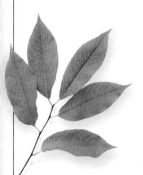

Wild cherry bark *Prunus serotina* has a powerful soothing effect on coughs.

COUGHS

Coughing helps to expel naturally congested phlegm or inhaled dust from the lungs. It may be caused by an infection or an irritant (*see page 158*).

❧ TREATMENT

Keep the child in a warm environment and offer a soothing linctus made from hot lemon juice, a teaspoonful of honey, and some glycerin (glycerol).

HERBAL MEDICINE Make an infusion of white horehound or wild cherry bark. Give half a teaspoonful three times a day.

AROMATHERAPY Add 2 to 3 drops of eucalyptus, thyme, cypress, or sandalwood oil to hot water. Use as an inhalation for 10 minutes.

DIET AND NUTRITION

Mucus-producing foods such as cows' milk and sugar are key culprits for this condition. Replace these foods with soybean milk or goats' milk, and introduce more fruit and vegetables into the diet.

HERBAL MEDICINE

Apply 2 to 3 drops of golden seal, Pulsatilla, or mullein oil three times daily to the ear.

HOMEOPATHY

Glue ear responds well to Pulsatilla 30c.

Consult a qualified practitioner/therapist for:
CRANIAL OSTEOPATHY
This can be helpful.

CAUTIONS AND CONTRAINDICATIONS

Always stay with a child during an inhalation. If a child has, or has had, eczema, do not give any homeopathic remedy in a high potency.

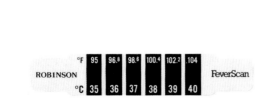

°F	95	96.8	98.6	100.4	102.2	104	
ROBINSON							FeverScan
°C	35	36	37	38	39	40	

To monitor fevers use a standard thermometer (top) for older children and a scanning type (left) that goes on the forehead for restless young babies.

Fresh lemon juice, combined with honey and glycerin is a simple but effective ingredient in a homemade linctus for children's coughs.

AROMATHERAPY *see page 50* ❧ DIETARY THERAPY *see page 74* ❧
HERBAL MEDICINE *see page 67* ❧ HOMEOPATHY *see page 83*

Colds, Croup, and Infestations

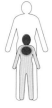

Common colds are caused by viruses, and are highly contagious. They are spread through coughing and sneezing, which, together with runny nose and sore throat, are the symptoms of the illness.

❧ TREATMENT

Ensure the child rests and drinks a lot of fluids, including hot water mixed with fresh lemon juice and a teaspoonful of honey.

DIET AND NUTRITION Offer plenty of fresh fruit and vegetables in the child's daily diet.

HERBAL MEDICINE Camomile, lemon balm, and rosehip teas will help reduce various symptoms.

HOMEOPATHY Belladonna, Pulsatilla, Natrum mur., and Euphrasia are available in drop form for children.

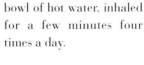

> **CAUTIONS AND CONTRAINDICATIONS**
>
> If croup persists for longer than 12 hours, or the child has difficulty breathing, call a physician immediately.

AROMATHERAPY Two drops of cinnamon oil in a bowl of hot water, inhaled for a few minutes four times a day.

CROUP

Croup usually affects children under five and manifests in a harsh barking cough with strained, heavy breathing. These symptoms are often accompanied by a high fever, irritability, and restlessness. It is caused by an inflammation of the main airways to the lungs.

❧ TREATMENT

Avoid a hot dry atmosphere by turning off the heating in the child's bedroom, but make sure the room is well ventilated. Use humidifiers if you have them.

HYDROTHERAPY Steam inhalation is a useful therapy.

HERBAL MEDICINE Make an infusion from 1 teaspoonful each of coltsfoot and vervain. Give 1 teaspoonful to a child aged under three, and 1 tablespoonful to older children, every few hours.

AROMATHERAPY Add two drops each of eucalyptus and sandalwood oils to a carrier oil and apply to the chest.

INFESTATIONS

THREADWORMS

Threadworms are one of the oldest known human infections. They usually infect the large intestine and may be visible around the anus or in the feces. They cause itching and sometimes inflammation around the anus.

TREATMENT

Threadworms are highly infectious: the whole household must be treated. Great attention should be paid to hygiene, especially before meals and after using the lavatory.

❧ **AROMATHERAPY** *An infusion of thyme may be helpful.* Consult a qualified practitioner/therapist for:

❧ **HERBAL MEDICINE** *An infusion of wormwood leaves may be prescribed.*

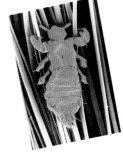

The head louse clings obstinately to hair shafts.

HEADLICE

Lice thrive on clean hair, where they lay their eggs (nits). These can be seen as tiny white flecks on individual hairs.

TREATMENT

Keep long hair tied back. If nits appear treat the whole household to prevent reinfection. Check the hair regularly for any sign of infestation.

❧ **AROMATHERAPY** *Make a mixture of ten drops each of geranium, eucalyptus, rosemary, and lavender, added to 4fl oz/10ml of almond oil. Rub into the hair and cover head with a plastic shower cap for 12 hours. Wash and comb to remove the dead nits.*

If anyone in the family picks up head lice, all members should be treated otherwise reinfestation will occur.

AROMATHERAPY *see page 50* ❧ DIETARY THERAPY *see page 74* ❧
HERBAL MEDICINE *see page 67* ❧ HOMEOPATHY *see page 83* ❧ HYDROTHERAPY *see page 26*

Infectious Diseases

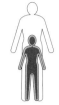

Infectious diseases spread very quickly among children. Mild bouts of diseases such as German measles or mumps early in life may be helpful as they establish immunity and prevent the child from suffering later in life when these diseases are more virulent and have a bad effect on fetal developments (German measles) or male fertility (mumps).

SORE THROAT

A virus or bacterium is usually the cause of a sore throat, which is often the first area of the body to respond to the infection. If a sore throat is recurring, or lasts for more than a few days, it may be the sign of a more serious illness and a physician should be consulted.

> ### CAUTIONS AND CONTRAINDICATIONS
>
> **WHOOPING COUGH**
> Immunization against whooping cough can be given in a course of three injections during the child's first year.
> If the child has a fever, immunization should be postponed until it has run its course. Check with your physician about other contrainidications.

◆ TREATMENT

DIET AND NUTRITION Offer fresh fruit juices, high in vitamin C. A diluted lemon juice gargle may help.

HOMEOPATHY Apis, Belladonna, or Hepar sulf. three times a day will help relieve symptoms.

HERBAL MEDICINE Give sage or thyme gargles with fresh lemon juice added.

WHOOPING COUGH (PERTUSSIS)

Caused by a bacterium, whooping cough attacks the mucous membranes that line the airways. The illness may last up to four months and can be extremely serious. Whooping cough symptoms include a "whoop", or noisy intake of breath, at the end of a cough, accompanied by a mild fever, runny nose, and loss of appetite.

> ### CAUTIONS AND CONTRAINDICATIONS
>
> **CHICKENPOX**
> Consult a physician if the child's eyes become affected, or there is high fever, excessive coughing, and vomiting. The spots will leave scars if they are scratched or infected.

◆ TREATMENT

DIET AND NUTRITION Give plenty of liquids, especially if the child is vomiting. Avoid dairy products and large meals.

HOMEOPATHY Drosera rotundifolia or Aconitum napellus will help, especially at night.

Consult a qualified practitioner/therapist for:
HERBAL MEDICINE White horehound, mullein flowers, thyme, and lavender may be prescribed.

CHICKENPOX

This highly infectious disease is caused by the herpes zoster virus. Symptoms include a rash of very itchy spots, usually on the body, which then spreads to the limbs, face, and head. The spots turn into watery blisters, which burst and after about five days form scabs. Try to avoid scratching, which spreads the infection.

◆ TREATMENT

NATUROPATHY Give plenty of fresh orange juice, lemon tea, or lemon juice sweetened with honey. Sponge the spots with tepid water. Three tablespoons of sodium bicarbonate added to a bath of lukewarm water should help ease itching.

HOMEOPATHY Rhus tox. will soothe the irritation; Antimonium tart. can help heal the scabs.

> ### CAUTIONS AND CONTRAINDICATIONS
>
> **GERMAN MEASLES**
> Avoid contact with pregnant women: German measles can damage the unborn baby, especially in early pregnancy. Immunization against German measles (MMR) is offered at between 12 and 15 months.

HERBAL MEDICINE An infusion of elderflower sponged onto the spots should relieve itching. For fever, offer yarrow, lime blossom, or meadowsweet herbal tea.

GERMAN MEASLES (RUBELLA)

Rubella is an acute viral disease whose symptoms include a slight pink rash of tiny spots, starting behind the ears or on the face and spreading down the body, and possibly watery eyes and swollen glands. *(See also page 138.)*

◆ TREATMENT

HERBAL MEDICINE A cool infusion of lavender, sponged onto the skin, should help relieve any itching.

ROSEOLA

This mild, infectious illness is similar to German measles and rarely needs treatment. It manifests in a pink rash with small spots, usually after a fever.

DIETARY THERAPY *see page 74* ◆ HERBAL MEDICINE *see page 67* ◆
HOMEOPATHY *see page 83* ◆ NATUROPATHY *see page 24*

Measles, Mumps, and Scarlet Fever

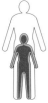

MEASLES
Caused by a virus, measles is an infectious disease. Symptoms include a high fever, a dry cough, sore eyes, and a pink rash over the entire body. White spots known as Koplik's spots may be visible on the inside of the cheeks a few days before the rash appears.

✑ TREATMENT
Ensure the child rests, and give additional fluids.

HOMEOPATHY Apis, Euphrasia, Sulfur, and Gelsemium should help relieve symptoms.

HERBAL MEDICINE Give an infusion of yarrow or elderflower with camomile added, every four hours. A cool infusion of lavender, sponged onto the skin, helps to relieve itching.

> **CAUTIONS AND CONTRAINDICATIONS**
> **MEASLES**
> Measles should always be reported to a physician even if treatment is not required. Immunization against measles (MMR) is offered at between 12 and 15 months.

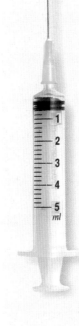

IMMUNIZATION
Alternative healthcare professionals are usually cautious about immunization against childhood diseases. Some believe that by giving tiny doses, about one tenth of the usual amount, complications can be avoided. Some homeopaths offer immunization counseling, and most will give alternative medical support should you decide not to immunize your child against certain diseases.

HOMEOPATHY *After the immunization, give Aconite for shock and Arnica for bruising.*

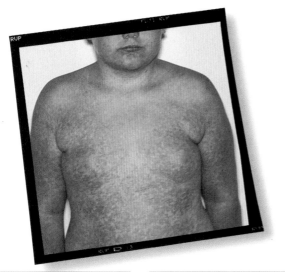

A typical measles rash spread across the upper chest and abdomen.

MUMPS
Caused by a virus, mumps is an infectious disease that mainly affects children over two years. Symptoms of mumps are swelling of the glands in front of the ear, and earache.

✑ TREATMENT
HOMEOPATHY Aconite, Belladonna, Rhus tox. and, Lachesis will help relieve symptoms. Jaborandi and Phytolacca are specifics for swollen glands.

HERBAL MEDICINE Infusions of yarrow or elderflower are helpful. Dandelion helps the liver to expel toxins.

SCARLET FEVER
This is a highly infectious, but rare, disease caused by the streptococcus bacterium. Symptoms include a sore throat, followed by a rash, vomiting, and fever.

✑ TREATMENT
Consult a qualified practitioner/therapist for:
HOMEOPATHY Remedies need to be prescribed for each stage of the disease.

> **CAUTIONS AND CONTRAINDICATIONS**
> **MUMPS**
> Consult a physician if symptoms are severe, or if the neck is stiff. Mumps measles, and rubella (MMR) immunization is offered at between 12 and 15 months.

> **CAUTIONS AND CONTRAINDICATIONS**
> **SCARLET FEVER**
> Scarlet fever is a serious disease. Notify a physician if it is suspected: antibiotics may be necessary. Keep the child in isolation for seven days from the start of the rash.

HERBAL MEDICINE *see page 67* ✑ HOMEOPATHY *see page 83*

FIRST AID • Minor Injuries

A N EMERGENCY is normally assumed to need expert medical help, and this is often the case. But sometimes there just isn't the time to wait for the experts, and if no action is taken it may be too late. On the other hand, there are plenty of less serious emergency situations that, with a little knowledge, most people can take care of perfectly safely and effectively themselves.

This section describes the many safe and effective self-help treatments and remedies for the most common emergency situations. A "Caution" indicates when you should get expert help as soon as possible. The most frequently used self-help remedies are listed below.

AN ALTERNATIVE FIRST AID KIT

The remedies listed below are highly effective for a number of common conditions and minor accidents.

REMEDY	CONDITION
Arnica cream	Bruises
Bach Rescue Remedy	Shock, stings, scalds, fainting, motion sickness, grief
Calendula ointment/cream	Stings, minor cuts, blisters
Essential oils	
Lavender	Jetlag, blisters, sunburn
Peppermint	Motion sickness
Rosemary	Sprains, jetlag, mental fatigue
Homeopathic tablets	
Arnica 6c	Bruises, nosebleeds, sprains, jetlag
Arsenicum alb. 6c	Diarrhea, fatigue, fainting, stomachache
Apis 6c	Insect bites, prickly heat
Belladonna 6c	Heatstroke, sunstroke
Carbo veg. 6c	Stomachache (caused by rich foods), fainting
Ledum 6c	Bruises, stings
Nux vomica 6c	Nausea, hangovers, stomachache, motion sickness
Phosphorus 6c	Nosebleeds, stomachache
Hypericum tincture/lotion	Bites (tincture), burns, blisters
Natrum mur. biochemic salts	Blisters, stings
Vitamins and minerals	
Vitamin C (1g tablets)	The common cold and influenza, hangovers
Vitamin E cream	Sunburn
Zinc (15mg tablets)	The common cold and influenza
Witch hazel	Bruises, stings, sunburn

NOSEBLEEDS

N osebleeds are a common form of bleeding since the blood vessels in the nose are very delicate. They are most often brought on by dry winter air. Other causes include high blood pressure, a severe common cold, or even a minor knock to the nose. They can be serious, especially in the elderly.

TREATMENT

Sit the person down with their head bent forward to prevent the blood from running down the back of the throat. Pinch nose firmly around the nostrils and hold position for 10 to15 minutes. Apply an icepack or cold compress over the bridge of the nose. To prevent recurrence, he or she should refrain from blowing the nose for a few hours to enable healing to start.

ACUPRESSURE *Press down on the area between the nose and the center of the top lip for up to one minute.*

HOMEOPATHY *Use Phosphorus 6c to speed up the clotting process. Use the same potency of Arnica if the nose has been hit. To prevent nosebleeds at night, use Sulfur 6c.*

HERBAL MEDICINE *To stem the flow of frequent nosebleeds, pour boiling water onto 3 teaspoonfuls of dried nettle and mix for ten minutes. Take three times a day.*

DIET AND NUTRITION *Strengthen blood vessels within the nose by increasing the amount of vitamin C-rich foods you eat (see pages 28 and 76). A daily dose of beet concentrate and 2g of vitamin C should also limit recurrent nosebleeds.*

> **CAUTIONS AND CONTRAINDICATIONS**
> If there is serious bleeding, call for medical help immediately.

ACUPRESSURE *see page 94* • DIETARY THERAPY *see page 74*
HERBAL MEDICINE *see page 67* • HOMEOPATHY *see page 83*

Cuts and Bruises

CUTS
Most minor bleeding can be treated effectively using self-help methods.

☙ TREATMENT
Apply firm pressure over the cut or wound to staunch the flow of blood. Clean the wound with warm water.

HERBAL MEDICINE Apply calendula ointment. Alternatively, douse the cut with calendula tincture.

BRUISES
Bruising occurs where there is bleeding under the skin, making the area painful and blue in color. If the skin has not been broken, follow the instructions given under the therapies below.

☙ TREATMENT
Place an icepack or cold facecloth over the affected area, applying light pressure for at least ten minutes.

HERBAL MEDICINE Apply a cold compress soaked in a comfrey infusion. Equally, comfrey can be used as a cream. Aloe vera gel will speed healing.

HOMEOPATHY Arnica is excellent for bruising. Take a tablet of 6c strength every hour up to four times a day, or apply as a cream. You can also apply a cold compress of diluted mother tincture. If the bruising does not disappear quickly, take Ledum 6c three times a day for four days. (It can also be used for puncture wounds.) Use Hypericum for severe bruising. When bones under the bruised region feel sore, Symphytum 6c is recommended. Ruta grav., or Bellis per. are also helpful here. For a black eye, Lachesis is the best remedy.

> **CAUTIONS AND CONTRAINDICATIONS**
>
> If the injured area is swollen, painful to use and/or misshapen, a broken bone may well be the cause. Call for immediate medical assistance.

DIET AND NUTRITION Naturopaths recommend an increase in vitamin K intake for those who bruise easily. A good way to achieve this is by eating 6oz/150g of yogurt a day. Fresh pineapple juice and green vegetables can also quicken the healing process.

Fractures and Sprains

FRACTURES
Fractures normally result from a hard blow or fall.

☙ TREATMENT
Support the injured area in whichever position it is found, and prepare a simple splint if appropriate.

HOMEOPATHY Take Arnica 6c or Calcarea 6c for pain relief. Eupatorium perf. can also help.

SPRAINS
Sprains affect ligaments rather than bones and can take several weeks to heal due to their poor blood supply. If serious, sprains produce similar symptoms to fractures.

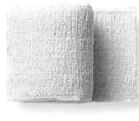

A crepe bandage will support a joint after a minor sprain.

☙ TREATMENT
Apply an icepack to the injured area, and bind appropriately.

HOMEOPATHY Take Arnica 6c (every half-hour, up to four doses), and Ruta grav. 6c (three times daily for a week).

AROMATHERAPY Add four drops of rosemary and sweet marjoram oils to a vessel of water, deep enough to immerse the injured area in. Keep submerged for around 15 minutes. Soak a cold compress in the same mixture. Hold it in place around injury, with Saran wrap, for several hours.

HYDROTHERAPY Treat affected area with a cold compress or icepack, then elevate and rest injured joint.

MASSAGE Concentrate on the muscles surrounding the injured area, working in toward the joint as it heals.

Consult a qualified practitioner/therapist for:
ACUPUNCTURE This can help relieve pain.

OSTEOPATHY OR CHIROPRACTIC Either of these may be helpful for more serious sprains.

> **SPLINT**
>
> Bring undamaged leg together with broken one, ensuring padding is placed between legs. Secure them together, tying bandages either side of the break.

ACUPUNCTURE *see page 90* ☙ AROMATHERAPY *see page 50* ☙ CHIROPRACTIC *see page 39* ☙
DIETARY THERAPY *see page 74* ☙ HERBAL MEDICINE *see page 67* ☙ HOMEOPATHY *see page 83* ☙
HYDROTHERAPY *see page 26* ☙ MASSAGE *see page 48* ☙ OSTEOPATHY *see page 42*

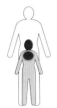

Burns and Scalds

BURNS

Burns are caused by excessive exposure to dry heat – for example, fire, electricity, or corrosive substances. First assess the severity of the burn. If it covers a small area of unbroken skin smaller than half the size of the victim's palm and only the surface layers, it is minor and can be treated as follows:

☙ TREATMENT

Place burned area under cold, running water for at least ten minutes. Do not apply ointments, butter, or other lotions to soothe the burn. Cover with a clean dressing.

HOMEOPATHY Mix ten drops of Hypericum in a glass of cold water and pour over wound.

HERBAL MEDICINE Place an ice-pack over burn for ten minutes, then apply fresh aloe vera.

SCALDS

Scalds are injuries resulting from wet heat – for example, corrosive/boiling liquids or steam. Only use self-help methods for minor injuries.

☙ TREATMENT

Same as for Burns (above).

BACH FLOWER REMEDIES Take a few drops of Bach Rescue Remedy in a glass of water.

SUNSTROKE/HEATSTROKE

Symptoms include headaches, dizziness, high temperature, and higher pulse, causing restlessness, and the possibility of circulatory collapse.

☙ PREVENTION

As with sunburn, take precautions to avoid the harmful effects of the sun.

☙ TREATMENT

Place sufferer in a cool room and wrap them in a sheet soaked in cool water. Use an electric fan to direct cold air toward the person, or fan manually. Body temperature

> **CAUTIONS AND CONTRAINDICATIONS**
>
> Seek urgent medical help for extensive deep injuries. Burns to the face and hands may require specialist advice.
> For advice on treatment of sunburn see *Travel First Aid, page 261*.

Gel from the aloe vera plant soothes burns and scalds.

should drop. Emergency medical help is required if body temperature fails to drop to normal levels: heat stroke is life-threatening.

HOMEOPATHY For a throbbing headache with high skin temperature take Belladonna 6c. If sufferer is also experiencing dizziness, take Glonoin 6c every 15 minutes, up to four doses. Use Cuprum if there is cramp and pallor.

PRICKLY HEAT

This condition often occurs when people are exposed to higher temperatures than they are used to. Symptoms include red, blotchy skin that becomes itchy in certain areas.

☙ TREATMENT

AROMATHERAPY Mix one drop of essential oil of sandalwood and four of lavender with 1fl oz/30ml of calendula carrier oil to make a soothing lotion.

DIET AND NUTRITION Increase intake of vitamin C to at least 500mg.

HOMEOPATHY Urtica 6c, Rhus tox. 6c, and Apis 6c all help. Take every 15 minutes, up to four doses as necessary. Repeat if required.

HERBAL MEDICINE Pour a mug of boiling water on to 4 teaspoonfuls of dried chickweed. Infuse for 15 minutes, leave to cool, then apply to the affected areas.

> **CAUTIONS AND CONTRAINDICATIONS**
>
> Babies and young children need particular care in hot weather. Make sure the head and neck are covered at all times and use sun creams with a high SPF (over 20) or total sunblock. Give plenty of fluids to drink.

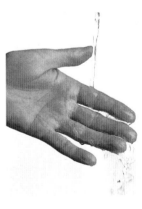

Run cold water over the burned area as quickly as possible after the accident to cool the skin and prevent further damage.

AROMATHERAPY *see page 50* ☙ BACH FLOWER REMEDIES *see page 86* ☙
DIETARY THERAPY *see page 74* ☙ HERBAL MEDICINE *see page 67* ☙ HOMEOPATHY *see page 83*

Bites and Stings

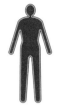

BITES

Bites from most domestic and farm animals are harmless but you should keep tetanus injections up to date if you come into contact with many animals.

⁓ TREATMENT

HOMEOPATHY For minor bites use Hypericum ointment. Pain and swelling can be eased by taking Apis 6c or Staphysagria.

STINGS

Stings may come from plants, insects, or fish.

⁓ TREATMENT

Apply calomine lotion.

NATUROPATHY Bee stings are acidic, wasp stings alkaline. Neutralize bee stings by bathing affected area in a mixture of 2 teaspoonfuls of sodium bicarbonate per cup of water. Dab a wasp sting with lemon juice or vinegar. Calendula ointment can reduce swelling. Witch hazel relieves symptoms.

HOMEOPATHY Use tincture of pyrethrum as a lotion.

BACH FLOWER REMEDIES Apply Bach Rescue Remedy as an ointment.

CAUTIONS AND CONTRAINDICATIONS

Insect stings can cause anaphylactic shock (*see page 159*). This is an extreme allergic reaction and calls for immediate medical assistance since it can cause coma leading to death. Apis 6c every ten minutes will help dampen the allergic reaction until help arrives.

CAUTIONS AND CONTRAINDICATIONS

Bites from creatures in the wild can often be extremely dangerous and expert medical help should always be sought as soon as possible. Even domestic and farm animal bites can be serious if the bite is deep enough to cause heavy bleeding, and medical help should be sought here too. In the United States, there is the additional danger of rabies from dog bites.

AROMATHERAPY Apply lavender oil and/or tea tree oil to the injured area every hour until symptoms subside.

An onion cut in half and rubbed on the area will soothe stung skin.

JELLYFISH STINGS

Stings from jellyfish may be more serious than insect stings, but should only cause painful burning and swelling. If the person stung goes into shock (*see page 159*), get medical help immediately.

⁓ TREATMENT

Scrape away remaining tentacles, but not with your hand. Treat injured area as for insect stings. A hot bath 100°–102°F/ 38°–39°C) is a good way to inactivate the toxins in jellyfish stings.

HOMEOPATHY To avoid a severe reaction take Apis 30c every hour until sting subsides. Ledum or Calendula can also help.

Yellow dock *Rumex crispus* is the effective folk remedy for nettle stings.

HOW TO PREVENT INSECT BITES AND STINGS

ALL INSECTS

⁓ **AROMATHERAPY** *Mix five drops of essential oil of eucalyptus or geranium in a cup of water and rub on skin.*

⁓ **HOMEOPATHY** *Ledum 6c serves a dual purpose. Taken twice a day, it helps prevent stings. If already stung, the same dose taken more frequently will relieve symptoms.*

⁓ **DIET AND NUTRITION** *Vitamin B1 (thiamine) repels insects when secreted from bodily pores. Take 100mg three times a day. In the same way, 60mg of zinc a day should keep insects away.*

⁓ **NATUROPATHY** *The odor of strong garlic can repel insects.*

MOSQUITOES

Oils, ointments, roll-ons, or sprays containing citrus juice, mint, and artemesia are particularly effective as repellents, as is cider vinegar. Apply to any exposed area of skin, particularly outside on warm evenings. At the same time, avoid wearing perfume, aftershave, or dark or colored clothing, all of which attract mosquitoes.

AROMATHERAPY *see page 50*
HOMEOPATHY *see page 83*

BACH FLOWER REMEDIES *see page 86*
NATUROPATHY *see page 24*

The Ailments

Emergencies • Breathing and Choking

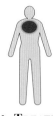

HICCUPS (OR HICCOUGHS)

Hiccups are caused by involuntary spasms of the large muscle (diaphragm) beneath the ribcage.

❧ TREATMENT

Several well-known methods allegedly stop short-term bouts of hiccuping, including holding your breath, drinking a glass of water from the upper rim of a glass, breathing into a paper bag (but for no longer than three minutes), and giving the sufferer a sudden shock.

HERBAL MEDICINE Sip lemon balm or peppermint tea.

TRADITIONAL CHINESE MEDICINE Ginger, rhubarb and berilla stems.

Consult a qualified practitioner/therapist for:
ACUPUNCTURE Recommended for long-term bouts.

CHOKING

Choking results from an obstruction in the throat that prevents the sufferer from breathing normally. It is usually a piece of food, but with babies and young children it could be a small toy or coin.

❧ TREATMENT

A firm slap on the back can dislodge food or other soft obstructions. Ask the person to bend forward, head lower than chest, and then give five sharp smacks with the heel of your hand between the shoulder blades. Repeat if necessary. If the obstruction is persistent an abdominal thrust should be used: place arms around sufferer from behind. With one hand form a fist. Hold the other hand over it and squeeze rapidly inward and upward, against underside of ribcage, several times. This maneuver should not be used on babies. More information is given in the box above.

CHOKING

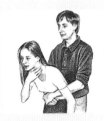

If back slapping has not dislodged the object, stand behind the person, clench your fist, put your arms around her and grasp your fist with your other hand. Pull inward and upward, the object should shoot out of the mouth.

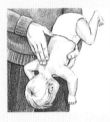

If a baby is choking, the method is gentler. Lay the baby along your arm, supporting the head and neck. Give five light slaps on the back between the shoulder blades. Hook the object out of the baby's mouth with your fingers if necessary.

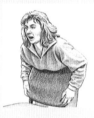

If you are choking yourself and there is no one around to help, find a high straight-backed chair. Lower yourself so that your stomach rests on the chair rail. Push down so that your diaphragm is pushed up and the force expels the obstruction.

Breathing into a paper bag two or three times can help cure hiccups.

CAUTIONS AND CONTRAINDICATIONS

HICCUPS
Seek medical help if hiccups persist for longer than 24 hours.

CAUTIONS AND CONTRAINDICATIONS

CHOKING
If victim does not resume normal breathing once obstruction is cleared, initiate resuscitation (see page 259), and seek medical help.

ACUPUNCTURE *see page* 90 ❧ HERBAL MEDICINE *see page* 67 ❧ TRADITIONAL CHINESE MEDICINE *see page* 30

Resuscitation and Recovery

In emergency situations it is essential to know how to give resuscitation in order to help someone to recover from breathing and heartbeat failure. In any case, always call for an ambulance or physician as soon as you can – the following measures are not a substitute for full emergency treatment.

THE RESUSCITATION PROCEDURE

If the casualty is unconscious, first check if they are breathing by listening and looking to see if the chest is rising or falling. If they are not, you must initiate resuscitation, which is a combination of artificial respiration and chest compression. If possible, use some kind of protection over your mouth to guard against infection while performing artificial respiration. Keep the casualty's head tilted back throughout and continue to remove obstructions from the mouth as they appear.

Artificial respiration helps the casualty to regain independent breathing. Chest compression should help to restore the heartbeat and is effective in maintaining sufficient circulation to protect the brain from death. Check the pulse every minute *(see page 260)*.

THE RECOVERY POSITION

Once you have established that the unconscious person is breathing and the heart is beating, place him or her in the recovery position. This allows the jaw and tongue to fall forward, keeping the airway clear and allowing any vomit or other obstructions to drain out freely. Check for broken bones and immobilize them before moving the person into the recovery position.

❀ Kneel beside casualty, lift the head and tilt the chin to open the airway, as for resuscitation. Straighten the legs; place the arm nearest to you at right angles to the body and bend it upward at the elbow. The palm of the hand should be uppermost.

❀ Lift the arm farthest from you and bring it across the chest. Hold the hand, palm outward against the cheek nearest to you.

❀ Holding the hands in place with one of your own, grasp the thigh farthest from you with your other hand; pull the knee up keeping the foot flat on the ground.

❀ Pull the thigh to roll the person over toward you onto his or her side. The hand pressed against the cheek will support the head.

❀ Tilt the head back again to clear the airway. Adjust the supporting hand if necessary.

❀ Adjust the upper leg. Both hip and knee should be bent at right angles.

RESUSCITATION PROCEDURE

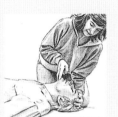

Clear the airways. The head should be tilted back and the jaw lifted forward to prevent the throat from being blocked by the tongue falling back.

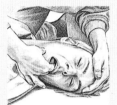

Turn the head to one side to remove any vomit, mucus or other visible obstructions from the mouth. Use your fingers to remove any obstructions from the mouth and throat.

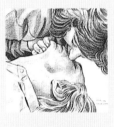

Tilt the head back, and place one hand against the chin to keep the mouth closed. Take a deep breath, securely place your mouth around the nose and breathe into it.

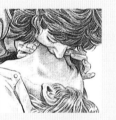

To initiate mouth-to-mouth respiration, clasp the nose shut with one hand. Breathe into the open mouth. Check that the chest is rising. Repeat breathing pattern 12 to 14 times a minute.

Locate the breastbone. Place the heel of the hand on chest, 1¼in/30mm from bottom of breastbone. Push down on the chest, then let it rise. For every 15 compressions, repeat artificial respiration for two breaths.

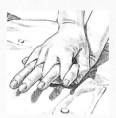

This shows the hand position for chest compression. Spread and raise fingers of one hand. Interlock the fingers of the other hand between them and clench it. One hand will be on top of the other, both palms facing down.

COMA *see page 218* ❧ HEART ATTACK *see page 168*

Fainting and Shock

A faint is caused by a sudden fall in blood supply to the brain, generally caused by a reflex slowing of the heart, which may be caused by emotional upset or distress. This is not serious, providing you do not injure yourself as you fall. Clinical shock, a physical response, is the result of a severe injury.

FAINTING

Fainting may be caused by shock, a sudden drop in blood pressure or a reduction in the body's blood sugar level. A faint feeling – dizziness, feeling cold and clammy – may be experienced without losing consciousness.

TREATMENT

Lay the patient down with feet raised slightly above the body. This increases the flow of blood back to the brain.

HOMEOPATHY Aconite can help someone who faints as a result of shock. Fainting from lack of air requires Carbo veg., and Arsenicum alb. is used in cases of fainting through exhaustion or cold.

ACUPRESSURE Gently stimulate the acupressure point two thirds of the way up between the top lip and the nose, using your fingernail.

BACH FLOWER REMEDIES Offer a few drops of Rescue Remedy in water or apply directly onto the tongue as soon as the patient comes round.

After fainting, lie down flat and raise the feet higher than the head to promote the flow of blood back to the top half of the body.

SHOCK

There are a number of reasons for someone going into clinical shock. The symptoms are similar to fainting, which is often a part of severe shock. Shock victims will look gray, pale, and clammy, and they may be incoherent.

TREATMENT

Put casualty in the position described for fainting. Loosen clothing to allow easy breathing, but ensure casualty is kept warm. Keep talking, offering reassurance.

CAUTIONS AND CONTRAINDICATIONS

Urgent medical assistance is needed when shock is brought about by a physical ordeal.

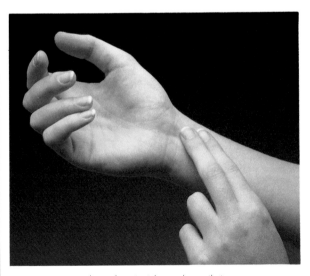
Learn how to take a pulse so that you can monitor the heartbeat of a person in shock.

PULSE AND BREATHING RATES

ADULTS Average 50–100 heartbeats and 12 breaths a minute.

CHILDREN Average 90–100 heartbeats and 20–40 breaths a minute.

BABIES Average 120–140 heartbeats and 20–40 breaths a minute.

HOW TO TAKE A PULSE

Use your fingers, not thumb. Place them either on inside of patient's wrist – 1in/25mm from bottom of hand and ¹/₂in/12.5mm in from side of wrist – or on neck (either side of windpipe, halfway up toward jawline).

Time pulse for 30 seconds. Leave fingers in place and time number of breaths for another 30 seconds.

Double both measurements for minute rates. Careful observation while measuring breathing rates is required because breathing patterns differ under scrutiny.

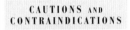

ACUPRESSURE *see page 94* • BACH FLOWER REMEDIES *see page 86* • HOMEOPATHY *see page 83*

Travel First Aid

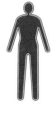

THE REMEDIES below are recommended for problems particularly associated with traveling and vacations.

MOTION SICKNESS

The sensation of motion when traveling affects the balance of the inner ear and can result in feelings of nausea, dizziness, and anxiety.

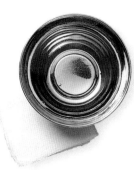

Cold water, with drops of lavender oil, soothes sunburned skin.

✌ TREATMENT

ACUPRESSURE Exert pressure using thumb on inside of either wrist, 1½ in/38mm up from bottom of hand. Massage firmly on this spot for a minute, then repeat on other wrist. Commercially-produced wristbands with nodules designed to rub on these exact spots are widely available and very effective.

BACH FLOWER REMEDIES Take Bach Rescue Remedy before and during journey.

AROMATHERAPY Essential oils of peppermint and ginger can be used to relieve symptoms. Add four drops to a lotion and rub into the chest. Further drops sniffed from a handkerchief may ease nausea.

HERBAL MEDICINE Either take two ginger root capsules half an hour before traveling or chew a piece of peeled ginger root during the journey.

HOMEOPATHY There are several measures to suit various travel ailments: Petroleum, Nux vomica, and Cocculus for vomiting and nausea; Tabacum for sweating and giddinesss; and Borax for anxiety. Sepia 6c may ease nausea brought on by the smell of food.

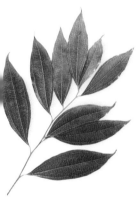

The Indian cockle, *Cocculus indicus*, supplies one of the homeopathic remedies for travel sickness.

JETLAG

An extra problem caused by flying to faraway places for exotic vacations is jetlag. Travel through different time zones confuses the body's natural day/night rhythm and can result in tiredness, loss of concentration, and general disorientation over when to eat or sleep.

✌ TREATMENT

AROMATHERAPY Use lavender to relax, or rosemary or lemon to stimulate and awaken.

HOMEOPATHY On arrival, take Cocculus 6c three times a day for three days. Arnica 6c, taken every three hours during the journey, then twice a day for three days on arrival, also helps.

Consult a qualified practitioner/therapist for:
CRANIAL ELECTRICAL STIMULATION This is occasionally used as part of craniosacral therapy.

SUNBURN

Sunburn results when the skin is overexposed to UV rays. Treat blistered or extremely reddened skin as for Burns, *see page 256.*

✌ PREVENTION

Sunburn can usually be avoided by taking some obvious precautions:
❉ keep out of the sun during the hottest part of the day
❉ build up your exposure slowly, especially if you have fair skin
❉ protect your skin with sunblock and suntan lotions
❉ cover your head and shoulders.

✌ TREATMENT

HYDROTHERAPY Take a cold bath or shower to soothe skin. Mix oatmeal, baking soda, or vinegar to water.

HERBAL MEDICINE Apply aloe vera gel to soothe and aid healing. Alternatively, bathe the affected area in cold water then add two drops of lavender oil, or make a cold compress of calendula infusion.

Ginger root *Zingiber officinale*, chewed raw, can prevent the onset of motion sickness.

> **CAUTIONS AND CONTRAINDICATIONS**
>
> In severe cases of sunburn, medical help should be sought. *(For information on sunstroke, see page 256.)*

NATUROPATHY Soak in cold water; apply vitamin E cream when dry. Eyes can be soothed by lying down and placing a slice of cucumber on each one for 15 minutes.

ACUPRESSURE *see page 94* ✌ AROMATHERAPY *see page 50* ✌ BACH FLOWER REMEDIES *see page 86* ✌
HERBAL MEDICINE *see page 67* ✌ HOMEOPATHY *see page 83* ✌ HYDROTHERAPY *see page 26* ✌ NATUROPATHY *see page 24*

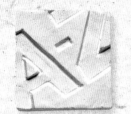

A–Z OF AILMENTS AND THERAPIES

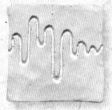

GLOSSARY

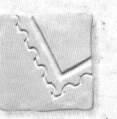

USEFUL ADDRESSES

FURTHER READING

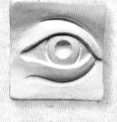

INDEX

PART THREE

QUICK REFERENCE LIBRARY

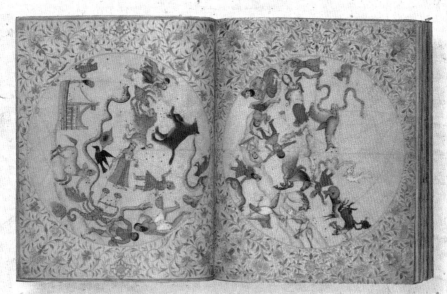

A–Z of Ailments • 1

This is a directory of common ailments and conditions. Each ailment is followed by a page number or numbers locating it in the book and is then followed by an alphabetical list of therapies that may be useful. Major therapies are covered in the first part of the book; for more information *see the A–Z of Therapies on pages 270–5.*

ACNE 200: useful therapies include acupuncture; diet and nutrition; herbal medicine; homeopathy

ADDICTIONS 226: useful therapies include acupuncture; aromatherapy; counseling; hypnotherapy; massage; meditation; psychotherapy; self-help groups; yoga

AIDS 136–7: useful therapies include acupuncture; aromatherapy; chi kung; counseling; diet and nutrition; herbal medicine; homeopathy; hypnotherapy; massage; meditation; reflexology; t'ai chi; Traditional Chinese Medicine; visualization; yoga

ALLERGIES 158–9: useful therapies include acupuncture; Alexander Technique; herbal medicine; homeopathy; reflexology; relaxation therapies

ALZHEIMER'S DISEASE 194: useful therapies include diet and nutrition; herbal medicine; homeopathy

ANEMIA 166: useful therapies include acupuncture; diet and nutrition; Traditional Chinese Medicine

ANGINA 168: useful therapies include acupuncture; *see also* **ATHEROSCLEROSIS** 169

ANKYLOSING SPONDYLITIS (AS) 177: useful therapies include acupuncture; herbal medicine; homeopathy; hydrotherapy; massage; osteopathy; TENS

ANOREXIA NERVOSA 225 *see also* **BULIMIA NERVOSA**

ANXIETY AND INSOMNIA 221: useful therapies include acupuncture; Alexander Technique; aromatherapy; Bach Flower Remedies; biofeedback; counseling; diet and nutrition; herbal medicine; homeopathy; hypnotherapy; massage; meditation; relaxation; visualization; yoga

APPENDICITIS 212: useful therapies include Bach Flower Remedies; homeopathy

ARTERIOSCLEROSIS *see* **ATHEROSCLEROSIS**

ASTHMA 160: useful therapies include acupuncture; Alexander Technique; aromatherapy; Bach Flower Remedies; chiropractic; diet and nutrition; herbal medicine; homeopathy; hydrotherapy; massage; osteopathy; reflexology

ATHEROSCLEROSIS 169: useful therapies include chelation therapy; counseling; diet and nutrition; herbal medicine; massage; relaxation therapies; yoga

AUTISM 230: useful therapies include behavioral therapy; diet and nutrition; massage; osteopathy; relaxation therapies

BACK PAIN/BACKACHE 174: useful therapies include acupuncture; chiropractic; hydrotherapy; massage; osteopathy; TENS

BACTERIAL INFECTIONS 130, 240: useful therapies include aromatherapy; homeopathy; Oriental herbal medicine

BACTERIAL VAGINOSIS 240: useful therapies include diet and nutrition; homeopathy; naturopathy

BAD POSTURE 176: useful therapies include Alexander Technique; chiropractic; diet and nutrition; osteopathy; Rolfing; yoga

BALDNESS 197: useful therapies include aromatherapy; diet and nutrition; herbal medicine

BEDWETTING 248: useful therapies include counseling; herbal medicine; homeopathy

BITES 257: useful therapies include aromatherapy; diet and nutrition; homeopathy

BLISTERS 198: useful therapies include aromatherapy; herbal medicine; homeopathy

BOILS 200: useful therapies include diet and nutrition; herbal medicine

BRONCHITIS/WHEEZING 157: useful therapies include aromatherapy; herbal medicine; homeopathy; Traditional Chinese Medicine

BRUISES 255: useful therapies include diet and nutrition; herbal medicine; homeopathy

BULIMIA NERVOSA 225: useful therapies include acupuncture; art therapy; counseling; dance therapy; group therapy; massage; psychotherapy; Traditional Chinese Medicine

BUNIONS/CORNS 185: useful therapies include diet and nutrition; homeopathy; hydrotherapy; massage; naturopathy

BURNS 256: useful therapies include aromatherapy; herbal medicine; homeopathy

CANCER 140–1: useful therapies include acupressure; acupuncture; aromatherapy; art, music, and drama therapy; Ayurvedic medicine; counseling; diet and nutrition; herbal medicine; homeopathy; hydrotherapy; hypnotherapy; macrobiotics; massage; meditation; naturopathy; psychotherapy; reflexology; relaxation therapies; t'ai chi; visualization; yoga

CARPAL TUNNEL SYNDROME 181: useful therapies include acupressure; acupuncture; diet and nutrition; hydrotherapy; osteopathy

CATARACTS 146–7: useful therapies include diet and nutrition; homeopathy

CATARRH 149: useful therapies include diet and nutrition; herbal medicine; homeopathy

CELIAC DISEASE 207: useful therapies include acupuncture; diet and nutrition; herbal medicine; homeopathy

CHICKENPOX 252: useful therapies include herbal medicine; homeopathy; naturopathy

CHILBLAINS 165: useful therapies include diet and nutrition; herbal medicine; homeopathy; hydrotherapy; naturopathy; Traditional Chinese Medicine; see also POOR CIRCULATION

CHOKING 258

CHRONIC FATIGUE SYNDROME (ME) 134–5: useful therapies include acupuncture; aromatherapy; counseling; diet and nutrition; herbal medicine; homeopathy; hypnotherapy; meditation; reflexology; relaxation; Traditional Chinese Medicine; yoga

COLD SORES 132: useful therapies include aromatherapy; diet and nutrition; herbal medicine; homeopathy

COLIC 248: useful therapies include aromatherapy; cranial osteopathy; diet and nutrition; herbal medicine; homeopathy

COLITIS 213: useful therapies include acupressure; acupuncture; diet and nutrition; herbal medicine; homeopathy

COMMON COLD AND INFLUENZA 132, 251: useful therapies include acupressure; acupuncture; aromatherapy; diet and nutrition; herbal medicine; homeopathy; naturopathy; Traditional Chinese Medicine

CONJUNCTIVITIS 146: useful therapies include herbal medicine; homeopathy

CONSTIPATION 209: useful therapies include acupuncture; herbal medicine; massage; reflexology

CORNS see BUNIONS

COUGHS 156, 250: useful therapies include acupressure; acupuncture; aromatherapy; diet and nutrition; herbal medicine; homeopathy; naturopathy

CRADLE CAP 248: useful therapies include aromatherapy; herbal medicine; naturopathy

CROHN'S DISEASE 213: useful therapies include aromatherapy; biofeedback; massage; meditation; yoga

CROUP 251: useful therapies include aromatherapy; herbal medicine; homeopathy; hydrotherapy

CUTS 255: useful therapies include herbal medicine; homeopathy

CYSTITIS AND URINARY TRACT INFECTION 216: useful therapies include acupressure; acupuncture; aromatherapy; diet and nutrition; herbal medicine; homeopathy

DANDRUFF 197: useful therapies include herbal medicine; naturopathy

DEAFNESS 148: useful therapies include acupuncture; homeopathy; naturopathy

DEPRESSION 228–9: useful therapies include aromatherapy; Bach Flower Remedies; cognitive therapy; color therapy; counseling; expression therapies; massage; psychotherapy

DIABETES 218–19: useful therapies include aromatherapy; autogenics; biofeedback; diet and nutrition; homeopathy; hypnotherapy; meditation; yoga

DIAPER RASH 249: useful therapies include aromatherapy; diet and nutrition; herbal medicine; homeopathy; naturopathy

DIARRHEA 209: useful therapies include acupressure; diet and nutrition; herbal medicine; homeopathy; naturopathy; Traditional Chinese Medicine

DIVERTICULITIS 212: useful therapies include acupuncture; diet and nutrition; herbal medicine; massage; reflexology

DROPPED ARCHES/FOOT PAIN 185: useful therapies include chiropractic; hydrotherapy; massage; osteopathy

DYSMENORRHEA (PAINFUL MENSTRUAL PROBLEMS) 244: useful therapies include aromatherapy; diet and nutrition; herbal medicine; homeopathy; shiatsu; yoga

EARACHE 148: useful therapies include acupuncture; aromatherapy; herbal medicine; homeopathy; osteopathy; reflexology

ECZEMA/DERMATITIS 202–3, 249: useful therapies include acupuncture; aromatherapy; diet and nutrition; herbal medicine; homeopathy; hydrotherapy; Traditional Chinese Medicine

EDEMA 214: useful therapies include acupressure; aromatherapy; herbal medicine; massage

EMPHYSEMA 162: useful therapies include acupuncture; aromatherapy; herbal medicine; homeopathy; reflexology

ERECTION PROBLEMS 235: useful therapies include aromatherapy; herbal medicine; hydrotherapy

EYESIGHT PROBLEMS 146: useful therapies include Bates method; homeopathy; yoga

FAINTING 260: useful therapies include acupressure; Bach Flower Remedies; homeopathy

FECAL INCONTINENCE 209: useful therapies include acupressure; diet and nutrition; homeopathy; yoga

FIBROSITIS 182: useful therapies include acupressure; acupuncture; aromatherapy; biochemic tissue salts; chiropractic; diet and nutrition; healing; herbal medicine; homeopathy; hypnotherapy; massage; myotherapy; osteopathy; Rolfing; Rosen method; shiatsu

A–Z of Ailments • 2

FLATULENCE 208: useful therapies include diet and nutrition; herbal medicine; reflexology

FRACTURES 255: useful therapies include acupuncture; homeopathy; osteopathy; reflexology

FRIGIDITY (LOSS OF SEXUAL DESIRE) 243: useful therapies include aromatherapy; counseling; Rolfing

FROZEN SHOULDER 180: useful therapies include acupressure; acupuncture; aromatherapy; chiropractic; herbal medicine; homeopathy; hydrotherapy; massage; osteopathy; TENS

FUNGAL INFECTIONS 130: Athlete's foot 199: useful therapies include aromatherapy; herbal medicine; homeopathy; Candida/thrush 240: useful therapies include aromatherapy; diet and nutrition; herbal medicine; homeopathy; naturopathy; Traditional Chinese Medicine; Ringworm 199: useful therapies include aromatherapy; herbal medicine; homeopathy

GALLSTONES 214: useful therapies include acupuncture; aromatherapy; diet and nutrition; herbal medicine

GASTROENTERITIS 206: useful therapies include diet and nutrition; herbal medicine; homeopathy

GENITAL HERPES 236: useful therapies include aromatherapy; herbal medicine; homeopathy; naturopathy

GENITAL WARTS 236: useful therapies include aromatherapy; herbal medicine; homeopathy

GERMAN MEASLES 138, 252: useful therapies include aromatherapy; herbal medicine; homeopathy

GINGIVITIS 152: useful therapies include herbal medicine; homeopathy

GLAUCOMA 147: useful therapies include the Bates method; homeopathy; hydrotherapy

GLUE EAR 250: useful therapies include aromatherapy; cranial osteopathy; diet and nutrition; herbal medicine; homeopathy; naturopathy; reflexology

GOITER 143: useful therapies include acupuncture; homeopathy; reflexology

GOUT 179: useful therapies include acupressure; chiropractic; diet and nutrition; herbal medicine; homeopathy; massage; osteopathy

GUILLAIN-BARRE SYNDROME 195: useful therapies include acupressure; acupuncture; Feldenkrais; hydrotherapy; massage; t'ai chi; yoga

HALITOSIS 152: useful therapies include diet and nutrition; herbal medicine; homeopathy; naturopathy

HANGOVERS 206: useful therapies include diet and nutrition; homeopathy; naturopathy

HAY FEVER 157: useful therapies include acupressure; aromatherapy; diet and nutrition; homeopathy

HEADLICE 251: useful therapies include aromatherapy

HEAT RASH 198, 256: useful therapies include aromatherapy; diet and nutrition; herbal medicine; homeopathy; naturopathy

HEMORRHOIDS *see* **VARICOSE VEINS**

HEPATITIS 139: useful therapies include acupuncture; diet and nutrition; herbal medicine; homeopathy; Traditional Chinese Medicine

HICCUPS 258: useful therapies include acupuncture; herbal medicine; Traditional Chinese Medicine

HIGH BLOOD PRESSURE 167: useful therapies include acupressure; acupuncture; aromatherapy; diet and nutrition; herbal medicine; homeopathy; hydrotherapy; hypnotherapy; t'ai chi; temperature biofeedback; Traditional Chinese Medicine; yoga

HIP COMPLAINTS 183: useful therapies include acupressure; acupuncture; Alexander Technique; chiropractic; diet and nutrition; homeopathy; hydrotherapy; massage; osteopathy; Rolfing

HOUSEMAID'S KNEE 183: useful therapies include acupressure; acupuncture; chiropractic; diet and nutrition; herbal medicine; homeopathy; hydrotherapy; massage; osteopathy

HYPERTHYROIDISM 143: useful therapies include herbal medicine; homeopathy

HYPOTHYROIDISM 143: useful therapies include herbal medicine; homeopathy

IMPETIGO 200: useful therapies include aromatherapy; herbal medicine; homeopathy

INDIGESTION/HEARTBURN 208: useful therapies include aromatherapy; diet and nutrition; herbal medicine; homeopathy; relaxation therapies; Traditional Chinese Medicine

INFERTILITY 233–4, 239: useful therapies include acupuncture; aromatherapy; autogenics; diet and nutrition; herbal medicine; homeopathy; reflexology; relaxation

IRRITABLE BOWEL SYNDROME 211: useful therapies include acupuncture; aromatherapy; biofeedback; counseling; diet and nutrition; herbal medicine; hypnotherapy; massage; meditation; yoga

JELLYFISH STINGS 257: useful therapies include homeopathy

JETLAG 261: useful therapies include aromatherapy; cranial electrical stimulation; herbal medicine; homeopathy

KIDNEY STONES 217: useful therapies include acupressure; acupuncture; diet and nutrition; herbal medicine

LABOR AND CHILDBIRTH 247: useful therapies include acupuncture; aromatherapy; herbal medicine; homeopathy; hydrotherapy; hypnotherapy; massage; relaxation therapies; TENS

LARYNGITIS 150: useful therapies include diet and nutrition; herbal medicine; homeopathy

LOW BLOOD PRESSURE 167: useful therapies include acupuncture; aromatherapy; Bach Flower Remedies; diet and nutrition; herbal medicine; massage; reflexology; yoga

LUMBAGO/LOWER BACK PAIN 174: useful therapies include acupressure; acupuncture; Alexander Technique; Bach Flower Remedies; chiropractic; massage; osteopathy

MANIC DEPRESSION *see* **SCHIZOPHRENIA**

ME *see* **CHRONIC FATIGUE SYNDROME**

MEASLES 253: useful therapies include herbal medicine; homeopathy

MENINGITIS 139: useful therapies include acupuncture; aromatherapy; diet and nutrition; herbal medicine; homeopathy; massage; Traditional Chinese Medicine; yoga

MENOPAUSE 245: useful therapies include acupuncture; aromatherapy; diet and nutrition; herbal medicine; homeopathy

MENORRHAGIA (HEAVY MENSTRUAL BLEEDING) 244: useful therapies include acupuncture; aromatherapy; diet and nutrition; homeopathy

MIGRAINE 144–5: useful therapies include acupuncture; Alexander Technique; aromatherapy; diet and nutrition; herbal medicine; massage; meditation; relaxation therapies; shiatsu; temperature biofeedback; yoga

MONONUCLEOSIS 133: useful therapies include aromatherapy; counseling; homeopathy; meditation; relaxation therapies; Traditional Chinese Medicine

MORNING SICKNESS 246: useful therapies include acupuncture; aromatherapy; diet and nutrition; herbal medicine; homeopathy

MOTION SICKNESS 261: useful therapies include acupressure; aromatherapy; Bach Flower Remedies; herbal medicine; homeopathy

MOTOR NEURONE DISEASE (MND) 195: useful therapies include diet and nutrition; massage; t'ai chi; yoga

MOUTH ULCERS 153: useful therapies include aromatherapy; diet and nutrition; herbal medicine; homeopathy

MULTIPLE SCLEROSIS (MS) 193: useful therapies include Alexander Technique; chiropractic; craniosacral therapy; diet and nutrition; herbal medicine; homeopathy; hydrotherapy; magnetic therapy; massage; meditation; osteopathy; yoga

MUMPS 253: useful therapies include herbal medicine; homeopathy

MUSCULAR DYSTROPHY 173: useful therapies include hydrotherapy; massage; osteopathy

NAUSEA 206: useful therapies include acupressure; aromatherapy; diet and nutrition; herbal medicine; homeopathy; naturopathy

NEURALGIA 190–1: useful therapies include acupressure; acupuncture; aromatherapy; biofeedback; chiropractic; homeopathy; hypnotherapy; naturopathy; osteopathy; Traditional Chinese Medicine

NEURITIS 190: useful therapies include aromatherapy; diet and nutrition; herbal medicine; homeopathy; naturopathy; yoga

NOSEBLEEDS 254: useful therapies include acupressure; diet and nutrition; herbal medicine; homeopathy; hydrotherapy

OBESITY 214: useful therapies include diet and nutrition; homeopathy; naturopathy

OBSESSIONS AND COMPULSIONS 226; *see also* **ANXIETY**

ORAL THRUSH 153: useful therapies include aromatherapy; Ayurveda; diet and nutrition; herbal medicine; homeopathy; naturopathy

OSTEOARTHRITIS 178: useful therapies include acupuncture; Ayurveda; chiropractic; diet and nutrition; herbal medicine; homeopathy; massage; osteopathy; Rolfing; yoga

OSTEOPOROSIS 177: useful therapies include acupuncture; cranial osteopathy; diet and nutrition; homeopathy; massage; naturopathy; osteopathy; Traditional Chinese Medicine

PAIN 186–7: useful therapies include acupressure; acupuncture; Alexander Technique; aromatherapy; autogenics; chiropractic; diet and nutrition; hypnotherapy; massage; meditation; osteopathy; psychotherapy; relaxation therapies; TENS; visualization; yoga

PANIC *see* **ANXIETY**

PARKINSON'S DISEASE 194: useful therapies include acupuncture; diet and nutrition; massage; Traditional Chinese Medicine; yoga

PELVIC INFLAMMATORY DISEASE (PID) 242: useful therapies include acupuncture; diet and nutrition

PHARYNGITIS 151: useful therapies include diet and nutrition; herbal medicine; homeopathy

PHOBIAS 227: useful therapies include homeopathy; psychotherapy

PILES *see* **VARICOSE VEINS**

PLEURISY 161: useful therapies include diet and nutrition; herbal medicine; homeopathy; hydrotherapy

PNEUMONIA 162: useful therapies include acupuncture; aromatherapy; diet and nutrition; herbal medicine; homeopathy

A–Z of Ailments • 3

POLIOMYELITIS 138: useful therapies include aromatherapy; counseling; diet and nutrition; homeopathy; hypnotherapy; massage

POOR CIRCULATION 164–5: useful therapies include acupuncture; diet and nutrition; herbal medicine; homeopathy; hypnosis/biofeedback; massage; reflexology; temperature biofeedback training

POSTNATAL DEPRESSION 229: useful therapies include acupuncture; aromatherapy; Bach Flower Remedies; counseling; diet and nutrition; herbal medicine; homeopathy; massage

PREMATURE EJACULATION 235: useful therapies include autogenics

PREMENSTRUAL SYNDROME (PMS) 245: useful therapies include acupuncture; aromatherapy; diet and nutrition; herbal medicine; homeopathy

PRICKLY HEAT/HEAT RASH 198, 256: useful therapies include aromatherapy; diet and nutrition; herbal medicine; homeopathy; naturopathy

PROSTATE ENLARGEMENT 234: useful therapies include acupuncture; diet and nutrition; herbal medicine; homeopathy

PROSTATITIS 234: useful therapies include diet and nutrition; herbal medicine; homeopathy

PSORIASIS 201: useful therapies include acupuncture; aromatherapy; diet and nutrition; herbal medicine; homeopathy; naturopathy; reflexology

RAYNAUD'S DISEASE (or Syndrome) 165: useful therapies include diet and nutrition; homeopathy; Traditional Chinese Medicine

REPETITIVE STRAIN INJURY (RSI) 181: useful therapies include acupressure; acupuncture; Alexander Technique; Bowen technique; chiropractic; homeopathy; hydrotherapy; massage; myotherapy; osteopathy; Rolfing

RESTLESS LEGS SYNDROME 184: useful therapies include acupuncture; diet and nutrition; herbal medicine; homeopathy; massage; osteopathy

RHEUMATOID ARTHRITIS 179: useful therapies include acupuncture; aromatherapy; diet and nutrition; healing; herbal medicine; homeopathy; hydrotherapy; massage; osteopathy

RINGWORM 199: useful therapies include aromatherapy; herbal medicine; naturopathy; *see also* **FUNGAL INFECTIONS**

ROSEOLA 252: useful therapies include diet and nutrition; herbal medicine; homeopathy; naturopathy

RUBELLA *see* **GERMAN MEASLES**

SCALDS 256: useful therapies include aromatherapy; Bach Flower Remedies; herbal medicine; homeopathy; *see also* **BURNS**

SCARLET FEVER 253: useful therapies include diet and nutrition; herbal medicine; homeopathy

SCHIZOPHRENIA, MANIC DEPRESSION 231: useful therapies include acupuncture; Bach Flower Remedies; counseling; group therapy; herbal medicine; homeopathy; psychotherapy; relaxation; *see also* **ANXIETY, DEPRESSION**

SCIATICA 191: useful therapies include acupressure; acupuncture; Alexander Technique; chiropractic; hydrotherapy; massage; moxibustion; osteopathy; Rolfing; Rosen method

SEASONAL AFFECTIVE DISORDER (SAD) 126, 229: useful therapies include aromatherapy; cognitive therapy; herbal medicine; light therapy; psychotherapy; relaxation therapies

SEIZURES/EPILEPSY 192: useful therapies include aromatherapy; Bach Flower Remedies; biofeedback; herbal medicine; homeopathy; meditation; naturopathy; yoga

SHINGLES 133: useful therapies include acupuncture; aromatherapy; diet and nutrition; herbal medicine; homeopathy

SHOCK: *see* 260 for treatment

SINUSITIS 149: useful therapies include acupuncture; diet and nutrition; herbal medicine; homeopathy; naturopathy

SLIPPED DISK 174: useful therapies include acupuncture; Bach Flower Remedies; chiropractic; homeopathy; hydrotherapy; osteopathy; TENS

SNEEZING 149: useful therapies include diet and nutrition; herbal medicine; homeopathy; yoga

SNORING 150: useful therapies include diet and nutrition; homeopathy; yoga

SORE BREASTS 246: useful therapies include aromatherapy; herbal medicine; homeopathy; massage

SORE THROAT 150, 252: useful therapies include acupuncture; aromatherapy; diet and nutrition; herbal medicine; homeopathy

SPRAINED ANKLE/ANKLE PAIN 184–5: useful therapies include acupressure; diet and nutrition; herbal medicine; homeopathy; hydrotherapy; osteopathy

SPRAINS 255: useful therapies include acupuncture; aromatherapy; chiropractic; homeopathy; hydrotherapy; massage; osteopathy; TENS

SQUINT 147: useful therapies include the Bates method; homeopathy; yoga

STAMMERING 222: useful therapies include Alexander Technique; counseling; hypnotherapy; psychotherapy; relaxation therapies

STIFF NECK 175: useful therapies include acupuncture; Alexander Technique; chiropractic; homeopathy; hydrotherapy; osteopathy; reflexology

STINGS 257: useful therapies include aromatherapy; Bach Flower Remedies; diet and nutrition; herbal medicine; homeopathy; naturopathy

STOMACHACHE 208: useful therapies include acupressure; diet and nutrition; herbal medicine; homeopathy; reflexology; relaxation therapies

STRESS 170, 223: useful therapies include aromatherapy; balance and movement therapy; diet and nutrition; expression therapy; energy therapy; herbal medicine; homeopathy; hydrotherapy; massage; meditation; psychotherapy/counseling; reflexology; relaxation therapies; vizualization

STRETCH MARKS 247: useful therapies include aromatherapy; diet and nutrition; homeopathy; massage

STROKE 168: useful therapies include acupuncture; biochemic tissue salts; chiropractic; diet and nutrition; herbal medicine; homeopathy; hydrotherapy; massage; osteopathy; Traditional Chinese Medicine; yoga

SUNBURN 261: useful therapies include aromatherapy; herbal medicine; homeopathy; hydrotherapy; naturopathy

SUNSTROKE/HEAT STROKE 256: useful therapies include aromatherapy; herbal medicine; homeopathy

TEARING OF THE PERINEUM 247: useful therapies include aromatherapy; herbal medicine; homeopathy

TEETHING 249: useful therapies include aromatherapy; cranial osteopathy; herbal medicine; homeopathy

TEMPOROMANDIBULAR JOINT (TMJ) **SYNDROME** 153: useful therapies include autogenics; cranial osteopathy; hydrotherapy

TENNIS ELBOW 180: useful therapies include acupressure; acupuncture; herbal medicine; homeopathy; hydrotherapy; myotherapy; osteopathy

THREADWORMS 251: useful therapies include aromatherapy; Ayurveda; diet and nutrition; herbal medicine; naturopathy

THRUSH 240: useful therapies include aromatherapy; diet and nutrition; herbal medicine; homeopathy; naturopathy

TICS/TWITCHING/PINS AND NEEDLES 191: useful therapies include acupuncture; behavioral therapy; homeopathy

TINNITUS 148: useful therapies include herbal medicine; homeopathy; osteopathy; yoga

TONSILLITIS 151: useful therapies include aromatherapy; Bach Flower Remedies; diet and nutrition; herbal medicine; homeopathy;

TOOTHACHE 153: useful therapies include acupuncture; herbal medicine; homeopathy

TUBERCULOSIS 163: useful therapies include aromatherapy; homeopathy; naturopathy

ULCERS 212: useful therapies include acupuncture; diet and nutrition; herbal medicine; homeopathy; naturopathy

URINARY INCONTINENCE 217: useful therapies include acupressure; diet and nutrition; homeopathy; Traditional Chinese Medicine

URTICARIA 203: useful therapies include aromatherapy; diet and nutrition; herbal medicine; homeopathy; naturopathy

UTERINE PROLAPSE 242: useful therapies include acupuncture; diet and nutrition

VAGINOSIS 240: useful therapies include aromatherapy; counseling; relaxation therapies

VAGINITIS 240: useful therapies include aromatherapy; herbal medicine; homeopathy; naturopathy

VARICOSE VEINS 210: useful therapies include aromatherapy; diet and nutrition; herbal medicine; homeopathy; hydrotherapy; yoga

VIRUSES 130: useful therapies include aromatherapy; Ayurveda; diet and nutrition; herbal medicine; homeopathy; naturopathy; Oriental herbal medicine

WARTS 199: useful therapies include aromatherapy; herbal medicine; homeopathy; naturopathy; visualization

WHIPLASH 175: useful therapies include acupuncture; Alexander Technique; aromatherapy; chiropractic; diet and nutrition; homeopathy; hydrotherapy; massage; osteopathy; Rolfing; Rosen method

WHOOPING COUGH (PERTUSSIS) 252: useful therapies include diet and nutrition; herbal medicine; homeopathy

A–Z of Therapies • 1

This is a directory of alternative therapies. Each therapy is followed by a page number or numbers locating it in the book and is then followed by an alphabetical list of complaints and conditions that it can help. The most common ailments are covered in the second part of the book; for more information *see the A–Z of Ailments on pages 264–9.*

ACUPRESSURE (applying pressure to acupuncture points) 31, 94–5; useful in the treatment of asthma; back pain; childhood illnesses; constipation; fatigue; headaches; joint problems; mental and emotional problems; organ imbalances

ACUPUNCTURE (inserting needles to improve health) 31, 90–3; useful in the treatment of allergies; anxiety; back pain; childhood illnesses; digestive disturbance; eye problems; headaches; insomnia; joint problems; labor pains; menstrual imbalances; mental and emotional problems; migraine; morning sickness; organ imbalances; respiratory problems; sinusitis; tinnitus; urinary infections

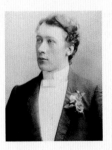

ALEXANDER TECHNIQUE (balance and movement therapy) 57; useful in the treatment of body tensions; headaches; neck pain; postural problems

AROMATHERAPY (therapeutic use of plant oils) 50–1; useful in the treatment of acne; anxiety; cellulite; colds; eczema; fungal infections; hay fever; headaches; indigestion; influenza; insect bites; insomnia; premenstrual tension/pain; postnatal illness; skin conditions

ART THERAPY (art as a therapeutic tool) 111; useful in the treatment of behavioral problems; digestive disorders; headaches; ME; some skin conditions; stress

AUTOGENIC TRAINING (relaxation therapy, using your mind to improve health) 117; useful in the treatment of Aids; depression; eczema; fatigue and tension; headaches; high blood pressure; indigestion; insomnia; irritable bowel syndrome; migraine; ulcers

AUTOMATIC COMPUTERIZED TREATMENT SYSTEM (ACTS) (computerized radionics) *see* **RADIONICS**

AYURVEDA (traditional Indian medicine, addressing the balance of mind, body, and spirit) 34; useful in the treatment of arthritis; diabetes; eczema; stress; tuberculosis; ulcers

BACH FLOWER REMEDIES (flower essences used to treat mental and physical disorders) 86; useful in the treatment of anxiety; depression; eczema; pain; shock; *see also* **FLOWER REMEDIES** 86–9

BATES METHOD (relaxation exercises for eyes) 147; useful in the treatment of eyesight problems; glaucoma; squint

BIOCHEMIC TISSUE SALTS (therapeutic use of tissue salts) 81; useful in the treatment of aching feet and legs; brittle nails; chilblains; colic; coughs; fibrositis; hair loss; hay fever; headaches; heartburn; indigestion; infants' teething pain; lumbago; menstrual pain; migraine; minor ailments; muscular pain; nervous exhaustion; neuralgia; piles; rheumatic conditions; sciatica; sinus disorders; stomach upsets; varicose veins

BIOENERGETICS (integrating the body and mind) 106; useful in the treatment of asthma; irritable bowel syndrome; migraine; stress and stress-related disorders; ulcers

BIOFEEDBACK (technologically supported relaxation therapy) 117; useful in the treatment of anxiety; headaches; high blood pressure; migraine; stress

BIORHYTHMS (identifying individual physical, intellectual, and emotional cycles to understand behavior) 29; useful in the treatment of depression; general ill-health

BOWEN TECHNIQUE (balance and movement therapy) 47; useful in the treatment of acute or chronic pain of musculoskeletal origin; back pain; muscle, joint, and bone problems; neck pain; sprains and strains resulting from sports activity

BREATHING (naturopathy) 25; useful in the treatment of anxiety; asthma; bronchitis; eczema; hiccups; panic; tension

CELLOID MINERALS (pharmacological doses of minerals) 81; useful in the treatment of anemia; diarrhea; goiter; high blood pressure; infertility; kidney problems; osteoporosis; premenstrual syndrome

CHI KUNG (development of internal energy) 59; useful in the treatment of Aids

CHINESE HERBAL MEDICINE
(treatment of conditions with Chinese
herbs and their extracts) 32, 72–3;
useful in the treatment of arthritis;
asthma; digestive disorders; digestive
disturbances; menstrual problems;
migraine; skin conditions

CHIROPRACTIC (therapeutic use of
joint manipulation) 39–41; useful in the
treatment of allergies; asthma; back
pain; general pain from pressure/injury;
headaches; joint sprains; muscular pain;
sciatica; stiffness; tennis elbow

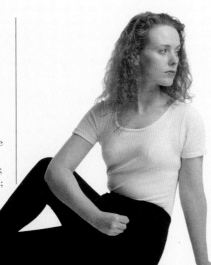

COGNITIVE THERAPY (boosting self-
confidence as a behavioral therapy) 109;
useful in the treatment of anxiety;
behavioral problems; depression;
insomnia

COLONIC IRRIGATION (colonic
hydrotherapy) 27; useful in the
treatment of candida; circulatory
disorders; constipation; diarrhea;
diverticulitis

COLOR THERAPY (the use of color and
light to enhance health) 126; useful in
the treatment of arthritis; asthma; blood
pressure; circulatory disorders;
depression; eczema; insomnia; migraine;
rheumatic pain; stress; tension

COUNSELING (talking to improve
health and well-being) 103; useful in the
treatment of Aids; anxiety; constipation;
depression; headaches; stress and stress-
caused disorders; and terminal illnesses
like cancer

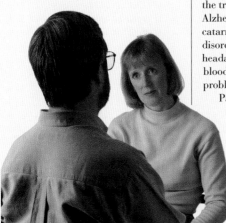

CRANIAL OSTEOPATHY (specialist
technique in which the bones of the skull
are manipulated) 44–5; useful in the
treatment of childbirth pains; child
hyperactivity; colic; digestive and
gynecological disorders; glue ear;
headaches; learning difficulties;
meningitis; painful sinuses; reduced jaw
mobility; tinnitus

CRANIOSACRAL THERAPY (CST)
(adapted form of cranial osteopathy) *see*
CRANIAL OSTEOPATHY

CRYSTAL HEALING (the use of crystals
and gemstones to enhance healing) 125;
useful in the treatment of anxiety;
chronic health conditions; depression

CUPPING (the use of suction cups to
remove impure energy from the body)
30; useful in the treatment of abscesses;
asthma; boils; bruising; colds; lumbago;
rheumatism; stiff joints

DIETARY THERAPY (altering diet to
prevent or treat illness) 74–5; useful in
the treatment of Aids; allergies;
Alzheimer's disease; arthritis; cataracts;
catarrh; cold sores; digestive and bowel
disorders; glandular fever; glue ear;
headache; heart disease; hepatitis; high
blood pressure; laryngitis; liver
problems; ME; MND; MS; pain;
Parkinson's disease; polio; sinusitis;
some cancers; sore throat, thrush

DREAMWORK (accurate dream
recall used therapeutically)
105; useful in the treatment of
chronic illnesses; depression

ELECTROCRYSTAL THERAPY (energy
restructuring) 125; useful in the
treatment of migraine; multiple sclerosis

ENCOUNTER GROUPS (group therapy)
107; useful in the treatment of anxiety;
behavioral problems; chronic illness;
depression; eating disorders

ENERGY THERAPIES (encouraging the
free flow of energy for good health)
121–7; useful in the treatment of
asthma; chronic illness; depression;
eczema; pain; stress

ENVIRONMENTAL THERAPIES 98–101;
useful in the treatment of asthma;
chronic ill health caused by
environment, such as cancer;
eczema

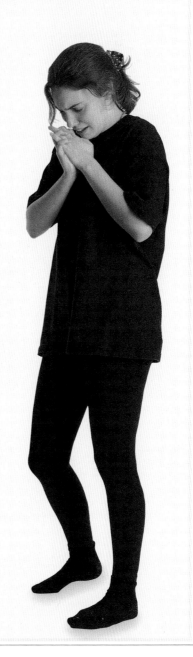

A–Z of Therapies • 2

EXPRESSION THERAPIES (using therapeutic activity to express emotions – for instance, dance movement therapy, 110; art therapy 111; sound therapy 127); useful in the treatment of anorexia and bulimia; anxiety; behavioral problems; depression; headaches; heart disorders; manic depression; schizophrenia; stress

EXTERNAL VISUALIZATION (encouraging therapeutic mental pictures for health) 120; useful in the treatment of anxiety; asthma; cancer; depression; heart disorders; pain; stress

FASTING (controlled abstinence from most or all solid foods) 29; useful in the treatment of asthma; chronic health conditions; diarrhea; digestive upsets; eczema; fevers; headaches; skin rashes

FELDENKRAIS (learning new patterns of movement) 56; useful in the treatment of arthritis; back pain; muscle injuries; physical problems including spasticity; stress; tension

FENG SHUI (Chinese art of balancing energies) 100; useful in the treatment of general ill-health; unhappiness, depression

FLOTATION THERAPY (relaxation through floating) 116; useful in the treatment of anxiety; arthritis; high blood pressure; insomnia; pain; stress

FLOWER REMEDIES (dealing with negative emotions) 86–9; useful in the treatment of anxiety; depression; exhaustion; fear and panic; lack of confidence; mental clarity; mood swings; shock and trauma; stress

FOOD COMBINING (combining foods for therapeutic effect) 28; useful for maintaining general health

GEM AND MINERAL ESSENCES (using stone vibrations to encourage emotional and spiritual well-being) 125; useful in the treatment of anxiety; depression; pain; stress

GEOPATHIC THERAPY (using the earth's energy to affect health) 100; useful in the treatment of cancer; insomnia; migraine; rheumatism; stress

GESTALT THERAPY (promoting personal growth through self-awareness) 107; useful in the treatment of anxiety; behavioral problems; hyperactivity; insomnia; tension

HEALING (using inner powers to encourage healing) 121; useful in the treatment of chronic conditions; infections; insomnia; pain

HELLERWORK (realigning the body to restore health) 58; useful in the treatment of aches, pains; posture; stress; tension

HERBAL MEDICINE (the use of herbs as medicine) 66–73; useful in the treatment of allergies; anxiety; arthritis; chronic illness; depression; digestive problems; earache; headache; high or low blood pressure; insomnia; kidney and urinary infections; menopausal problems; menstrual problems; migraine; skin diseases; tinnitus

HOMEOPATHY (using natural remedies to boost the body's own healing ability) 82–5; useful in the treatment of allergies; anxiety; arthritis; asthma; bruising; burns; cold sores; colds, influenza; constipation; cramp; cystitis; deafness; depression; diarrhea; dizziness; earache; eczema; eye conditions; fear, panic; fever; food poisoning; headaches; heat exhaustion; indigestion; insomnia; irritable bowel syndrome; joint problems; low blood pressure; ME; menopausal problems; muscular problems; nausea; rheumatic pain; sciatica; shock; skin problems; stings; swelling; tinnitus

HYDROTHERAPY (the therapeutic use of water) 26–7; useful in the treatment of anemia; arthritis; asthma; back pain; blood/circulation problems; gallstones; glaucoma; headaches; labor pain and childbirth; menstrual problems; muscle problems; pain; rheumatism; stress and tension

HYPNOTHERAPY (the use of hypnosis to encourage healing and well-being) 112–15; useful in the treatment of addictions; anxiety; asthma; behavioral problems; childbirth and labor pain; insomnia; irritable bowel syndrome; migraine; phobias; stress; ulcers

INTERNAL VISUALIZATION (imagining the workings of one's own body to encourage healing and well-being) 120; useful in the treatment of anxiety; arthritis; headaches; migraine; pain; rheumatism; stress-related disorders; tension

LIGHT THERAPY (the therapeutic use of light) 126; useful in the treatment of anxiety; depression; hyperactivity in children; overeating; SAD; tiredness

MACROBIOTIC DIET (balancing foods for health) 75; useful in the treatment of arthritis; cancer; depression; digestive disorders; skin problems; stress

MAGNETIC/ELECTROMAGNETIC THERAPY (balancing the body's energy to encourage healing) 101; useful in the treatment of anxiety; back, neck, and shoulder pain; bruising; depression; inflammation; lumbago; rheumatic pain; sciatica; stress; whiplash

MASSAGE (relaxing the body and encouraging healing and well-being through touch) 48–9; useful in the treatment of anxiety; back pain; cancer; circulation problems; colic; depression; headaches; heart disorders; high blood pressure; hyperactivity; insomnia; sinusitis; tension

MEDITATION (reaching a tranquil mental state that refreshes the mind and body) 118–19; useful in the treatment of addictions; anger and aggression; anxiety; chilblains; chronic pain; circulatory disorders; depression; headaches; hyperactivity; insomnia; nervousness; physical tension

MEGAVITAMIN THERAPY (taking large doses of vitamins for health) 80; useful in the treatment of acne; addictions; aging; anemia; cancer; common cold; depression; diabetes; hyperactivity; premenstrual syndrome; schizophrenia; viruses

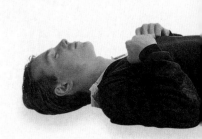

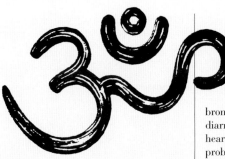

METAMORPHIC TECHNIQUE
(manipulating the foot to come to terms
with and overcome physical and mental
problems) 54; useful in the treatment of
anxiety; colic; depression; hyperactivity;
insomnia; long-standing health
problems; night terrors and sleep
disorders

MOXIBUSTION (application of heat to
acupuncture points) 31, 90; useful in the
treatment of arthritis; chronic illnesses
like eczema and asthma; fatigue; frozen
shoulder; ME; pain; stiff neck; weak
back

MYOTHERAPY (diffusion of trigger
points in muscles to retrain muscles and
relieve pain) 46; useful in the treatment
of addictions; arthritis; backache;
chronic recurrent pain of
musculoskeletal origin; colic; Epstein-
Barr; headaches; migraine; sinusitis;
sports injuries; tinnitus; TMJ

NATUROPATHY (a philosophy
incorporating a number of
therapies. which aims to help
the body cure itself) 24–5;
useful in the treatment of
allergies; anxiety; arthritis;
asthma; bacterial infections;
bronchitis; colds; deafness; depression;
diarrhea; digestive disorders; fatigue;
heart disorders; influenza; kidney
problems; skin problems;   ulcers;
viruses

NUTRITIONAL THERAPY (adding
specific nutrients to, or altering, the diet
to improve health) 76; useful in the
treatment of Alzheimer's disease;
anemia; arthritis; cancer; cataracts;
catarrh; colds and general infections;
conjunctivitis and other eye conditions;
coronary heart disease; coughs; glue ear;
headache; indigestion; infertility;
influenza; joint/bone problems;
laryngitis; low blood sugar; MND; MS;
osteoporosis; Parkinson's disease;
pregnancy; premenstrual syndrome;
sinusitis; sore throat; stress; tiredness

ORIENTAL HERBAL MEDICINE (Far-
Eastern therapy using herbs for health)
72; useful in the treatment of allergies;
anemia; bronchitis; chronic hepatitis;
cirrhosis of the liver; common cold;
coughs; depression; digestive problems;
endometriosis; fever; hangover; hysteria;
infertility; inflammation; influenza;
menopausal problems; menstrual
problems; motion sickness; muscular
spasm; nervous disorders; peptic ulcer;
postoperative weakness; stiff shoulders;
swelling; tonsillitis; tuberculosis

OSTEOPATHY (manipulative therapy
which treats mechanical problems in the
framework) 42–5; useful
in the treatment of aches
and pains following
childbirth; arthritic
pain; back pain; digestive
and respiratory
difficulties; gynecological
problems; headache; joint
sprains; muscular pain;
osteoarthritis; painful sinuses;
recurrent strain injuries;
reduced jaw mobility; sciatica;
sports injuries; stress

POLARITY THERAPY (balancing the
vital energy force in the body) 55; useful
in the treatment of respiratory problems;
tension and stress

PSIONIC MEDICINE (helping the body
to heal itself)124; useful in the
treatment of many chronic illnesses,
including Aids; arthritis; asthma; cancer;
eczema

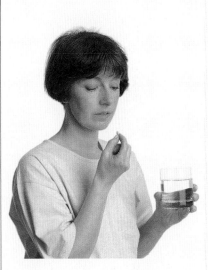

A–Z of Therapies • 3

PSYCHODRAMA (acting out feelings as an emotional release) 107; useful in the treatment of anxiety; behavioral problems; depression; insomnia; stress and stress-related disorders

PSYCHOSYNTHESIS (developing a harmonious and balanced personality through self-development) 108; useful in the treatment of chronic health problems; headaches; migraine; phobias; stress

RADIONICS (analyzing and measuring energy patterns to determine and treat disease) 124; useful in the treatment of chronic illnesses; emotional problems; physical pain

REFLEXOLOGY (massage of reflex points on feet and hands to encourage health and well-being) 52–4; useful in the treatment of back pain; digestive disorders; heart disease; infertility; insomnia; liver problems; menstrual problems; migraine; multiple sclerosis; pain; sinusitis; stress

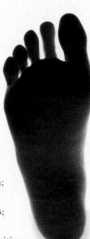

RELAXATION (calming the mind and body for health) 116; useful in the treatment of anxiety; asthma; depression; digestive disorders; eczema; infertility; insomnia; mental tension; pain; physical tension; pins-and-needles; psoriasis; respiratory disorders; stress

ROLFING (treating the tissues to improve posture) 46; useful in the treatment of anxiety; arthritis; breathing difficulties; depression; musculoskeletal pain resulting from mechanical stress; poor posture

ROSEN TECHNIQUE (combining touch and verbal communication to evoke muscular relaxation) 47; useful in the treatment of addictions; anxiety; body tension; chronic health conditions; circulatory problems; general injuries

SCHUESSLER SALTS (mineral remedies for everyday ailments) 81; useful in the treatment of anemia; anxiety; asthma; boils; bronchitis; chilblains; circulation; cold sores; colds; colic; coughs; cramp; depression; digestive problems; fevers; headaches; heartburn; hemorrhoids; hiccups; indigestion; inflammation; influenza; insomnia; loss of taste and smell; menstrual pains; morning sickness; muscular disorders; slow healing skin and wounds; sore throat; spasms; spots; tonsillitis; toxic accumulation; varicose veins

SHAMANISM (traditional spiritual medicine, in which healing is encouraged through the power of nature and the Divine) 37; useful in the treatment of conditions like asthma; cancer; eczema; Epstein-Barr

SHIATSU (stimulating the vital points along the body's meridians in order to encourage healing, and good health, and well-being) 96–7; useful in the treatment of back/neck pain; circulatory disorders; constipation; depression; diarrhea; headaches; immune problems; insomnia; menstrual problems; mental problems; migraine; nervous problems; nervous system problems; osteoporosis; stiff joints; stress; tension; toothache

SOUND THERAPY (the therapeutic use of sound vibrations) 127; useful in the treatment of arthritis; back pain; fibrositis; fractures; migraine; neuralgia; postsurgical recovery; rheumatism; sinusitis; sprains; stress and stress-related disorders

SPIRITUAL HEALING (the use of a healer to channel divine healing energies) 122; useful in the treatment of chronic conditions such as Aids; cancer; insomnia; psoriasis

T'AI CHI (development of life force in body through a series of slow-moving, circular movements) 60; useful in the treatment of anxiety; blood pressure; chronic health problems; circulatory disorders; insomnia; postural problems; stress and stress-related disorders; tension

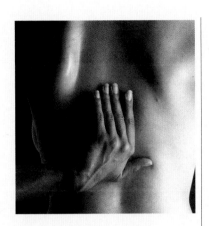

TEMPERATURE BIOFEEDBACK TRAINING (relaxation therapy involving the use of temperature to train responses) 170; useful in the treatment of chilblains; circulation problems; high blood pressure; Raynaud's Syndrome

THALASSOTHERAPY (use of the healing powers of the sea and seaweed) 26; useful in the treatment of abdominal pain; allergies; digestive disorders

THERAPEUTIC TOUCH (healing with the hands) 122; useful in the treatment of chronic health conditions, like Aids; asthma; cancer; psoriasis

TRADITIONAL CHINESE MEDICINE 30–2; *see also* **ACUPRESSURE** 31, 94–5, **ACUPUNCTURE** 31, 90–3, **CHINESE HERBAL MEDICINE** 32, 72–3, **CUPPING** 30, **MOXIBUSTION** 31, 90

TRAGER APPROACH (light, non-intrusive hand and mind movements to release deep-seated physical and mental problems and imbalances) 58; useful in the treatment of asthma; back pain; emphysema; high blood pressure; migraine; neuromuscular disorders; polio; posture problems; sciatica; severe restriction of movement

TRANSCENDENTAL MEDITATION (form of meditation) 119; useful in the treatment of anger and aggression; anxiety; depression; insomnia; nervousness; physical tension; stress and stress-related disorders

TRANSCUTANEOUS ELECTRICAL NERVE STIMULATION (TENS or TNS) (noninvasive pain relief that works by stimulating the endorphins) 101; useful in the treatment of arthritis; back pain; circulatory problems; labor pains; lumbago; sciatica; sports injuries

TRANSACTIONAL ANALYSIS (psychotherapy which provides fast, practical help with problems) 108; useful in the treatment of anxiety; depression; headaches; insomnia; migraines; stress

TREE REMEDIES (the therapeutic use of the essential oil of trees) 89; useful in the treatment of breathing difficulties; negative emotions; *see also* **FLOWER REMEDIES** 86–9

VISUALIZATION (forming positive mental pictures to encourage good health) 120; useful in the treatment of anxiety; asthma; cancer; eating disorders; heart disorders; insomnia; pain; phobias; stress and stress-related disorders

YOGA (spiritual and physical exercises to encourage health and well-being) 61–5; useful in the treatment of anxiety; arthritis; backache; blood pressure; body tension; diabetes; headaches; migraine; multiple sclerosis; osteoporosis; pain; postnatal illness; pregnancy problems; premenstrual syndrome; rheumatism; rheumatoid arthritis; squint; stress; tinnitus; ulcers

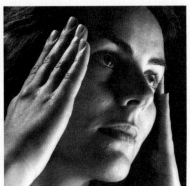

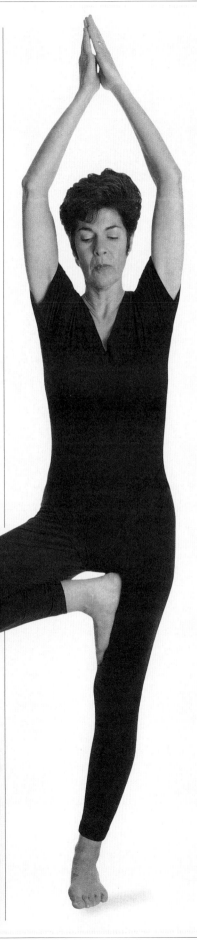

Glossary

ACUTE a condition that sets in quickly and requires immediate treatment.

AGGRAVATION the exacerbation of symptoms that can occur when taking homeopathic remedies, particularly in the case of chronic ailments.

ALLERGEN a substance that causes an allergic reaction.

ALLOPATHIC Western medicinal treatment, based on treating symptoms rather than the underlying condition.

ANALGESIC pain relieving.

ANTIBACTERIAL acts against bacteria.

ANTIBIOTIC any drug used to treat bacterial infections; i.e. penicillin.

ANTIBODIES produced by our immune system to attack what it considers to be an invader, such as bacteria, a virus, or an allergen.

ANTI-INFLAMMATORY reducing inflammation.

ANTISPASMODIC prevents contractions of the muscles.

ARTICULATION range of movement of the joints.

ASTRINGENT constricts the blood vessels or membranes in order to reduce irritation, inflammation, and swelling.

AURA every person, animal, and plant is said to have a visible aura, or magnetic field. These are said to indicate the state of health, emotions, mind, and spirit.

AUTOGENIC DISCHARGE sensations or muscle movements that accompany the release of stored tensions.

AUTOIMMUNE DISORDER when the body creates antibodies against itself.

AVERSION THERAPY a part of behavioral therapy in which you learn through punishment.

BENIGN tumor that is not cancerous or dangerous.

BIOPSY removal of fluid or tissue from the body for examination.

BODYWORK manipulation by the hands to release tension; used in many therapies, such as Hellerwork and osteopathy.

CAUTERY burning tissue in the body.

CHANNELS invisible pathways in which chi or qi travels; also called meridians. They appear in and on the body.

CHEST BREATHING one of two ways of breathing that should be used only as a fast response to shock or stress; addressed in breathing or relaxation therapy. *See* **DIAPHRAGMATIC BREATHING.**

CHI (or qi) the life force of the body which circulates through its meridians or channels.

CHRONIC a condition that is deep-seated, often recurrent, and usually of a long duration.

COMPRESS a pad that is soaked in hot or cold substances and applied to the body.

COMPLEMENTARY the term used to describe alternative forms of medical treatment – emphasizing the fact that they support rather than replace orthodox medicine.

CONSTITUTIONAL homeopathic term relating to the physical and mental constitution of a person, including hereditary factors and underlying health issues.

DEFICIENT condition in Chinese medicine; any disorder that is caused by the body's inability to maintain balance, through improper function of the Zangfu.

DEGENERATIVE a condition in which there is irreversible and progressive decomposition.

DETOXIFICATION the removal of toxins from the body.

DHEA (DEHYDROEPIANDROSTERONE) a hormone; deficiency may be implicated in ME, MS, Alzheimer's disease, and other problems of the nervous system.

DIALOGUE discussion on how habitual ideas and emotions can affect your mind, body, and spirit; a central part of Hellerwork therapy.

DIAPHRAGMATIC BREATHING the natural rhythmic breathing that allows full expansion of the lungs; taught in breathing or relaxation therapy. *See* **CHEST BREATHING.**

DIURETIC reduces the fluid level of the body.

DU the channel that runs up the spine, from the coccyx, over the head to the upper lip.

DYSFUNCTION abnormal functioning of a system or organ within the body.

EFFLEURAGE slow, rhythmic massage.

EGO STATE three different types of ego state, called parent, adult and child, are described in TA (transactional analysis) therapy; the aim of TA is to gain autonomy over the ego states.

EMPIRICAL POINTS points on the body that are effective for particular symptoms and conditions; used in acupuncture.

ESSENCE the pure energy extracted from food that is transformed into chi by the body. Also the integral part of a plant, its life force, as used in flower remedies, herbalism, and aromatherapy.

ESSENTIAL OIL pure, concentrated essence taken from the plant; said to be its life force.

ETIOLOGY investigation of the cause of disease.

EXCESS CONDITION a condition in which chi, blood, or body fluids are imbalanced, accumulating in parts of the body.

EXPECTORANT promoting the expulsion of phlegm from the lungs.

FAST abstention from most or all foods for a given period.

FRICTION small circular movements used in massage.

GANGLION swelling within a tendon or joint; also a group of nerves.

H-FACTOR the basic sound present in the cells and organs in the body. Important term in sound therapy.

HIGH–VELOCITY THRUST spinal adjustment used in chiropractic and osteopathy, involving speedy movements without force.

INFLAMMATION swelling and redness in the body, as a result of injury or illness.

INFUSION immersion of herbs in boiling water.

INHALANT a remedy or drug that is breathed in through the nose or mouth.

INTENTIONAL EXERCISES exercises used in autogenic training and therapy that have the specific intention of relieving suppressed tension, sadness, and anger.

JINGLUO Chinese term for the channels, or meridians, which run invisibly through the body carrying the chi, or life force.

KAPHA the moon force, which is a basic life force or element in Ayurvedic medicine.

LESION a term used to explain an abnormality or damage to the body.

MALIGNANT cancerous and possibly life-threatening.

MANIPULATION chiropractic, osteopathic, and other therapies use manipulations to adjust the spine, joints, and tissues.

MANTRA uplifting sentence used in meditation.

MERIDIANS channels that run through the body, beneath the skin, in which the life force or chi is carried. There are 14 main meridians running to and from the hands and feet to the body and head.

MOBILIZATION chiropractic technique to increase range of movement.

MOXA dried mugwort, which is burned on the end of needles, or rolled into a stick, and then heated in moxibustion. It is said to warm the chi in the body in order to increase its flow.

MOXABUSTION *see* **MOXA**

NEEDLING the process used by acupuncturists to stimulate points along the meridians in order to alter or encourage the flow of chi in the body. Thin needles are used, hence the term.

NEGATIVE deep, dissipating touch used in polarity therapy to release and polarize blocked energy.

NEUROMUSCULAR MASSAGE massage that encourages nerve and muscle activity.

NEUTRAL a type of touch used in polarity therapy, which is light and balancing.

ORTHODOX the term for conventional medicine.

PALPATION examination with the hands.

PASSIVE movement of the joint that is the result of gentle pressure; used in chiropractic, among other manipulative therapies.

PERCUSSION vigorous drumming massage.

PETRISSAGE kneading massage movement.

PITTA the sun force, one of the three basic life forces or elements controlling all physical and mental processes in Ayurvedic medicine.

POLARITY stretching exercises to release stagnation and encourage healing and good health; used in polarity therapy.

POLYCREST a homeopathic remedy that has a broad spectrum of actions, and can therefore be used for a variety of different conditions.

POSITIVE a type of touch used in polarity therapy, which is energizing and stimulating.

POTENCY the dilution of a homeopathic remedy; the higher the number, the higher the strength, and the greater the dilution.

PROVING the process used in homeopathy for testing a remedy; it can occur when the wrong remedy is prescribed and taken over a period of time, and the symptoms of the condition it is aimed at manifest themselves.

REFERRED PAIN pain that is felt in a different part of the body from the area that is actually affected.

REN the Chinese meridian that runs down the front of the body, from the lower lip to behind the genitalia.

SELF-LIMITING a condition that lasts a set length of time and usually clears of its own accord.

SHEN the spirit of the person, in Traditional Chinese Medicine.

SOFT TISSUES tissues of the body, including muscles, tendons, ligaments, and organs.

STAGNANT when the flow of chi or qi is blocked in the meridians.

STRETCHING TECHNIQUES techniques used to stretch or ease tension in the muscles in massage.

SUCCUSSION the shaking method used in preparing homeopathic remedies.

SYMPTOM PICTURE homeopathic term for the overall pattern of symptoms characterizing each individual person.

SYSTEMIC desensitization encouraging you to dwell on the worst dread or fear and then introducing relaxation to counteract the fear; used in behavioral therapy.

TONIFICATION a process in Chinese medicine that involves strengthening and supporting the blood and chi.

TOXIN a substance that is poisonous to the body.

TRAUMA physical or emotional injury.

TYPE term used by Bach and other flower remedy therapists to describe your general personality and approach to life.

UNDERCURRENTS the tug of emotions, such as anger and jealousy, that influence you; a fundamental part of encounter group therapy.

VATA the wind force in Ayurvedic medicine – one of the three basic life forces or elements that must be in balance for physical and mental processes to be balanced.

YIN/YANG Chinese philosophy that explains the interdependence of all elements of nature. These contrasting aspects of the body and mind must be balanced before health and well-being can be achieved. Yin is the female force, and yang is the male.

ZANGFU the term in Traditional Chinese Medicine for internal organs (different from those of Western medical science).

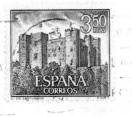
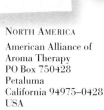
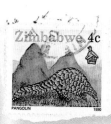

Acupuncture

AUSTRALASIA

New Zealand Register of
Acupuncturists Inc.
PO Box 9950
Wellington 1
New Zealand
Tel/Fax: 64 4 476 8578

EUROPE

British Acupuncture
Council
Park House
206–8 Latimer Road
London W10 6RE
Great Britain
Tel: 44 181 964 0222
Fax: 44 181 964 0333

NORTH AMERICA

American Association for
Acupuncture and Oriental
Medicine
4101 Lake Boone Trail
Suite 201
Raleigh
North Carolina 27607
USA
Tel: 1 919 787 5181

National Acupuncture
and Oriental Medicine
Alliance
PO Box 77511
Seattle
Washington 98177–0531
USA
Tel: 1 206 524 3511

National Acupuncture
and Oriental Medicine
Alliance (National
Alliance)
14637 Starr Road, SE
Olalla
Washington 98359 USA
Tel: 1 206 851 6896
Fax: 1 206 851 6883

National Commission for
the Certification of
Acupuncturists (NCCA)
PO Box 97075
Washington, DC
20090–7075 USA
Tel: 1 202 232 1404
Fax: 1 202 462 6157

Alexander technique

AUSTRALASIA

Australian Society of
Teachers of the Alexander
Technique (AUSTAT)
PO Box 716
Darlinghurst
New South Wales 2010
Australia
Tel: 61 8339 571

EUROPE

Society of Teachers of the
Alexander Technique
20 London House
266 Fulham Road
London SW10 9EL
Great Britain
Tel: 44 171 351 0828
Fax: 44 171 352 1556

NORTH AMERICA

Canadian Society of
Teachers of the Alexander
Technique
PO Box 47025
No.19–555 West 12th
Avenue
Vancouver
British Columbia V5Z
3XO
Canada

North American Society
of Teachers of the
Alexander Technique
(NASTAT)
PO Box 517
Urbana
Ilinois 61801–0517 USA
Tel: 1 217 367 6956

Aromatherapy

EUROPE

Academy of
Aromatherapy and
Massage
50 Cow Wynd
Falkirk
Sterlingshire FK1 1PU
Great Britain
Tel: 44 1324 612658

International Federation
of Aromatherapists
Stamford House
2–4 Chiswick High Road
London W4 1TH
Great Britain
Tel: 44 181 742 2605
Fax: 44 181 742 2606

International Society of
Professional
Aromatherapists
ISPA House
82 Ashby Road
Hinckley
Leics OE10 1SN
Great Britain
Tel: 44 1455 637987
Fax: 44 1455 890956

Tisserand Institute
65 Church Road
Hove
East Sussex BN3 2BD
Great Britain
Tel: 44 1273 206640
Fax: 44 1273 329811

NORTH AMERICA

American Alliance of
Aroma Therapy
PO Box 750428
Petaluma
California 94975–0428
USA
Tel: 1 707 778 6762
Fax: 1 707 769 0868

American Aromatherapy
Association
PO Box 3679
South Pasadena
California 91031 USA
Tel: 818 457 1742

National Association of
Holistic Aromatherapy
PO Box 17622
Boulder
Colorado 80308–0622
USA
Tel: 1 303 258 3791

Autogenic training

EUROPE

British Association for
Autogenic Training and
Therapy
Heath Cottage
Pitch Hill
Ewnhurst
Near Cranleigh
Surrey GU6 7NP
Great Britain

Ayurveda

EUROPE

Maharishi Ayur-Veda
Health Centre
24 Linhope Street
London NW1 6HT
Great Britain
Tel: 44 171 724 6267

Maharishi Ayur-Veda
Health Centre
The Golden Dome
Woodley Park
Skelmersdale
Lancashire WN8 6UQ
Great Britain
Tel: 44 1695 51008

NORTH AMERICA

American Association of
Ayurvedic Medicine
PO Box 598
South Lancaster
Massachusetts 01561
USA
Tel: 1 800 843 8332
Fax: 1 201 777 1197

Canadian Association of
Ayurvedic Medicine
PO Box 541
Station B
Ottawa
Ontario K1P 5P8
Canada
Tel: 1 613 837 5737

Bach flower remedies

AUSTRALASIA

Martin & Pleasance
137 Swan Street
Richmond
Victoria 3121
Australia
Tel: 61 39 427 7422

EUROPE

Dr. Edward Bach Centre
Mount Vernon
Sotwell
Wallingford
Oxon OX10 0PZ
Great Britain
Tel: 44 1491 834678
Fax: 44 1491 825022

NORTH AMERICA

Nelson Bach USA Ltd.
Wilmington Technology
Park
100 Research Drive
Wilmington
Massachusetts
01887–4406 USA
Tel: 1 508 988 3833

Biofeedback

NORTH AMERICA

Association for Applied
Psychophysiology and
Biofeedback
10200 West 44th Avenue
Apt 304
Wheat Ridge
Colorado 80033–8436
USA
Tel: 1 303 422 8894
Fax: 1 303 422 8894

Bowen technique

AUSTRALASIA

Bowen Therapy Academy
of Australia
PO Box 733
Hamilton 3300
Victoria
Australia

Chiropractic

ASIA

Chiropractic Association
(Singapore)
Box 23
Tanglin Post Office
Singapore
Tel: 65 293 9843/734
8584
Fax: 65 733 8380

Chiropractic Council of
Japan
2621–5
Noborito Tama-ku
Kawasaki 214
Japan
Tel: 81 44 933 9547
Fax: 81 44 933 4449

Hong Kong
Chiropractors'
Association
GPO Box 5588
Hong Kong
Tel: 852 375 5785
Fax: 852 537 5487

Manu R. Shah, D.C.
Sheikh Ismail Building
Aquem Alto
Margao
Goa 403 601
India
Tel: 91 83 422 3707

Thailand Chiropractic
Association
Medico-Chiro Center
Sukumvit 24 Road
Bangkok
Thailand
Tel: 66 2 258 8694

AUSTRALASIA

Chiropractors'
Association of Australia
PO Box 241
Springwood
New South Wales 2777
Australia
Tel: 61 47 515 644
Fax: 61 47 515 856

New Zealand
Chiropractors'
Association
PO Box 7144
Wellesley Street
Auckland
New Zealand
Tel: 64 9 373 4343
Fax: 64 9 373 5973

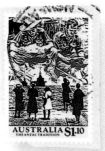
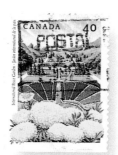
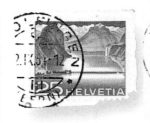
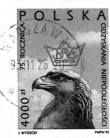
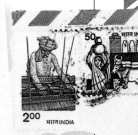

EUROPE

Anglo-European College
of Chiropractic
13–15 Parkwood Road
Bournemouth BH5 2DF
Great Britain
Tel: ++ 1202 436275
Fax: ++ 1202 436312

British Chiropractic
Association
29 Whitley Street
Reading
Berks RG2 0EG
Great Britain
Tel: ++ 1734 757557
Fax: ++ 1734 757257

Chiropractic Association
of Ireland
28 Fair Street
Drogheda
County Louth
Irish Republic
Tel: 353 41 305999
Fax: 353 41 51863

European Chiropractors'
Union
The Waldegrave Clinic
82 Waldegrave Road
Teddington
Middx TW11 8LG
Great Britain
Tel: ++ 181 943 2424
Fax: ++ 181 977
6626/287 6626

NORTH AMERICA

American Chiropractic
Association
1701 Clarendon
Boulevard
Arlington
Virginia 22209 USA
Tel: 1 703 276 8800
Fax: 1 703 243 2593

Canadian Chiropractic
Association
1396 Eglinton Avenue
West
Toronto
Ontario M6C 2E4
Canada
Tel: 1 416 781 5656
Fax: 1 416 781 7344

International
Chiropractors'
Association
Suite 100
1110 Glebe Road
Arlington
Virginia 22201 USA
Tel: 1 703 528 5000
Fax: 1 703 528 5023

World Chiropractic
Alliance
2950 North Dobson Road
Suite One
Chandler
Arizona 85224-1802
USA
Tel: 1 800 347 1011

Cognitive therapy
EUROPE
Association of Cognitive
Analytic Therapists
Munro Clinic
Guy's Hospital
London SE1 9RT
Great Britain
Tel: ++ 171 955 2906
Fax: ++ 171 955 2984

British Association for
Behavioural and
Cognitive
Pyschotherapies
Dept of Clinical
Psychology
Northwick Park Hospital
Watford Road
Harrow HA1 3UJ
Great Britain
Tel: ++ 181 869 2325
Fax: ++ 1 869 2317

**Colonic irrigation
(colonic
hydrotherapy)**
EUROPE
Colonic International
Association (CIA)
16 Englands Lane
London NW3 4TG
Great Britain
Tel/Fax: ++ 171 483
1595

NORTH AMERICA

International Association
for Colon Hydrotherapy
2051 Hilltop Drive
Suite A-11
Redding
California 96002 USA
Tel: 1 916 222 1498
Fax: 1 916 222 1497

Color therapy
EUROPE
Colour and Reflexology
9 Wyndale Avenue
Kingsbury
London NW9 9PT
Great Britain
Tel: ++ 181 204 7672

Hygeia College of Colour
Therapy
Brook House
Minchinhampton Hill
Avening
Near Tetbury
Glos GL8 8NS
Great Britain
Tel: ++ 1453 832150
Fax: ++ 1453 835757

Counseling
EUROPE
British Association for
Counselling
1 Regent's Place
Rugby
Warwicks CV21 2PJ
Great Britain
Tel: ++ 1788
550899/578328
Fax: ++ 1788 562189

NORTH AMERICA

American Counseling
Association
5999 Stevenson Avenue
Alexandria
Virginia 22304-9800
USA
Tel: 1 703 823 0988

**Craniosacral therapy
(cranial osteopathy)**
EUROPE
Cranosacral Association
Monomark House
27 Old Gloucester Street
London WC1N 3XX
Great Britain
Tel: ++ 1285 821 648

Crystal healing
EUROPE
Affiliation of Crystal
Healing Organizations
(ACHO)/International
College of Crystal Healing
46 Lower Green Road
Esher
Surrey KT10 8HD
Great Britain
Tel: ++ 181 398 7252
Fax: ++ 181 398 4237

School of Electro-crystal
Therapy
117 Long Drive
South Ruislip
Middx HA4 0HL
Great Britain
Tel/Fax: ++ 181 841
1716

School of White Crystal
Healing
Grylls Rose
Court Mill Lane
Wadeford
Chard
Somerset TA20
Great Britain
Tel: ++ 1460 65815
Fax: ++ 1460 52346

Spiritual Venturers
Association
72 Pasture Road
Goole
North Humberside DN14
6HE
Great Britain
Tel/Fax: ++ 1405 769119

Dreamwork
NORTH AMERICA
Association for the Study
of Dreams
PO Box 1600-NY
Vienna
Virginia 22183 USA
Tel: 1 703 242
0062/8888

Expression therapies
EUROPE
British Psychodrama
Association
8 Rahere Road
Cowley
Oxford OX4 3QG
Great Britain
Tel/Fax: ++ 1865 715055

Institute for Arts in
Therapy and Education
2–18 Britannia Row
Islington
London N1 8QG
Great Britain
Tel: ++ 171 704 2534
Fax: ++ 171 354 1761

Laban Centre for
Movement and Dance
Laurie Grove
New Cross
London SE14 6NH
Great Britain
Tel: ++ 181 682 4070
Fax: ++ 181 694 8749

NORTH AMERICA

American Art Therapy
Association
1202 Allanson Road
Mundelein
Illinois 60060 USA
Tel: 1 708 949 6064

American Association of
Music Therapy
PO Box 80012
Valley Forge
Pennsylvania 19484 USA
Tel: 1 215 265 4006

American Dance Therapy
Association
2000 Century Plaza
Suite 108
Columbia
Maryland 21044 USA
Tel: 1 410 997 4040
Fax: 1 410 997 4048

International Dance
Exercise Association
(IDEA)
6190 Cornerstone Court
East
Apt 204
San Diego
California 92121–3773
USA
Tel: 1 619 535 8979
Fax: 1 619 535 8234

Laban/Bartenieff
Institute of Movement
Studies
11 East Fourth Street
3rd Floor
New York 10003 USA
Tel: 1 212 477 4299
Fax: 1 212 477 3702

National Association of
Music Therapy
8455 Colesville Road
Suite 930
Silver Springs
Maryland 20910 USA
Tel: 1 301 589 3300

National Coalition of Arts
Therapy Organizations
505 11th Street, South
East
Washington, DC 20003
USA
Tel: 1 202 543 6864

Feldenkrais
AUSTRALASIA
Australian Feldenkrais
Guild INc.
Locked Bag Number 19
Post Office 2037
Glebe
New South Wales
Australia
Tel/Fax: 61 2 597 6561

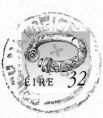
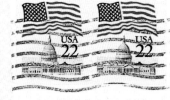

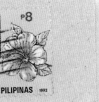

New Zealand
Practitioners and
Students Association
PO Box 90091
Auckland Mail Centre
Auckland
New Zealand
Tel/Fax: 64 9 479 6529

EUROPE

Feldenkrais Guild UK
PO Box 370
London N10 3XA
Great Britain

NORTH AMERICA

Feldenkrais Guild
524 Ellsworth Street
PO Box 489
Albany
Oregon 97321–1043 USA
Tel: 1 503 926 0981
Fax: 1 503 926 0572

Flower therapy

EUROPE

Flower Essence
Fellowship
Laurel Farm Clinic
17 Carlingcott
Peasedown St John
Bath BA2 8AN
Great Britain
Tel: 44 1761 434098
Fax: 44 1761 434905

Flower Remedy
Programme
PO Box 65
Hereford HR2 0UW
Great Britain
Tel: 44 1873 890218
Fax: 44 1873 890314

Gem and mineral essences

EUROPE

Earthworks
43 Wessex Trade Centre
Poole
Dorset BH12 3PG
Great Britain
Tel: 44 1202 717127
Fax: 44 1202 717128

Guild of Vibrational
Medicine
Waveney Lodge
Hoxne
Suffolk IP21 4AS
Great Britain
Tel/Fax: 44 1379 668848

Gestalt therapy

EUROPE

Gestalt Centre London
64 Warwick Road
St Albans AL1 4DL
Great Britain
Tel: 44 1727 864806
Fax: 44 1727 838891

NORTH AMERICA

Gestalt Center for
Psychotherapy and
Training
510 East 89th Street
New York 10128 USA
Tel: 1 212 879 3669

Gestalt Therapy Institute
of Los Angeles
Faculty Training Office
1460 Seventh Street
Suite 301
Santa Monica
California 90401 USA
Tel: 1 909 629 9935

Hellerwork

EUROPE

Hellerwork Inc. (Rose-
Marie Amoroso)
1 Finsbury Avenue
Broadgate
London EC2M 2PA
Great Britain
Tel: 44 171 247 9982
Fax: 44 171 247 0082

NORTH AMERICA

Hellerwork International
406 Berry Street
Mount Shasta
California 96067 USA
Tel: 1 916 926 2500
Fax: 1 916 926 6839

Herbalism

AUSTRALASIA

National Herbalists
Association of Australia
Suite 305
BST House
3 Smail Street
Broadway
New South Wales 2007
Australia
Tel: 61 2 211 6437
Fax: 61 2 211 6452

EUROPE

School of Herbal
Medicine/Phytotherapy
Bucksteep Manor
Bodle Street Green
Near Hailsham
Sussex BN27 4RJ
Great Britain
Tel: 44 1323 833 812/4
Fax: 44 1323 833 869

NORTH AMERICA

American Herbalists
Guild
PO Box 1683
Soquel
California 95073 USA

Holistic medicine

EUROPE

British Holistic Medical
Association
Trust House
Royal Shrewsbury
Hospital South
Shrewsbury
Shropshire SY3 8XF
Great Britain
Tel: 44 1743 261155
Fax: 44 1743 353637

Holistic and Creative
Therapy Association
2A Burston Drive
St Albans
Herts AL2 2HR
Great Britain
Tel: 44 1727 674567

Holistic Health
Foundation
2 De La Hay Avenue
Plymouth
Devon PL3 4HH
Great Britain
Tel: 44 1752 671 485
Fax: 44 1345 251759

NORTH AMERICA

American Holistic Health
Association
PO Box 17400
Anaheim
California 90017–7100
USA
Tel: 714 779 6152/777
2917

American Holistic
Medical Association
4101 Lake Boone Trail
Suite 201
Raleigh
North Carolina 27607
USA
Tel: 1 919 787 5181
Fax: 1 919 787 4916

Association of Holistic
Healing Centers
109 Holly Crescent
Suite 201
Virginia Beach
Virginia 23451 USA
Tel: 1 804 422 9033
Fax: 1 804 422 8132

Canadian Holistic
Medical Association
491 Eglington Avenue
West
Apt 407
Toronto
Ontario M5N 1A8
Canada
Tel: 1 416 485 3071

International Association
of Holistic Health
Practitioners
5020 West Spring
Mountain Road
Las Vegas
Nevada 89102 USA
Tel: 1 702 873 4542

Homeopathy

AUSTRALASIA

Australian Federation for
Homeopathy
PO Box 806
Spit Junction
New South Wales 2088
Australia

Australian Institute of
Homeopathy
21 Bulah Heights
Berdwra Heights
New South Wales 2082
Australia

Institute of Classical
Homeopathy
24 West Haven Drive
Tawa
Wellington
New Zealand

EUROPE

British Homoeopathic
Association
27A Devonshire Street
London W1N 1RJ
Great Britain
Tel: 44 171 935 2163

Centre d'Etudes
Homeopathiques de
France
228 Boulevard Raspail
75014 Paris
France

Société Medical de
Biotherapie
62 rue Beaubourg
75003 Paris
France

Society of Homoeopaths
2 Artisan Road
Northampton NN1 4HU
Great Britain
Tel: 44 1604 21400
Fax: 44 1604 22622

NORTH AMERICA

American Foundation for
Homeopathy
1508 S. Garfield
Alhambra
California 91801 USA

American Institute of
Homeopathy
1585 Glencoe Street
Suite 44
Denver
Colorado 80220-1338
USA
Tel: 1 303 321 4105

Foundation for
Homeopathic Education
and Research
2124 Kittredge Street
Berkeley
California 94704 USA

Homeopathic Council for
Research and Education
50 Park Avenue
New York 10016 USA

International Foundation
for Homeopathy
2366 Eastlake Avenue
East
Suite 301
Seattle
Washington 98102 USA

National Center for
Homeopathy
801 North Fairfax Street
Suite 306
Alexandria
Virginia 22314 USA

Hydrotherapy

EUROPE

UK College of
Hydrotherapy
515 Hagley Road
Birmingham B66 4AX
Great Britain
Tel: 44 121 429 9191
Fax: 44 121 478 0871

NORTH AMERICA

Aquatic Exercise
Association
PO Box 1609
Nokomis
Florida 34274 USA
Tel: 1 813 486 8600

Hypnotherapy

EUROPE

British Hypnotherapy
Association
67 Upper Berkeley Street
London W1H 7DH
Great Britain
Tel: 0171 723 4443

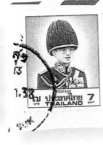
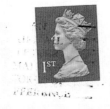
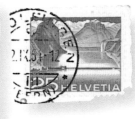
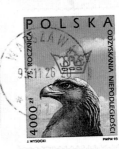
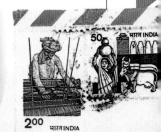

National Register of
Hypnotherapists and
Pyschotherapists
12 Cross Street
Nelson
Lancs BB9 7EN
Great Britain
Tel: 44 1282 699378
Fax: 44 1282 698633

NORTH AMERICA

American Association of
Professional
Hypnotherapists
PO Box 29
Boones Mill
Virginia 24065 USA
Tel: 1 703 334 3035

American Guild of
Hypnotherapists
2200 Veterans Boulevard
New Orleans
Louisiana 70062 USA

National Society of
Hypnotherapists
2175 North West 86th
Suite 6A
Des Moines
Iowa 50325 USA
Tel: 1 515 270 2280

Massage

AUSTRALASIA

Society of Clinical
Masseurs
PO Box 483
9 Delhi Street
Mitchum 3131
Victoria
Australia
Tel: 61 3 874 6973

EUROPE

Academy of
Aromatherapy and
Massage
50 Cow Wynd
Falkirk
Sterlingshire FK1 1PU
Great Britain
Tel: 44 1324 6126598

London College of
Massage
5 Newman Passage
London W1P 3PF
Great Britain
Tel: 44 171 323 3574
Fax: 44 171 637 7125

Massage Training
Institute
24 Highbury Road
London N5 2DQ
Great Britain
Tel: 44 171 226 5313

NORTH AMERICA

American Massage
Therapy Association
820 Davis Street
Suite 100
Evanston
Illinois 60201-4444 USA
Tel: 1 708 864 0123
Fax: 1 708 864 1178

Associated Bodyworkers
and Massage
Professionals
28677 Buffalo Park
Evergreen
Colorado 80439-7347
USA
Tel: 1 303 674 8478
Fax: 1 303 674 0859

International Association
of Infant Massage
PO Box 438
Elma
New York 14059-0438
USA
Tel: 1 716 652 9789
Fax: 1 716 652 1990

International Massage
Association
3000 Connecticut Avenue
NW
Apt 102
Washington, DC 20008
USA
Tel: 1 202 387 6555
Fax: 1 202 332 0531

National Association of
Massage Therapy
PO Box 1400
Westminster
Colorado 80030–1400
USA
Tel: 1 800 776 6268

Skilled Touch Institute of
Chair Massage
584 Castro Street
Suite 555
San Francisco
California 94114–2588
USA
Tel: 1 415 861 4746
Fax: 1 415 861 0443

Naturopathy

AUSTRALASIA

Australian Natural
Therapists Association
(ANTA)
PO Box 308
Melrose Park
South Australia 5039
Australia
Tel: 61 8 371 3222
Fax: 61 8 297 0003

Federation of Natural and
Traditional Therapists
(FNTT)
238 Ballarat Road
Footscray
Victoria 3011
Australia
Tel: 61 3 9318 3057

New Zealand Natural
Health Practitioners
Accreditation Board
PO Box 37–491
Auckland
New Zealand
Tel: 64 9 625 9966

EUROPE

British College of
Naturopathy and
Osteopathy
Frazer House
6 Netherhall Gardens
London NW3 5RR
Great Britain
Tel: 44 171 435 6464
Fax: 44 171 431 3630

General Council and
Register of Naturopaths
Goswell House
2 Goswell Road
Street
Somerset BA16 0JG
Great Britain
Tel: 44 1458 840072
Fax: 44 1458 840075

NORTH AMERICA

American Association of
Naturopathic Physicians
PO Box 20386
Seattle
Washington 98102 USA
Tel: 1 206 323 7610

American Naturopathic
Medical Association
PO Box 19221
Las Vegas
Nevada 89132 USA
Tel: 1 702 796 9067

Canadian Naturopathic
Association
205, 1234 17th Avenue
South West
PO Box 4143
Station C
Calgary
Alberta
Canada
Tel: 1 413 244 4487

Nutritional and diet
therapy

EUROPE

British Nutrition
Foundation
High Holborn House
52–4 High Holborn
London WC1V 6RQ
Great Britain
Tel: 44 171 404 6504
Fax: 44 171 404 6747

College of Natural
Therapy
133 Gatley Road
Gatley
Cheadle
Cheshire SK8 4PD
Great Britain
Tel: 44 161 491 4314
Fax: 44 161 491 4190

Institute for Optimum
Nutrition
13 Blades Court
Deodor Road
London SW15 2NU
Great Britain
Tel: 44 181 877 9993
Fax: 44 181 877 9980

NORTH AMERICA

American Association of
Nutrition Consultants
1641East Sunset Road,
Apt B-117
Las Vegas
Nevada 89119 USA
Tel: 1 709 361 1132

American Dietetics
Association
216 West Jackson
Boulevard
Apt 800
Chicago
Illinois 60606–6995 USA
Tel: 1 800 877 1600

Oriental medicine

ASIA

World Academic Society
of Medical Qigong
No.11 Heping Jie Nei Kou
Beijing 100029
China

AUSTRALASIA

Australian Traditional
Medicine Society Limited
ATMS
PO Box 1027
(mailing)/12/27 Bank
Street (office)
Meadowbank
New South Wales 2114
Australia
Tel: 61 2 809 6800

Qigong Association of
Australia
458 White Horse Road
Surrey Hills
Victoria 3127
Australia
Tel: 61 3 9836 6961
Fax: 61 3 830 5608

Shiatsu Therapy
Association of Australia
PO Box 1
Balaclava
Victoria 3183
Australia
Tel/Fax:61 03 530 0067

EUROPE

British Complementary
Medicine Association
39 Prestbury Road
Cheltenham
Glos GL52 2PT
Great Britain
Tel: 44 1242 226770
Fax: 44 1242 226778

College of Integrated
Chinese Medicine
19 Castle Street
Reading
Berks RG1 7SB
Great Britain
Tel: 44 1734 508880
Fax: 44 1734 508890

Feng Shui Network
PO Box 2133
London W1A 1RL
Great Britain
Tel: 44 171 935 8935
Fax: 44 171 935 9295

Register of Chinese
Herbal Medicine
PO Box 400
Wembley
Middx HA9 9NZ
Great Britain
Tel: 44 181 904 1357

Dr Yves Requena
Institut Européen de Qi
Gong
La Ferme des Vences
13122 Ventabren
France
Tel: 33 42 92 56 10
Fax: 33 42 92 56 40

Shiatsu Society
31 Pullman Lane
Godalming
Surrey GU7 1XY
Great Britain
Tel/Fax: 44 1488 860771

Useful Addresses • 3

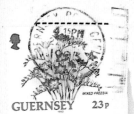
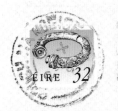
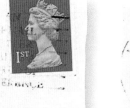
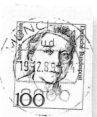

Tse Qigong Centre
Qi Magazine
PO Box 116
Manchester M20 3YN
Great Britain
Tel: ++ 161 434 5289

NORTH AMERICA

American Association of
Oriental Medicine
(AAOM)
433 Front Street
Catasauqua
Pennsylvania 18032 USA
Tel: 1 610 266 1433
Fax: 1 610 264 2768

American Shiatsu
Association
PO Box 718
Jamaica Plain
Massachusetts 02130
Tel: 1 617 236 5867

Chi Kung School at the
Body-Energy Center
PO Box 19708
Boulder
Colorado 80308 USA
Tel: 1 303 442 2250
Fax: 1 303 442 3141

International Chi
Kung/Qigong Directory
PO Box 19708
Boulder
Colorado 80308 USA
Tel: 1 303 442 3131
Fax: 1 303 442 3141

Qigong Academy
8103 Marlborough
Avenue
Cleveland
Ohio 44129 USA
Tel/Fax: 1 216 842 8042

Osteopathy

AUSTRALASIA

Chiropractors and
Osteopaths' Registration
Board of Victoria
PO Box 59
Carlton South
Victoria 3053
Australia
Tel: 61 3 349 3000
Fax: 61 3 349 3003

NSW Chiropractors and
Osteopathic Registration
Board
PO Box K599
Haymarket
New South Wales 2000
Australia
Tel: 61 2 281 0884
Fax: 61 2 281 2030

EUROPE

General Register and
Council of Osteopaths
56 London Street
Reading
Berks RG1 4SQ
Great Britain
Tel: ++ 1734 576585
Fax: ++ 1734 566246

NORTH AMERICA

American Academy of
Osteopathy
3500 DePauw Boulevard
Suite 1080
Indianopolis
Indiana 46268-139 USA
Tel: 1 317 879 1881
Fax: 1 317 879 0563

American Association of
Colleges of Osteopathic
Medicine
6110 Executive
Boulevard, Apt 405
Rockville
Maryland 20852 USA
Tel: 1 301 468 0990

American Osteopathic
Association
142 East Ohio Street
Chicago
Illinois 60611 USA
Tel: 1 312 280 5800
Fax: 1 312 280 3860

Polarity therapy

EUROPE

UK Polarity Therapy
Association
Monomark House
27 Old Gloucester Street
London WC1N 3XX
Great Britain
Tel: ++ 1483 417714

Zero Balancing
Association UK
36 Richmond Road
Cambridge CB4 3PU
Great Britain
Tel/Fax: ++ 1233 315480

NORTH AMERICA

American Polarity
Therapy Association
2888 Bluff Street
Suite 149
Boulder
Colorado 80301 USA
Tel: 1 303 545 2080
Fax: 1 303 545 2161

Zero Balancing
Association
PO Box 1727
Capitola
California 95010 USA
Tel: 1 408 476 0665

Psychosynthesis

EUROPE

Institute of
Psychosynthesis
65A Watford Way
London NW4 3AQ
Tel: ++ 181 202 4525

Psychotherapy

EUROPE

European Association for
Psychotherapy (EAP)
Rosenbursenstrasse
8/3/7
A-1010 Vienna
Austria
Tel: 43 1 512 7090
Fax: 43 1 512 7091

UK Council for
Psychotherapy
167–9 Great Portland
Street
London W1N 5FB
Great Britain
Tel: ++ 171 436 3002
Fax: ++ 171 436 3013

Radionics

EUROPE

Radionic Association
Barelein House
Goose Green
Deddington
Banbury
Oxon OX15 0SZ
Great Britain
Tel/Fax: ++ 1869 338852

Reflexology

ASIA

China Reflexology
Association
PO Box 2002
Beijing 100026
China
Fax: 86 1 5068309

Chinese Society of
Reflexologists
Xuanwu Hospital
Capital Institute of
Medicine
Chang Chun Street
Beijing
China

Rwo-Shr Health Institute
International
Room 1902
Java Commercial Centre
128 Java Road
North Point
Hong Kong

Rwo-Shr Health Institute
International
1–11 Wilayah Shopping
Centre
Jalan Campbell 50100
Kuala Lumpur
Malaysia

AUSTRALASIA

New Zealand Institute of
Reflexologists Inc.
253 Mt Albert Road
Mt Roskill
Auckland
New Zealand

New Zealand Reflexology
Association
PO Box 31 084
Auckland 4
New Zealand

Reflexology Association of
Australia
15 Kedumba Crescent
Turramurra 2074
New South Wales
Australia

Victorian School of
Reflexology and Herbal
Studies
19 Dickson Street
Sunshine
Victoria 3020
Australia
Tel: 61 03 312 5573
Fax: 61 03 311 3501

EUROPE

Association of
Reflexologists
27 Old Gloucester Street
London WC1N 3XX
Great Britain
Tel: ++ 990 673320

Association of Vacuflex
Reflexology
PO Box 93
Tadworth
Surrey KT20 7YB
Great Britain
Tel/Fax: ++ 1737 842961

British School of
Reflexology and Holistic
Association of
Reflexologists
92 Sheering Road
Old Harlow
Essex CM17 0JW
Great Britain
Tel: ++ 1279 429060
Fax: ++ 1279 445234

Bond van Europese
Reflexologen (Society of
European Reflexologists)
Netherlands Section
PO Box 9009
1006 AA Amsterdam
Netherlands
Fax: 31 34 20 22178/31
20 61 76918

International Federation
of Reflexologists
76–8 Edridge Road
Croydon
Surrey CR01EF
Great Britain
Tel: ++ 181 667 9458
Fax: ++ 181 649 9292

International Institute of
Reflexology
15 Hartfield Close
Tonbridge
Kent
Great Britain
Tel/Fax: ++ 1732 350629

Irish Reflexologists
Institute
c/o 11 Fitzwilliam Place
Dublin 2
Irish Republic
Tel: 353 1 760137
Fax: 353 1 610 466

Scottish School of
Reflexology
2 Wheatfield Road
Ayr KA7 2XB
Scotland
Tel: ++ 1292 287142

NORTH AMERICA

Association of Vacuflex
Reflexology
1951 Glenarie Avenue
North Vancouver
V7P 1XP
Canada
Tel: 1 604 986 7121

Association of Vacuflex
Reflexology
2222 Kilkare Parkway
Pt. Pleasant
New Jersey 08742 USA
Tel: 1 908 892 7566

Foot Reflex Awareness
Association
PO Box 7622
Mission Hills
California 91346 USA

International Institute of
Reflexology
PO Box 12042
Saint Petersberg
Florida 33733 USA
Tel: 1 813 343 4811

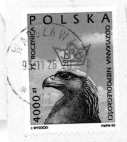
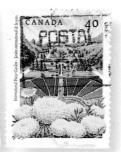
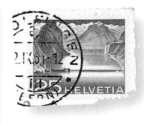
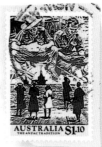

Reflexology Association of
America
4012 S. Rainbow
Boulevard
Box K585
Las Vegas
Nevada 89103-2509 USA

Reflexology Association of
Canada (RAC)
11 Glen Cameron Road
Unit 4
Thornhill
Ontario L8T 4NB
Canada
Tel: 1 905 889 5900

Reiki
NORTH AMERICA

Center for Reiki Training
29209 Northwestern
Highway #592
Southfield
Michigan 48034–9841
USA
Tel: 1 810 948 9534

Rolfing
AUSTRALASIA

Rolf Institute: Pacific
Basin Branch Office
28 Davies Street
Brunswick 3056
Victoria
Australia
Tel: 61 3 383 5045

EUROPE

Rolf Institute: European
Branch Office
Herzogstrasse 40
D-800 Munich 40
Germany
Tel: 49 89 39 68 02

NORTH AMERICA

The Rolf Institute
205 Canyon Boulevard
Boulder
Colorado 80302-4920
USA
Tel: 1 303 449 5903/800
530 8875
Fax: 1 303 449 5978

Shamanism
EUROPE

Sacred Hoop
28 Cowl Street
Evesham
Worcs WR11 4PL
Great Britain
Tel/Fax: 44 1386 49680

NORTH AMERICA

Cross-Cultural
Shamanism Network
PO Box 430
Willits
California 95490 USA
Tel: 1 707 459 0486

Foundation for Shamanic
Studies
PO Box 1939
Mill Valley
California 94942 USA
Tel: 1 415 380 8282
Fax: 1 415 380 8416

Sacred Circles Institute
PO Box 733
Mukilteo
Washington 98275
USA
Tel: 1 206 353 8815

The South and Meso
American Information
Center
PO Box 28703
Oakland
California 94604 USA
Tel: 1 510 834 4263
Fax: 1 510 834 4264

Spiritual healing
AUSTRALASIA

Australian Spiritual
Healers Association
PO Box 4090
Race View
Queensland 4305
Australia
Tel: 61 7 329 40027

National Federation of
Healers Inc.
PO Box 112
Oxonford
Queensland 4210
Australia
Tel: 61 7 821 3922

EUROPE

National Federation of
Spiritual Healers
Old Manor Studio
Church Street
Sunbury on Thames
Middx TW16 6RG
Great Britain
Tel: 44 1932 783164

Stress therapy
EUROPE

Association of Stress
Therapists
5 Springfield Road
Palm Bay
Cliftonville
Kent CT9 3EA
Great Britain
Tel: 44 1843 291255

Trager Approach
NORTH AMERICA

The Trager Institute
21 Locust Avenue
Mill Valley
California 94941-2806
USA
Tel: 1 415 388 2688
Fax: 1 415 388 2710

Transactional analysis
EUROPE

Institute of Transactional
Analysis
BM Box 4104
London WC1 3XX
Tel: 44 171 404 5011

Transcendental meditation
AUSTRALASIA

Maharishi Foundation of
New Zealand
3 Adam Street
Greenlane
Auckland 1105
New Zealand
Tel: 64 9 523 3324

Maharishi Vedic College
PO Box 81
Bundoora 3083
Victoria
Australia
Tel: 61 3 9467 8911

EUROPE

Transcendental
Meditation
Freepost
London SW1P 4YY
Great Britain
Tel: 44 990 143733

NORTH AMERICA

Maharishi University of
Management
Fairfield
Iowa 52557 USA
Tel: 1 515 472 1134

Maharishi Vedic College
500 Wilbrod Street
Ottawa
Ontario K1N 6N2
Canada
Tel: 1 613 565 2030

Yoga
AUSTRALASIA

BKS Iyengar Association
of Australia
1 Rickman Avenue
Mosman 2088
New South Wales
Australia

International Yoga
Teachers' Association
c/o 14/15 Huddart
Avenue
Normanhurst
New South Wales 2076
Australia

EUROPE

British Wheel of Yoga
1 Hamilton Place
Boston Road
Sleaford
Lincs NG34 7ES
Great Britain
Tel: 44 1529 306851

Institute of Iyengar Yoga
223A Randolph Avenue
London W9 1NL
Great Britain
Tel/Fax: 0171 624 3080

Israeli Yoga Teachers'
Association
c/o PO Box 48087
Tel Aviv 61480
Israel

Patanjali Yoga Centre &
Ashram
The Cott
Marley Lane
Battle
Sussex TN33 0RE
Great Britain

Sivananda Yoga Vedanta
Centre
51 Felsham Road
London SW15 1AZ
Great Britain

NORTH AMERICA

BKS Iyengar Yoga
National Association of
the US
8223 West Third Street
Los Angeles
California 90088 USA
Tel: 1 213 653 0357

International Association
of Yoga Therapists
109 Hillside Avenue
Mill Valley
California 94941 USA
Tel: 1 415 383 4587
Fax: 1 415 381 0876

Sivananda Yoga Vedanta
Center
243 West 24th Street
New York 10011 USA

Sivananda Yoga Vedanta
Centre
5178 St Lawrence
Boulevard
Montreal
Quebec H2T 1R8
Canada

Sivananda Yoga Vedanta
Centre
77 Harbord Street
Toronto
Ontario M5S 1G4
Canada

Unity in Yoga
303 2495 West 2nd
Avenue
Vancouver
British Columbia VGK
1J5
Canada

Unity in Yoga
International
PO Box 281004
Lakewood
Colorado 80228 USA

Unity Yoga International
7918 Bolling Drive
Alexandria
Virginia 22308 USA

Yogaville
Buckingham
Virginia 23921 USA

Further Reading

All books on this list have been published in the UK, unless otherwise noted.

A–Z of Natural Healthcare, by Belinda Grant (Optima, 1993)

Acupressure Techniques, by Dr. Julian Kenyon (Thorsons, 1987)

Acupuncture: Energy Balancing for Body, Mind and Spirit, by Peter Mole (Element Books, 1992)

Acupuncture for Everyone, by Dr. Ruth Lever (Penguin, 1987)

Against Therapy, by Jeffrey Masson (Collins, 1989)

The Alexander Technique: Natural Poise for Health, by Richard Brennan (Element Books, 1991)

All Day Energy, by Kathryn Marsden (Bantam Books, 1995)

The Alternative Dictionary of Symptoms and Cures, by Dr. Caroline Shreeve (Century, 1987)

The Alternative Health Guide, by Brian Inglis & Ruth West (Michael Joseph, 1983)

Anorexia and Bulimia, by Julia Buckroyd (Element Books, UK/USA, 1996)

Anxiety, Phobias & Panic Attacks, by Elaine Sheehan (Element Books, UK, 1996)

Aromatherapy, by Christine Wildwood (Element Books, 1991)

Aromatherapy: Massage with Essential Oils, by Christine Wildwood (Element Books, 1991)

The Art of Chi Kung: Making the Most of Your Vital Energy, by Wong Kiew Kit (Element Books, 1993)

The Art of Shiatsu: A Step-by-Step Guide, by Oliver Cowmeadow (Element Books, 1992)

Arthritis & Rheumatism: A Comprehensive Guide to Effective Treatment by Pat Young (Element Books, 1995)

Awareness Through Movement, by Moshe Feldenkrais (Penguin, 1987)

Back to Eden, by Jethro Kloss (Woodbridge Press, USA, 1981)

Beat PMT through Diet, by Maryon Stewart (Ebury Press, 1988)

Beat Psoriasis, by Sandra Gibbons (Thorsons, 1992)

Better Health through Natural Healing, by Ross Tratler (McGraw-Hill, USA, 1987)

Body and Soul, Sara Martin (Arkana, 1989)

Bodywise by Joseph Heller and William A. Henkin (Tarcher, 1986)

Cancer and Complementary Therapies (BACUP, 1994)

Choices in Healing, by Michael Lerner (MIT Press, USA/UK, 1994)

Clinical Ecology, by Dr. George Lewith and Dr. Julian Kenyon (Thorsons, 1985)

The Complete Family Guide to Homeopathy, by Dr. Christopher Hammond (Element Books, UK/USA, 1996)

The Complete Guide to Food Allergy and Environmental Illnesses, by Dr. Keith Mumby (Thorsons, 1993).

The Complete Illustrated Guide to Reflexology, by Inge Dougans (Element Books, UK/US, 1996)

The Complete Illustrated Holistic Herbal, David Hoffman (Element Books, UK/USA, 1996)

The Complete Relaxation Book, by James Hewitt (Rider, 1987)

The Complete Yoga Course, by Howard Kent (Headline Press, 1993)

Depression, by Sue Breton (Element Books, UK, 1996)

Diabetes: A Comprehensive Guide to Effective Treatment, by Catherine Steven (Element Books, 1995)

The Elements of Yoga, by Godfrey Devereux (Element, 1994)

The Encyclopaedia of Alternative Health Care, by Kristen Olsen (Piatkus, 1989)

Encyclopaedia of Natural Medicine, by Brian Inglis and Ruth West (Michael Joseph, 1983)

Encyclopaedia of Natural Medicine, by Michael Murray and Joseph Pizzorno (Macdonald Optima, 1990)

Flower Remedies: Natural Healing with Flower Essences, by Christine Wildwood (Element Books, 1991)

The Fountain of Health: An A–Z of Traditional Chinese Medicine, by Dr. Charles Windrige/Dr. Wu Xiaochun (Mainstream Publishing, 1994)

Gentle Medicine, by Angela Smyth (Thorsons, 1994)

The Greening of Medicine, by Patrick Pietroni (Gollancz, 1990)

Guide to Complementary Medicine and Therapies, by Anne Woodham (Health Education Authority, 1994)

The Handbook of Complementary Medicine, by Stephen Fulder (Oxford Medical Publications, 1988)

Headaches, by Dr. John Lockie with Karen Sullivan (Bloomsbury, 1992)

Healing the Heart, by Elizabeth Wilde McCormick (Optima, 1992)

Heart Disease: A Comprehensive Guide to Effective Treatment, by Richard Thomas (Element Books, 1994)

Herbs for Common Ailments, by Anne McIntyre (Gaia, 1992)

The Home Herbal, by Barbara Griggs (Pan Books, 1995)

How to Live Longer and Feel Better, by Linus Pauling (W. H. Freeman, USA, 1986)

The Illustrated Encyclopaedia of Essential Oils, by Julia Lawless (Element Books, UK/USA, 1995)

Job's Body: A Handbook For Bodywork, by Deane Juhan (Station Hill, 1987)

Life, Health and Longevity, by Kenneth Seaton (Scientific Hygiene, USA, 1994)

Living with ME, by Charles Shepherd (Cedar, 1992)

Massage: A Practical Introduction, by Stewart Mitchell (Element Books, 1992)

Maximum Immunity, by Michael Wiener (Gateway Books, 1986)

Medicine and Culture, by Lynn Payer (Gollancz, 1990)

Migraine: A Comprehensive Guide to Effective Treatment, by Eileen Herzberg (Element Books, 1994)

Miracles Do Happen, by C. Norman Shealy (Element Books, UK/USA, 1995)

Multiple Sclerosis: A Comprehensive Guide To Effective Treatment, by Richard Thomas (Element Books, 1995)

The Natural Way Colds and Flu, by Penny Davenport (Element Books, 1995)

The Natural Way Migraine, by Eileen Herzberg (Element Books, 1994)

Nutritional Medicine, by Stephen Davies and Alan Stewart (Pan Books, 1987)

The Polarity Process: Energy as a Healing Art, by Franklyn Sills (Element Books, 1989)

Raw Energy, by Leslie & Susannah Kenton (Arrow Books, 1985)

Reader's Digest Family Guide to Alternative Medicine, ed. Dr. Patrick Pietroni (The Reader's Digest Association, UK/USA/South Africa/Australia, 1991)

Red Moon: Understanding and Using the Gifts of the Menstrual Cycle, by Miranda Gray (Element Books, 1994)

The Reflexology and Colour Therapy Workbook, by Pauline Wills (Element Books, 1992)

The Rowland Remedy, by John Rowland (Javelin Books, 1986)

Stress: An Owner's Manual by Arthur Rowshan (Element Books, 1993)

Teach Yourself Meditation, by James Hewitt (Hodder and Stoughton, 1978)

Trager Mentastics: Movement as a Way to Agelessness, by Milton Trager, M.D., with Cathy Guadagno-Hammond, Ph.D. (Station Hill Press, 1987)

Understanding Cancer, ed. Edith Rudinger (Consumers' Association, 1986)

The Vitamin Guide: Using Vitamins for Optimum Health, by Hasnain Walji (Element Books, 1992)

Will to be Well, by Neville Hodgkinson (Hutchinson, 1984)

The Women's Guide to Homoeopathy, by Andrew Lockie and Nicola Geddes (Hamish Hamilton, 1992)

You Can Heal Your Life, by Louise Hay (Eden Grove, USA, 1988)

You Don't Have To Die, by Leon Chaitow (Future Medicine Publishing, USA, 1994)

You Don't Have to Feel Unwell, by Robin Needes (Gateway Books, 1994)

Index • 1

A

abdominal touch diagnosis 18
Abrams, Albert 124
acne 200
acupressure 31, 94–5
acupuncture 31, 90–3
acute, definition 276
acuyoga 95
addictions 226
age regression 114
Aids 136–7
ailments 129–61
air purifiers 25
Alexander, F. Matthias 57
Alexander Technique 57
allergens 158–9, 276
allergic reactions 202–3
allergic rhinitis see hay fever
allergies 134, 158–9
allergy testing methods 99
Alzheimer's disease 194
America, herbal medicine 71
analytical theory 102, 105, 114
anaphylactic shock 159
anemia 166
angelica 69
angina 168
ankle pain 184–5
ankylosing spondylitis (AS) 177
anorexia nervosa 224, 225
anthroposophical medicine 23
anti-Candida diet 75
anxiety 221
appendicitis 212
applied kinesiology 20, 41, 99
Arabic medicine 36
arm pain 180
arnica 69
aromatherapy 50–1
art therapy 111
arterial disease 164
arteriosclerosis 168, 169
arthritis 178–9
Ashtanga yoga 62
Assagioli, Roberto 108
assumption of responsibility 109
asthma 160
astringent, definition 276
atherosclerosis 168, 169
athlete's foot 199
atopy 158
aura 126
    definition 276
    diagnosis 21
auricular cardiac reflex (ACR) 99
auricular therapy 92

autism 230
autogenic
    definition 276
    training 117
autoimmune, definition 276
Automated Computerized Treatment System (ACTS) 124
autosuggestion therapy 114
aversion conditioning 109
aversion therapy 276
Avicenna see Ibn Sina
Awareness Through Movement 56
Ayurveda 34

B

babies' colic 248
baby massage 48
Bach, Dr. Edward 86
Bach Flower Remedies 86
back problems 174
bacterial infections 130, 200
bacterial vaginosis 240
bad breath 152
balance therapies 56–65
baldness 197
balm of Gilead 69
Bates method 146, 147
baths 26
bedwetting 248
behavior rehearsal 109
behavioral therapy 102, 109
Benor, Dan 122
Bensen, Herbert 119
Benveniste, Jacques 84
Berne, Eric 108
biochemic tissue salts 81
biodynamic massage 48, 106
bioenergetics 106
biofeedback 117, 145, 170
biorhythms 29
bites 257
bladder problems 216
blisters 198
blood pressure 167, 170
blood problems 164–71
bodywork 38, 276
boils 200
bone problems 172–82
borage 69
Bouchardon, Patrice 89
bowels 208
Bowen techniques 47
Bowen, Tom 38, 47
Boyesen, Gerda 106
Braid, James 112
brain 188
breasts, sore 246
breathing 25, 258
    problems 154–7
    rate 260
brittle bones 177

bronchitis 157
bruises 255
bulimia nervosa 224, 225
bunions 185
burns 256
bursitis of the knee 183

C

camomile 51, 69
cancer 140–1
    cervical 241
    massage 49
candle posture 65
carcinoma 140
carcinoma in situ 241
carpal tunnel syndrome 181
cataracts 146–7
catarrh 149
cautery, definition 276
celiac disease 207
cell command therapy 114
celloid minerals 81
cervical cancer 241
chakras 20, 55, 121, 126
channels, definition 276
chelation therapy 169
Cherokee medicine 71
chest breathing 25, 276
chi 11, 30, 31, 90, 277
chi kung 59
chickenpox 252
chilblains 165
child allergies 158
childbirth 246, 247
children's ailments 248–53
Chinese herbalism 32, 72–3
chiropractic 17, 38, 39–41
chlamydia 237
choking 258
cholesterol 169
chronic, definition 276
chronic fatigue syndrome (CFS) 134–5
circulation 164, 165
cocounseling 103
cobalt 80
cognitive analytic therapy 109
cognitive restructuring 109
cognitive therapy 109
cold sores 132
colds 132, 251
colic 248
colitis 213
colon hydrotherapy 24
colonic cleansing 27
colonic hydrotherapy 27
colonic irrigation 24, 27
color therapy 126
coma 218
comfrey 69

Complete Posture 65
complete therapeutic systems 23–37
compresses 27, 68, 276
conjunctivitis 146
constipation 209
contraception 238
copper 80
corns 185
coughs 156, 250
counseling 103–4
counter conditioning 109
crabs 237
cradle cap 248
cranial osteopathy 44–5
craniosacral therapy (CST) 44–5
creative arts therapies 110
Crohn's disease 213
croup 251
crystal therapies 125
cumulative trauma disorder 181
cupping 30, 90
cuts 255
Cymatics 127
cystitis 216
cytotoxic testing 99

D

dance movement therapy 110
dandelion 69
dandruff 197
deafness 148
decoctions 68
dehumidifiers 25
depression 228–9, 231
dermatitis 202
desensitization 98, 109
detoxification, definition 276
developmental counseling 103
diabetes 218–19
diagnostic techniques 16–22
diaper rash 249
diaphragmatic breathing 25, 276
diarrhea 209
diet 28, 171
dietary therapy 74–5
digestive system 204–19
direct-suggestion therapy 114
diuretic, definition 276
diverticulitis 212
Do In 95
Doctrine of Signatures 67
douches 26
Dougans, Inge 54
dowsing 20

Index • 2

dreamwork 105
dropped arches 185
Duchenne muscular
    dystrophy 173
dynamic psychology 106
dysfunction, definition 276
dysmenorrhea 244

E
ear problems 148
earache 148
eating disorders 224–5
eczema 202–3, 249
edema 214
effleurage, definition 276
ego state, definition 276
electrical testing 99
electrocrystal therapy 125
electromagnetic therapy 101
elimination diets 28, 99, 159
emotional problems 220–31
emphysema 162
empirical 276
encounter groups 107
enemas 27
energetic tree oils 89
energy therapies 12, 121–6
environmental therapies
    98–101
epilepsy 192
erection problems 235
essence, definition 276
essential oils 50–1, 276
Estimated Average
    Requirement (EAR) 79
eucalyptus 51
excess condition 276
exclusion diets 75
exercise 170
expectorant, definition 276
eye problems 146–7
eyesight problems 146

F
facio-scapulo-humeral
    muscular dystrophy 173
fainting 260
fast, definition 276
fasting 29, 74
fecal incontinence 209
feet 183–5
Feldenkrais method 56
Feldenkrais, Moshe 56
feng shui 100
fennel 69
fibromyalgia 182
fibrositis 182
first aid 254–61
fish oil 76
Fitzgerald, William 52
five elements 30
flat feet 185
flatulence 208

flotation therapy 116
flower essences 88–9
flower remedies 86–9
fluid retention 214
folic acid 76
fomentations 27
food 28
    combining 28, 75
    supplements 78–9
    therapies 66, 74–80
fractures 255
Freud, Sigmund 105, 112
friction, definition 276
frigidity 243
frozen shoulder 180
fruit mono diets 29
fungi 130

G
gallstones 214
ganglion, definition 276
garlic 69, 163
gastroenteritis 206
Gattefosse, René-Maurice 50
gem therapies 125
genital herpes 236
genital problems 240
genital warts 236
geopathic stress 100
geopathic therapy 100
geranium 51
German measles 138, 252
germanium 80
Gerson therapy 141
Gestalt therapy 107
gingivitis 152
glaucoma 147
glue ear 250
goiter 143
gonorrhea 237
Goodheart, George 41
gout 179
Green, Elmer 170
Guelpa fast 29
Guillain-Barre syndrome 195
gut bacteria 24

H
H-factor, definition 276
Hahnemann, Samuel 23, 82
hair
    loss 197
    mineral analysis 20, 99
    problems 197
halitosis 152
hand pain 180
hangover prevention 206
Hatha yoga 62
Hay diet 28, 75
Hay, Dr. William 28
hay fever 157, 158
Hayashi, Chujiro 123
head problems 142–53

headache 144–5
headlice 251
healing 121–2
heart attack 168
heart disease 168–9, 170
heart problems 164–71
heartburn 208, 246
heat rash (prickly heat) 198,
    256
heatstroke 256
height, weight calculation
    215
Hellerwork 58
hemorrhoids 210
hepatitis 139
herb gardens 69
herbalism 32, 33, 66–73
hernia 234
herpes 133
hiccups 258
high-velocity thrust 276
hips 183–5
HIV 136–7, 237
hives 203
"holding" therapy 230
homeopathy 17, 23, 66,
    82–5
Hopi ear candle therapy 148
housemaid's knee 183
human immunodeficiency
    virus see HIV
humanistic psychology 102,
    104, 107
hydrotherapy 26–7
hypertension 167
hyperthyroidism 143
hypnoanethesia 114
hypnohealing 114
hypnosis 112–15
hypnotherapy 112–15
hypotension 167
hypothyroidism 143
hyssop 69

I
Ibn Sina 36
immune system 131, 135,
    158
immunity 130–41
immunization 253
impetigo 200
impotence 235
incontinence
    fecal 209
    urinary 217
indigestion 208
infections 130–41, 199–200
infective endocarditis 171
infertility 233, 234, 239
inflammation, definition 276
inflammatory bowel disease
    213
influenza 132

infusions 68, 276
Ingham, Eunice 52
inhalant, definition 276
insect bites/stings 257
insomnia 221
integrative psychology 102
intradermal testing 99
iodine 80
ionizers 25
iridology 20, 22
iris diagnosis 20, 22
iron 76, 79, 80
irritable bowel syndrome 211

J
Janet, Pierre 112
Japan, herbal medicine 72
Japanese medicine 33
jasmine 51
jaw problems 152–3
jellyfish stings 257
Jensen, Bernard 22
jetlag 261
Jin Shen 95
jingluo, definition 277
joint problems 172–82
Jung, Carl Gustav 105

K
kanpo 33
kapha, definition 277
Katz, Richard 89
kidney stones 217
kidneys 204–5
kinesiology 99
Kirlian photography 21
Kneipp, Father 24
Krieger, Dolores 122
Kundalini yoga 62
Kushi, Michio 28
kyphosis 176

L
Laban, Rudolf von 110
labor 247
laryngitis 150
laser therapy 93
Laurence, George 124
lavender 51, 69
legs 183–5
lemon balm 69
leukemia 140
life force 12, 34
light therapies 126
limb girdle muscular
    dystrophy 173
Lindlahr, Henry 24, 28
Ling, Per Henrik 48
listening 19
liver diet 75
lordosis 176
low blood sugar diet 75

Lower Reference Nutrient
  Intake (LRNI) 79
lumbago 174
Lust, Benedict 24
lymphoma 140

M
McCollum, Elmer 76
macrobiotic diet 75
macrobiotics 28
macronutrients 76
magnesium 80, 160
magnetic therapy 101
male sexual problems 233–7
malignant, definition 277
malnutrition 215
manic depression 231
manipulation 38, 277
Manners, Peter Guy 127
mantra, definition 277
marigold 69
marjoram 51
Maslow, Abraham 104
massage 48–9
ME see myalgic
  encephalomyelitis
meadowsweet 69
measles 253
meditation 118–19
Mediterranean diet 171
megavitamin therapy 76, 80
meningitis 139
menopause 245
menorrhagia 244
menstruation 244
mental health problems
  220–31
meridians 18, 30, 31, 90,
  121, 277
Mermet, Abbé 20
Mesmer, Anton 112
Metamorphic technique 54
micronutrients 76
migraine 144–5
miliaria 198
mind-body relationship 102
mineral essences 125
mineral salts 81
mineral therapies 66
minerals 77–9
mobilization, definition 277
moles 198
mononucleosis 133
MORA 21
Moreno, Jacob 107
morning sickness 246
mosquitoes 257
motion sickness 261
motor neurone disease
  (MND) 195
mouth problems 150–1
mouth ulcers 153
movement therapies 56–65

moxa, definition 277
moxibustion 31, 90
multiple sclerosis 193
mumps 253
muscle problems 172–82
muscle-testing 20
muscular dystrophy 173
music therapy 111, 127
myalgic encephalomyelitis
  (ME) 134–5
myotherapy 46

N
Nature Cure 23, 24
naturopathy 23–9
nausea 206
neck injuries 175
neoplasm 140
neroli 51
nerves 188, 189
nervous system 40, 188–95
nettle 69
nettle rash 203
neuralgia 190–1
neuritis 190
nonspecific urethritis 236
nose 149
nose bleeds 254
nutrition 66
nutritional therapy 28, 66,
  76

O
obesity 214
observational diagnosis 18
obsessions 226
obsessive compulsive
  disorder 226
Oldfield, Harry 21, 125
oral thrush 153
oregano 69
Oriental diagnosis 16–17,
  18–19
Oriental systems 30–3
orthodox, definition 277
orthomolecular psychiatry 76
osteoarthritis 178
osteopathy 17, 38, 42–5
osteoporosis 177

P
pain 186–7
Palmer, Bartlet Joshua 39
Palmer, Daniel David 38, 39
palpation, definition 277
palpitations 222
panic 222
Parkinson's disease 194
parts therapy 114
passive, definition 277
past life therapy 115
Pasteur, Louis 163
Pauling, Linus 76

Peckzely, Ignatiz von 22
pelvic inflammatory disease
  (PID) 242
peppermint 69
percussion, definition 277
perineum, tearing of 247
peripheral ischemia 164
Perls, Fritz 107
perspiration 19
pertussis 252
petrissage, definition 277
pharyngitis 151
phobias 227
phosphorus 80
physical diagnostic methods
  20
physical therapies 12, 38–55
physiomedicalism 68
phytotherapy 68
piles 210
pins and needles 191
PIP see polycontrast
  interface photography
pitta, definition 277
plant therapies 66–73, 82–9
pleurisy 161
pneumonia 162
polarity, definition 277
polarity therapy 55
polio 138
pollution 98
polycontrast interface
  photography (PIP) 21
postnatal depression 229
posture 176
potassium 80
potency, definition 277
potentization 82
poultices 68
prana 11, 34
pregnancy 246
Preissnitz, Vincent 24, 26
premature ejaculation 235
premenstrual syndrome 245
prenatal therapy 54
prickly heat 198, 256
problem-focused counseling
  103
prostate enlargement 234
prostatitis 234
proving, definition 277
Prudden, Bonnie 46
psionic medicine 124
psoriasis 201
psychic diagnostic methods
  20
psychic healing 122
psychodrama 107
psychodynamic therapies
  109
psychological problems 235
psychological therapies 12,
  102–20

psychosexual problems 243
psychosynthesis 108
psychotic illness 231
pubic lice 237
pulse 260
pulse diagnosis 91
pulse-taking 18

Q
qi see chi
questioning 19

R
radiesthesia 20
radionics 21, 124
Raja yoga 62
rational-emotive approach
  109
Raynaud's disease 165
recovery position 259
Reference Nutrient Intake
  (RNI) 79
referred pain, definition 277
reflex zone therapy 52
reflexology 48, 52–4
regression 115
Reich, Wilhelm 106
reiki 123
Reilly, David 84
relaxation 114, 116, 120
ren, definition 277
Rentsch, Oswald 47
repetitive strain injury 181
reproductive problems
  232–46
Rescue Remedy 87
respiratory system 154–5
restless legs syndrome 184
resuscitation 259
rheumatism 178
rheumatoid arthritis 179
ringworm 199
Rogers, Carl 104
role playing 109
Rolf, Ida 38, 46, 58
Rolfing 46
rose 51
rosemary 51, 69
Rosen, Marion 38, 47
Rosen techniques 47
roseola 252
rubella 138, 252
ryodoraku 93

S
sage 69
St. John, Robert 54
St. John's wort 69
Salute to the Sun 64
sandalwood 51
sarcoma 140
scabies 199
scalds 256

Index • 3

scarlet fever 253
schizophrenia 231
Schroth cure 29
Schuessler salts 81
Schultz, Johannes 117
sciatica 191
scoliosis 176
Scottish douche 26
Seasonal Affective Disorder
  (SAD) 126, 229
seizures 192
selenium 80
self-help 254–61
self-limiting, definition 277
semaphore method 114
sexual desire 243
sexual problems 232–46
sexually transmitted diseases
  (STDs) 236–7
shamanism 37
shen, definition 277
Shen Tao 95
shiatsu 31, 48, 95, 96–7, 145
shingles 133
shock 260
showers 26
sickle cell anemia 166
Siddha meditation 119
sinusitis 149
sitz baths 26
skin problems 196–203
skin rashes 249
sleep apnea 150
sleep patterns 19
slipped disk 174
Smith, Fritz 55
Smith, Gordon 124
sneezing 149
snoring 150
solution-focused therapy 109
sore breasts 246
sore throat 150, 252
sound therapies 111, 127
spas 26
spiritual growth 120
spiritual healing 122
splints 255
sports massage 48

sprained ankle 184–5
sprains 255
squint 147
stagnant, definition 277
stammering 222
Steiner, Rudolf 23
Still, Andrew Taylor 38, 42
stings 257
stomach 208
stomachache 208
Stone, Randolph 55
stress 120, 170, 223
stretch marks 247
stroke 168
sublingual drop testing 99
subluxation 41
succussion, definition 277
suggestion therapy 114
sunburn 261
sunstroke 256
Sutherland, William Garner
  44, 45
synergism 68
syphilis 237

T
t'ai chi 60
Tantric yoga 62
taste 19
teeth 152–3, 171
teething 249
temperature biofeedback
  145, 170
temporomandibular joint
  (TMJ) syndrome 153
tennis elbow 180
therapeutic touch 122
threadworms 251
throat problems 150–1
thrush 153, 240
thyme 69
thyroid disorders 143
Tibetan medicine 35
tics 191
tinctures 68
tinnitus 148
tissue salts 81
tongue diagnosis 18, 19

tonification, definition 277
tonsillitis 151
toothache 153
toxin, definition 277
Traditional Chinese Medicine
  30–2, 72
Trager approach 58
Trager, Milton 58
transactional analysis 108
transcendental meditation
  119
transcutaneous electrical
  nerve stimulation (TENS)
  101
transpersonal therapies 108
trauma, definition 277
travel first aid 261
Travell, Janet 46
tree remedies 86, 89
Trigger Point Injection
  Therapy (TPIT) 46
Tsubo 95
tuberculosis 163
tumors 140
twitching 191
type, definition 277

U
ulcers 153, 212
Unani-Tibb 36
undercurrents, definition 277
Upledger, John E. 45
urethritis 216
urinary incontinence 217
urinary system 204–19
urinary tract infection 216
urine analysis 19
urticaria 203
Usui, Dr. Mikao 123
uterine prolapse 242

V
Vacuflex Reflexology System
  (VRS) 54
vaginismus 243
vaginitis 240
valerian 69
varicose veins 210

vata, definition 277
VEGA 21
vegan diet 75
vegetable juice fasts 29
vegetarian diet 28, 75
verrucas 199
viral infections 132, 138,
  199
viruses 130
visual meditation 119
visualization 120
vitamin C 76, 80, 215
vitamins 76–80
vomiting 206

W
walking in water 27
warrior posture 65
warts 199
water birth 247
water fasts 29
weight, calculation from
  height 215
Western diagnosis 17, 20–2
wheezing 157
whiplash injury 175
whooping cough 252
witch hazel 69
women's sexual problems
  238–46

X
X-rays, chiropractic 41

Y
yang 11, 30
  definition 277
  foods 28, 75
yarrow 69
yellow dock 69
yin 11, 30
  definition 277
  foods 28, 75
yoga 61–5

Z
zangfu, definition 277
Zero Balancing (ZB) 55
zinc 80